STUDY GUIDE
for
KINN'S THE ADMINISTRATIVE MEDICAL ASSISTANT

Seventh Edition

Alexandra Patricia Young-Adams, BBA, RMA, CMA (AAMA), MA
Adjunct Instructor
Everest College, Arlington Midcities Campus
Arlington, Texas
Professional Writer
Grand Prairie, Texas

ELSEVIER
SAUNDERS

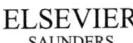

ELSEVIER
SAUNDERS

3251 Riverport Lane
St. Louis, Missouri 63043

STUDY GUIDE FOR KINN'S THE ADMINISTRATIVE MEDICAL ASSISTANT   ISBN: 978-1-4160-5442-9

Copyright © 2011, 2007, 2003, 1999, 1993, 1988, 1982 by Saunders, an imprint of Elsevier Inc.

All rights reserved. No part of this publication may be reproduced or transmitted in any form or by any means, electronic or mechanical, including photocopy, recording, or any information storage and retrieval system, without permission in writing from the publisher.

Notices

Knowledge and best practice in this field are constantly changing. As new research and experience broaden our understanding, changes in research methods, professional practices, or medical treatment may become necessary.

Practitioners and researchers must always rely on their own experience and knowledge in evaluating and using any information, methods, compounds, or experiments described herein. In using such information or methods they should be mindful of their own safety and the safety of others, including parties for whom they have a professional responsibility.

With respect to any drug or pharmaceutical products identified, readers are advised to check the most current information provided (i) on procedures featured or (ii) by the manufacturer of each product to be administered, to verify the recommended dose or formula, the method and duration of administration, and contraindications. It is the responsibility of practitioners, relying on their own experience and knowledge of their patients, to make diagnoses, to determine dosages and the best treatment for each individual patient, and to take all appropriate safety precautions.

To the fullest extent of the law, neither the Publisher nor the authors, contributors, or editors, assume any liability for any injury and/or damage to persons or property as a matter of products liability, negligence or otherwise, or from any use or operation of any methods, products, instructions, or ideas contained in the material herein.

Executive Editor: Susan Cole
Associate Developmental Editors: Jennifer Presley and Jamie Augustine
Publishing Services Manager: Julie Eddy
Project Manager: Rich Barber

Printed in the United States

Last digit is the print number: 9 8 7 6 5 4 3 2 1

To the Student

This study guide was created to help you to achieve the objectives of each chapter in *Kinn's: The Medical Assistant: An Applied Learning Approach* and to establish a solid base of knowledge in medical assisting. Completing the exercises in each chapter in this guide will help reinforce the material studied in the textbook and learned in class.

Study Hints for All Students

Ask Questions!

There are no stupid questions. If you do not know something or are not sure about it, you need to find out. Other people may be wondering the same thing but may be too shy to ask. The answer could mean life or death to your patient. That is certainly more important than feeling embarrassed about asking a question.

Chapter Objectives

At the beginning of each chapter in the textbook are learning objectives that you should have mastered by the time you have finished studying that chapter. Write these objectives in your notebook, leaving a blank space after each. Fill in the answers as you find them while reading the chapter. Review to make sure your answers are correct and complete. Use these answers when you study for tests. You should also do this for separate course objectives that your instructor has listed in your class syllabus.

Vocabulary

At the beginning of each chapter in the textbook are vocabulary terms that you will encounter as you read the chapter. These terms are in bold type the first time they appear in the chapter.

Summary of Learning Objectives

Use the Summary of Learning Objectives at the end of each chapter in the textbook to help you review for exams.

Reading Hints

As you read each chapter in the textbook, look at the subject headings to learn what each section is about. Read first for the general meaning and then reread parts you did not understand. It may help to read those parts aloud. Carefully read the information given in each table and study each figure and its legend.

Concepts

While studying, put difficult concepts into your own words to determine whether you understand them. Check this understanding with another student or the instructor. Write these concepts in your notebook.

Class Notes

When taking lecture notes in class, leave a large margin on the left side of each notebook page and write only on right-hand pages, leaving all left-hand pages blank. Look over your lecture notes soon after each class, while your memory is fresh. Fill in missing words, complete sentences and ideas, and underline key phrases, definitions, and concepts. At the top of each page, write the topic of that page. In the left margin, write the key word for that part of your notes. On the opposite left-hand page, write a summary or outline that combines material from the textbook and the lecture. These can be your study notes for review.

Study Groups

Form a study group with some other students so that you can help one another. Practice speaking and reading aloud. Ask questions about material you find unclear. Work together to find answers.

References for Improving Study Skills

Good study skills are essential for achieving your goals in medical assisting. Time management, efficient use of study time, and a consistent approach to studying are all beneficial. Various methods can be used for reading a textbook and taking class notes. Some methods that have proven helpful can be found in *Saunders Health Professional's Planner*.

Additional Study Hints for English as a Second Language (ESL) Students

Vocabulary
If you find a nontechnical word you do not know (e.g., drowsy), try to guess its meaning from the sentence (e.g., With electrolyte imbalance, the patient may feel fatigued and drowsy.). If you are not sure of the meaning or if it seems particularly important, look it up in the dictionary.

Vocabulary Notebook
Keep a small alphabetized notebook or address book in your pocket or purse. Write down new nontechnical words you read or hear, along with their meanings and pronunciations. Write each word under its initial letter so that you can find it easily, as in a dictionary. For words you do not know or for words that have a different meaning in medical assisting, write down how each word is used and how it is pronounced. Look up the meanings of these words in a dictionary or ask your instructor or first-language buddy (see the following section). Then write the different meanings or uses that you have found in your book, including the medical assisting meaning. Continue to add new words as you discover them.

First-Language Buddy
English as a second language (ESL) students should find a first-language buddy—another student who is a native speaker of English and who is willing to answer questions about word meanings, pronunciations, and culture. Maybe, in turn, your buddy would like to learn about your language and culture; this could be useful for his or her medical assisting career.

Contents

Chapter 1 Becoming a Successful Student, **1**
Chapter 2 The Healthcare Industry, **5**
Chapter 3 The Medical Assisting Profession, **13**
Chapter 4 Professional Behavior in the Workplace, **19**
Chapter 5 Interpersonal Skills and Human Behavior, **25**
Chapter 6 Medicine and Ethics, **33**
Chapter 7 Medicine and Law, **39**
Chapter 8 Computer Concepts, **47**
Chapter 9 Telephone Techniques, **53**
Chapter 10 Scheduling Appointments, **63**
Chapter 11 Patient Reception and Processing, **71**
Chapter 12 Office Environment and Daily Operations, **77**
Chapter 13 Written Communications and Mail Processing, **85**
Chapter 14 The Paper Medical Record, **93**
Chapter 15 The Electronic Medical Record, **99**
Chapter 16 Health Information Management, **103**
Chapter 17 Privacy in the Physician's Office, **111**
Chapter 18 Basics of Diagnostic Coding, **117**
Chapter 19 Basics of Procedural Coding, **127**
Chapter 20 Basics of Health Insurance, **135**
Chapter 21 The Health Insurance Claim Form, **141**
Chapter 22 Professional Fees, Billing, and Collecting, **155**
Chapter 23 Banking Services and Procedures, **165**
Chapter 24 Financial and Practice Management, **173**
Chapter 25 Medical Practice Management and Human Resources, **179**
Chapter 26 Medical Practice Marketing and Customer Service, **185**
Chapter 27 Emergency Preparedness and Assisting With Medical Emergencies, **191**
Chapter 28 Career Development and Life Skills, **199**

Procedure Checklists

Procedure 5-1	Recognize and Respond to Verbal Communications, 209	Work Product 10-7	Scheduling Inpatient and Outpatient Admissions and Procedures, 267
Procedure 5-2	Recognize and Respond to Nonverbal Communications, 211	Work Product 10-8	Scheduling Inpatient and Outpatient Admissions and Procedures, 269
Procedure 6-1	Respond to Issues of Confidentiality, 213	Work Product 10-9	Scheduling Inpatient and Outpatient Admissions and Procedures, 271
Procedure 6-2	Develop a Plan for Separation of Personal and Professional Ethics, 215	Work Product 10-10	Scheduling Inpatient and Outpatient Admissions and Procedures, 273
Procedure 7-1	Perform Within the Scope of Practice, 217	Procedure 11-1	Organize a Patient's Medical Record, 275
Procedure 7-2	Practice Within the Standard of Care for a Medical Assistant, 219	Procedure 11-2	Register a New Patient, 277
Procedure 7-3	Incorporate the Patients' Bill of Rights into Personal Practice and Medical Office Policies and Procedures, 221	Procedure 12-1	Explain General Office Policies, 279
		Procedure 12-2	Instruct Individuals According to Their Needs, 281
Procedure 7-4	Complete an Incident Report, 223	Procedure 12-3	Inventory Office Supplies and Equipment, 283
Procedure 7-5	Apply Local, State, and Federal Healthcare Laws and Regulations That Affect the Medical Assisting Practice Setting, 225	Procedure 12-4	Prepare a Purchase Order, 285
		Procedure 12-5	Perform and Document Routine Maintenance of Office Equipment, 287
Procedure 7-6	Report Illegal and/or Unsafe Behaviors That Affect the Health, Safety, and Welfare of Others to Proper Authorities, 227	Procedure 12-6	Use the Internet to Access Information Related to the Medical Office, 289
		Procedure 12-7	Make Travel Arrangements, 291
Work Product 7-1	Complete an Incident Report, 229	Procedure 12-8	Develop a Personal (Patient and Employee) Safety Plan, 293
Procedure 8-1	Use Office Hardware and Software to Maintain Office Systems, 231	Procedure 12-9	Equipment Maintain a Current List of Community Resources for Emergency Preparedness, 295
Procedure 9-1	Demonstrate Telephone Techniques, 233		
Procedure 9-2	Take a Telephone Message, 235		
Procedure 9-3	Call the Pharmacy with New or Refill Prescriptions, 237	Procedure 12-10	Use Proper Body Mechanics, 297
		Procedure 12-11	Develop and Maintain a Current List of Community Resources Related to Patients' Healthcare Needs, 299
Procedure 10-1	Manage Appointment Scheduling Using Established Procedures, 239		
Procedure 10-2	Schedule and Monitor Appointments, 241	Work Product 12-1	Equipment Inventory, 301
Procedure 10-3	Schedule New Patients, 243	Work Product 12-2	Supply Inventory, 303
Procedure 10-4	Schedule Appointments with Established Patients or Visitors, 245	Work Product 12-3	Maintenance Log, 305
		Work Product 12-4	Travel Expense Report, 307
Procedure 10-5	Document Appropriately and Accurately, 247	Work Product 12-5	Develop a Personal (Patient and Employee) Safety Plan, 309
Procedure 10-6	Schedule Outpatient Admissions and Procedures, 249	Procedure 13-1	Compose Professional Business Letters, 311
Procedure 10-7	Schedule Inpatient Admissions, 251	Procedure 13-2	Report Relevant Information to Others Succinctly and Accurately, 313
Procedure 10-8	Schedule Inpatient Procedures, 253		
Work Product 10-1	Advance Preparation and Establishing a Matrix, 255	Procedure 13-3	Receive, Organize, Prioritize, and Transmit Information Expediently, 315
Work Product 10-2	Scheduling Appointments, 257		
Work Product 10-3	Scheduling Appointments, 259	Procedure 13-4	Address an Envelope According to Postal Service Optical Character Reader Guidelines, 317
Work Product 10-4	Scheduling Appointments, 261		
Work Product 10-5	Scheduling Appointments, 263		
Work Product 10-6	Document Appropriately and Accurately, 265	Work Product 13-1	Addressing an Envelope, 319
		Work Product 13-2	Initiating Correspondence, 321

Work Product 13-3	Initiating a Memo, 323	Work Product 21-2	Completing a CMS-1500 Claim Form, 383
Work Product 13-4	Responding to Correspondence, 325	Work Product 21-3	Completing a CMS-1500 Claim Form, 385
Work Product 13-5	Responding to a Memo, 327		
Work Product 13-6	Initiating a Fax, 329	Work Product 21-4	Completing a CMS-1500 Claim Form, 387
Procedure 14-1	Organize a Patient's Medical Record, 331		
		Work Product 21-5	Completing a CMS-1500 Claim Form, 389
Procedure 14-2	Prepare an Informed Consent for Treatment Form, 333	Procedure 22-1	Use Computerized Office Billing Systems, 391
Procedure 14-3	Add Supplementary Items to Patients' Records, 335	Procedure 22-2	Post Entries on a Day Sheet, 393
Procedure 14-4	Prepare a Record Release Form, 337	Procedure 22-3	Post Adjustments, 395
Procedure 14-5	File Medical Records Using an Alphabetic System, 339	Procedure 22-4	Process a Credit Balance, 397
		Procedure 22-5	Process Refunds, 399
Procedure 14-6	File Medical Records Using a Numeric System, 341	Procedure 22-6	Post Non-Sufficient Funds Checks, 401
Procedure 14-7	Maintain Organization by Filing, 343	Procedure 22-7	Explain Professional Fees and Make Credit Arrangements with a Patient, 403
Procedure 14-8	Document Patient Care Accurately, 345		
Work Product 14-1	Document Patient Care Accurately, 347		
Procedure 15-1	Document Patient Education Accurately, 349	Procedure 22-8	Perform Billing Procedures, 405
		Procedure 22-9	Perform Collection Procedures, 407
Procedure 15-2	Execute Data Management Using Electronic Healthcare Records such as the EMR, 351	Procedure 22-10	Post Collection Agency Payments, 409
		Work Product 22-1	Perform Billing Procedures, 411
Work Product 15-1	Document Patient Education Accurately, 353	Work Product 22-2	Perform Billing Procedures, 413
		Work Product 22-3	Perform Billing Procedures, 415
Procedure 17-1	Apply HIPAA Rules for Privacy and Release of Information, 355	Work Product 22-4	Posting to Patient Accounts, 417
		Work Product 22-5	Posting to Patient Accounts, 419
Procedure 17-2	Perform Risk Management Procedures, 357	Work Product 22-6	Posting to Patient Accounts, 421
		Work Product 22-7	Proof of Posting, 423
Procedure 18-1	Perform ICD-9-CM Coding, 359	Work Product 22-8	Perform Collection Procedures, 425
Procedure 19-1	Perform Procedural Coding: CPT Coding, 361	Work Product 22-9	Perform Collection Procedures, 427
		Procedure 23-1	Write Checks in Payment of Bills, 429
Procedure 19-2	Perform Procedural Coding: Evaluation and Management (E&M) Coding, 363	Procedure 23-2	Prepare a Bank Deposit, 431
		Procedure 23-3	Reconcile a Bank Statement, 433
		Work Product 23-1	Prepare a Bank Deposit, 435
Procedure 19-3	Perform Procedural Coding: Anesthesia Coding, 365	Procedure 24-1	Perform Accounts Receivable Procedures, 437
Procedure 19-4	Perform Procedural Coding: HCPCS Coding, 367	Procedure 24-2	Perform Accounts Payable Procedures, 439
Procedure 20-1	Apply Managed Care Policies and Procedures, 369	Procedure 24-3	Account for Petty Cash, 441
		Procedure 24-4	Process an Employee Payroll, 443
Procedure 20-2	Apply Third-Party Guidelines, 371	Procedure 25-1	Interview Effectively, 445
Procedure 20-3	Verify Eligibility for Managed Care Services, 373	Procedure 25-2	Conduct a Performance Review, 447
		Procedure 25-3	Arrange a Group Meeting, 449
Procedure 20-4	Perform Preauthorization (Precertification) and/or Referral Procedures, 375	Procedure 26-1	Design a Presentation, 451
		Procedure 26-2	Prepare a Presentation Using PowerPoint, 453
Procedure 20-5	Perform Deductible, Co-Insurance, and Allowable Amount Calculations, 377	Procedure 27-1	Develop a Patient Safety Plan: Order the Correct Medication from the Pharmacy, 455
Procedure 21-1	Gathering Data to Complete CMS-1500 Form, 379	Procedure 27-2	Evaluate the Work Environment to Identify Safe and Unsafe Working Conditions: Develop an Environmental Safety Plan, 457
Work Product 21-1	Completing a CMS-1500 Claim Form, 381		

Procedure 27-3	Develop an Employee Safety Plan: Manage a Difficult Patient, 459	**Procedure 27-10**	Perform First Aid Procedures: Administer Oxygen, 475
Procedure 27-4	Demonstrate the Proper Use of a Fire Extinguisher, 461	**Procedure 27-11**	Perform First Aid Procedures: Respond to an Airway Obstruction in an Adult, 477
Procedure 27-5	Participate in a Mock Environmental Exposure Event: Evacuate a Physician's Office, 463	**Procedure 27-12**	Perform First Aid Procedures: Care for a Patient Who Has Fainted, 479
Procedure 27-6	Maintain an Up-to-Date List of Community Resources for Emergency Preparedness, 465	**Procedure 27-13**	Perform First Aid Procedures: Control Bleeding, 481
		Procedure 28-1	Organize a Job Search, 483
Procedure 27-7	Maintain Provider/Professional-Level CPR Certification: Use an Automated External Defibrillator, 467	**Procedure 28-2**	Prepare a Résumé, 485
		Procedure 28-3	Complete a Job Application, 487
		Procedure 28-4	Interview for a Job, 489
Procedure 27-8	Perform Patient Screening Using Established Protocols: Telephone Screening and Appropriate Documentation, 469	**Procedure 28-5**	Negotiate a Salary, 491
Procedure 27-9	Maintain Provider/Professional-Level CPR Certification: Perform Adult Rescue Breathing and One-Rescuer CPR; Perform Pediatric and Infant CPR, 471		

1 Becoming a Successful Student

VOCABULARY REVIEW

Match the following terms and definitions.

1. _____ The constant practice of considering all aspects of a situation when deciding what to believe or what to do
2. _____ Actions that identify the medical assistant as a member of a healthcare profession, including dependability, respectful patient care, initiative, positive attitude, and teamwork
3. _____ The way an individual looks at information and sees it as real
4. _____ The manner in which an individual perceives and processes information to learn new material
5. _____ The way an individual internalizes new information and makes it his or her own
6. _____ The process of considering new information and internalizing it to create new ways of examining information
7. _____ Sensitivity to the individual needs and reactions of patients

A. Learning style
B. Reflection
C. Professional behaviors
D. Processing
E. Empathy
F. Perceiving
G. Critical thinking

SKILLS AND CONCEPTS

Time Management

Answer the following questions.

1. List five time management skills.

    a. _____
    b. _____
    c. _____
    d. _____
    e. _____

    Which of these do you think will require the most effort on your road to becoming a medical assistant? How can you better prepare yourself for the challenges ahead?

    _____
    _____

2. Describe five strategies for breaking the cycle of procrastination.

    a. _____
    b. _____
    c. _____
    d. _____
    e. _____

3. What barriers cause you to procrastinate? How can you prepare yourself to avoid procrastination?

_____

_____

_____

_____

Problem Solving and Conflict Management

True and False: Indicate which statements are true (T) and which are false (F).

1. _____ The best way to deal with conflict situations is through open, honest, assertive communication.
2. _____ The first step in conflict resolution is examination of the pros and cons.
3. _____ Conflicts should be resolved immediately.
4. _____ Sometimes you will not be able to solve problems, or a conflict may not be important enough for you to act to change the situation.
5. _____ It is best if you attempt to solve the conflict in a private place at a prescheduled time.
6. _____ You need to understand the problem and gather as much information about the situation as possible before you decide to act.
7. _____ As a future member of the healthcare team, you will frequently face problems and conflict.

Assertive Behaviors

True and False: Indicate which statements are true (T) and which are false (F).

1. _____ We are born either assertive or passive, and there is nothing we can do to change those behaviors.
2. _____ Assertive communication will get you what you want.
3. _____ A person who responds to conflict passively really is not bothered by the situation.
4. _____ Nonassertive individuals ultimately may respond with anger or an emotional outburst if pushed too far.
5. _____ Aggressive individuals ignore the needs of others.

Briefly answer the following questions.

6. Describe four different nonassertive behaviors.

   a. _____

   b. _____

   c. _____

   d. _____

7. Describe four different aggressive behaviors.

   a. _____

   b. _____

   c. _____

   d. _____

8. Explain the process of developing and delivering an assertive message.

STUDY SKILLS

1. Examine your own note-taking ability. Review the note-taking strategies in Chapter 1 and record the ideas you plan to incorporate into your academic goals for this term.

CASE STUDIES

Read the case studies and answer the questions.

1. Dr. Weaver is running late seeing patients this afternoon. Sara Kline has been waiting in the examination room for Dr. Weaver for 30 minutes. She peeks her head out of the examination room doorway and demands to know what is taking so long. How should you, the medical assistant, approach this patient? How do you calm her down and explain the physician's situation without compromising other patients' confidentiality? What are some things you can do for the patient to make the wait not seem so long?

2. Victoria Graham, a 68-year-old woman with diabetic retinopathy, arrives today for diabetes disease management education. How might the medical assistant approach Ms. Graham's learning style? What are some possible barriers and how can the medical assistant help Ms. Graham overcome them?

3. You have been working with another student to prepare for your next exam. The student asks to borrow your notes but has yet to return them so you can study for the exam. You are usually a nonassertive person, but you know that you have to get your notes back or you will not do well on the test. How can you formulate an assertive message? Summarize the steps to take and exactly what "I" message you will deliver.

WORKPLACE APPLICATIONS

1. You are the office manager for a busy family practice office. Over the past week, you have noticed that one of your employees has been 15 minutes late every day. Should you approach this employee? If so, how would you manage the situation? What are the main points you would want to stress to this employee? Are there any consequences? What follow-up, if any, should be done?

2. Physicians' offices are extremely busy and must deal with many daily demands. How should one prepare for proper time management? Why is it necessary to prioritize tasks? What are some ideas the medical assistant can use to get the most out of the day and stay organized?

3. Connie is the manager of a busy family practice office. The insurance clerk has complained that the receptionist takes too many smoking breaks and accepts too many personal calls while at work. What type of information should Connie obtain before approaching the receptionist? How should this situation be handled? Where? Who should be present?

4. After being on vacation for a week, Laura returns to the office to find her desk piled high with the following tasks. Laura decides to get organized and make a list of the items that need attention. Prioritize the tasks from "most important and urgent" to "needs to be done later today" and "may be done later this week." Explain your answers.

    a. Make staff schedule for next week

    b. Pull patients' charts for the laboratory results the office received this morning for the physician's review

    c. Call and order immunization vaccines (the staff has informed you they are on the last vial)

    d. Call and confirm the patient appointments for tomorrow

    e. Order general stock supplies (e.g., bandages, gauze, needles, and sharps containers)

    f. Review the insurance reimbursements the practice received for last month and address any claims that have not been paid

    g. File charts

    h. Edit the physician's schedule for a meeting scheduled next month

2 The Healthcare Industry

VOCABULARY REVIEW

Fill in the blanks with the correct vocabulary terms from this chapter.

1. A nurse sees several patients in a hospital emergency department and determines which patient is the most ill and should be seen by the physician first. The process the nurse is using is called _____.

2. An administrative assistant in a large clinic must write a letter to another state to determine whether a physician whom the clinic wants to hire has ever had his license revoked. This action is part of a process called _____.

3. A patient arrives at a physician's office and sees the physician. This event is called a(n) _____.

4. Accrediting agencies look for _____ or _____ to determine whether a healthcare facility is following required policies and regulations.

5. A physician who has been _____ has been charged with a crime but has not yet been tried in a court of law.

6. A person who is unable to pay for medical expenses is often called _____, and most hospitals will provide such patients with emergency care.

7. A group of healthcare practitioners involved in reviewing the charts of patients with a certain disease to determine the medical necessity of procedures might be serving in a(n) _____ organization.

8. When families look for an assisted living facility for a relative, they often consider the _____ that will add to the comfort and convenience of the patient.

9. Physicians who conduct a great amount of research are often _____ in medical journals and articles within their field of study.

10. A new hospital contacts The Joint Commission (formerly JCAHO) to begin the _____ process, which verifies that the facility meets or exceeds standards.

11. Dr. Robertson uses mostly herbs and natural supplements in his practice of medicine. Although he could be any type of physician, he probably practices _____.

12. Dr. Wray combines conventional medicine with manipulative techniques when treating his patients. This type of medicine is called _____.

13. Dr. Stern treats patients by locating slight misalignments of the vertebrae and corrects them using manipulative techniques. He practices _____ medicine.

14. Dr. Margolis practices _____, which is a medical discipline in which treatments and medications are used to counteract the signs and symptoms of disease. Most of the physicians in the United States practice this type of medicine.

15. Susan works for Dr. Burns and has forwarded information about his medical license, medical training, and experience to Mercy Hospital. He is applying for _____ at the hospital.

SKILLS AND CONCEPTS

Part I: Pioneers in Medicine

Fill in the blanks.

1. The surgical research technician who contributed to the success of the Blalock-Taussig procedure was _____.

2. _____ presented rules of health to the Jews around 1205 BC, making him the first advocate of preventive medicine and the first public health officer.

3. _____, known as the father of medicine, was the most famous of the ancient Greek physicians, best remembered for an oath that has been taken by many physicians for more than 2,000 years.

4. _____ was a Greek physician who migrated to Rome in AD 162 and became known as the "Prince of Physicians."

5. _____ was a Belgian anatomist who is known as the "Father of Modern Anatomy."

6. In 1628 _____ announced his discovery that the heart acts as a muscular pump, forcing and propelling the blood throughout the body.

7. _____ was the first to observe bacteria and protozoa through a lens.

8. English scientist, _____, is known as the "Founder of Scientific Surgery."

9. _____ observed that those who had contracted cowpox never contracted smallpox.

10. _____ directed that in his wards, the students were to wash and disinfect their hands before examining women in labor and delivering infants.

11. _____ saved the dairy industry of France from disaster in the nineteenth century by developing a process now called *pasteurization*.

12. _____ reasoned that microorganisms must be the cause of infection and should be kept out of wounds.

13. _____ was the first to use ether as an anesthetic agent.

14. Marie and Pierre _____ discovered radium in 1898, and they were awarded the 1902 Nobel Prize in Physics for their work on radioactivity.

15. _____, the founder of nursing, is known as "The Lady With the Lamp."

16. In 1881 _____ organized a committee in Washington that became the American Red Cross.

17. _____ became the American leader of the birth control movement.

18. _____ wrote about death and dying.

19. Salk and _____ almost eradicated polio, which was once a killer and crippler of thousands in the United States.

20. David _____, MD, considered by many to be one of the most brilliant minds today, is helping to piece together the puzzle of the human immunodeficiency virus (HIV).

21. During his terms as the Surgeon General of the United States, _____ became a proponent of tobacco awareness, insisting that tobacco advertisements must be made less attractive to the youth of today.

Part II: Word Find

Using the answers from the previous section, find the names of past and present leaders in the healthcare industry.

```
S  K  H  U  N  T  E  R  Q  T  W  L
E  E  O  S  S  G  R  E  N  N  E  J
M  O  L  O  H  M  E  I  B  C  V  M
M  H  I  P  P  O  C  R  A  T  E  S
E  N  S  C  Y  S  X  U  R  C  S  A
L  E  T  K  E  E  P  C  T  E  A  N
W  W  E  H  V  S  D  K  O  G  L  G
E  U  R  I  R  T  C  V  N  X  I  E
I  E  J  G  A  L  E  N  O  Z  U  R
S  E  E  K  H  W  B  P  B  X  S  K
S  L  O  N  G  V  S  A  B  I  N  M
E  L  A  G  N  I  T  H  G  I  N  Y
P  A  S  T  E  U  R  Z  F  M  G  E
F  Y  Z  S  A  M  O  H  T  X  M  O
K  U  B  L  E  R  R  O  S  S  C  T
O  B  T  S  K  O  O  P  L  D  N  C
```

Part III: National Healthcare Organizations

Spell out the following acronyms.

1. WHO

___

2. DHHS

___

3. USAMRIID

___

4. CDC

___

5. NIH

___

6. CLIA

___

7. OSHA

___

Part IV: Healthcare Professionals

Use the appropriate terms to complete the sentences.

1. Dr. Hazlehurst bears responsibility for her practice 7 days a week. This practice is called a(n) _____.

2. A(n) _____ is formed when two or more physicians elect to associate in the practice of medicine without incorporating.

3. Dr. Sorrow and Dr. Wester sold their practice to a large artificial entity with legal and business status, and now they work for a(n) _____.

4. A(n) _____ is trained to locate subluxations of the spine and repair them, using x-ray examinations and adjustments.

5. _____ physicians, or DOs, complete requirements similar to those for MDs to graduate and practice medicine.

6. Duncan wants to become a(n) _____, who treats and prevents problems related to the teeth and gums and the tissue surrounding them.

7. The professional who is trained and licensed to examine the eyes, test visual acuity, and treat defects of vision by prescribing correctional lenses is called a(n) _____.

8. A(n) _____ is educated in the care of the feet, including surgical treatment.

9. _____ and medical laboratory technicians perform diagnostic testing on blood, body fluids, and other types of specimens to assist the physician in obtaining a diagnosis.

10. _____ provide direct patient care services under the supervision of licensed physicians and are trained to diagnose and treat patients as directed by the physician.

11. _____ are registered nurses who provide anesthetics to patients during procedures performed by surgeons, physicians, dentists, or other qualified healthcare professionals.

12. _____ assist patients in regaining their mobility and improving their strength and range of motion, which may have been impaired by an accident or injury or as a result of disease.

Part V: Healthcare Facilities

Fill in the blanks.

1. Roger's hands were injured in an accident, and he must undergo rehabilitation. He is obtaining treatment at a(n) _____ health center so that he can prepare to return to work.

2. Susan's son, Brandon, had his tonsils removed at the _____ unit of their local hospital and went home later that evening.

3. _____ facilities have become very popular because they give the residents a sense of independence while still providing supervision and various amenities.

4. _____ centers provide patients an alternative to hospital emergency departments.

5. _____ diagnose and treat people who have sleep disorders.

Part VI: Matching Patients with Physicians

Match the following patients with the physician who should treat them. The specialties are based on the divisions of medicine recognized by the American Board of Medical Specialties. Write the corresponding letter for the physician on the blank next to the patient's name.

1. _____ Mr. West has complained of problems with excessive gas and bloating after meals. He also has some pain in his lower abdominal area.

2. _____ Ms. Jindra has suffered from severe acne most of her adult life. She hopes to find a treatment that will give her more confidence in her appearance.

a. Dr. Stayer
b. Dr. Quincy
c. Dr. Haskins

3. _____	The results of Ms. Robles' amniocentesis are abnormal, and her obstetrician suspects that she may be carrying a child who will be born with a birth defect.	d. Dr. Marrs
4. _____	Ms. O'Neal is pregnant with her first child.	e. Dr. Cantrell
5. _____	Ms. Sklaar had gastric bypass surgery 2 years ago and now wants to undergo abdominoplasty to remove excess skin.	f. Dr. DuBois
6. _____	Mr. Taylor experiences pain in his left eye when he is exposed to bright sunlight. He is concerned, because his mother and grandmother both lost their eyesight in their later years.	g. Dr. Gleaton
		h. Dr. Kirkham
7. _____	Jack Monroe is the lead singer for a popular rock band. He experienced laryngitis during a world tour and needs to see a physician quickly to help him get back on the road.	i. Dr. Jones
		j. Dr. Faught
8. _____	Sarah is 1 year old and needs several immunizations.	k. Dr. Martin
9. _____	Jimmie suffers from asthma related to reactions that occur when he is around grass, shrubs, and some animals.	l. Dr. Rowinski
10. _____	Mrs. Downey had a stroke and needs surgery to remove a small clot that has lodged in her brain.	m. Dr. Antonetti
11. _____	Andrea is having a hysterectomy and will be given a general anesthetic. While in the hospital, she meets the physician who will administer the anesthetic during surgery.	n. Dr. Jackson
		o. Dr. Tips
12. _____	Mrs. Ballard had an ovarian cyst, which was removed after a visit to the emergency department. She received a bill later from the physician who evaluated the cyst for malignancies.	p. Dr. Roberts
13. _____	Mrs. Harris had several polyps in her gastrointestinal tract. She was referred for surgery by her family physician.	q. Dr. Skylar
14. _____	Mrs. Richardson has had migraine headaches for about 6 months. Her family physician thinks she should see a specialist.	r. Dr. Burns
		s. Dr. True
15. _____	Bobbie broke his arm and was taken to the emergency department. X-ray films were taken, and they were read by a physician.	t. Dr. Williams
16. _____	Mr. Oldman periodically suffers from kidney stones and may need surgery.	
17. _____	Rhonda was taken to the emergency department after a car accident.	
18. _____	Mr. Anton contacted a physician for removal of a minor cyst on his back.	
19. _____	The entire Blair family sees one physician.	
20. _____	Mr. Saxton will have surgery tonight to treat a punctured lung.	

Part VII: Short Essay Questions

Answer the following questions using complete sentences.

1. Why was the education offered by Johns Hopkins University Medical School so effective in training physicians?

   _____

   _____

   _____

2. Explain the differences between the two medical symbols discussed in the chapter and what each icon represents.

_____
_____
_____

3. Why is the history of medicine important to us today?

_____
_____
_____

4. Which ancient cultures contributed to the medical terminology we use today?

_____
_____
_____

5. Which medical pioneer do you feel contributed the most to medicine?

_____
_____
_____

6. Explain the role of the hospitalist.

_____
_____
_____

Part VIII: Healthcare Occupations
Match the following descriptions with the appropriate healthcare occupation.

1. _____ Provides services such as injury prevention, assessment, and rehabilitation
2. _____ Is qualified to implement exercise programs designed to reverse or minimize debilitation and enhance the functional capacity of medically stable patients
3. _____ Practices medicine under the direction and responsible supervision of a medical doctor or doctor of osteopathy
4. _____ Performs diagnostic examinations and therapeutic interventions of the heart and/or blood vessels, both invasive and noninvasive
5. _____ Assists licensed pharmacists by performing duties that do not require the expertise of a pharmacist
6. _____ Assists in developing and implementing the anesthesia care plan
7. _____ Helps improve patient mobility, relieve pain, and prevent or limit permanent physical disabilities

a. Audiologist

b. Cardiovascular technologist

c. Therapeutic recreation specialist

d. Physical therapist

e. Pharmacy technician

f. Dietetic technician

g. Anesthesiology assistant

h. Specialist in blood bank technology

i. Diagnostic medical sonographer

8. _____ Helps patients use their leisure in ways that enhance health, functional abilities, independence, and quality of life

9. _____ Identifies patients who have hearing, balance, and related ear problems

10. _____ Integrates and applies the principles from the science of food, nutrition, biochemistry, food management, and behavior to achieve and maintain health

11. _____ Evaluates, treats, and manages patients of all ages with respiratory illnesses and other cardiopulmonary disorders

12. _____ Evaluates disorders of vision, eye movement, and eye alignment

13. _____ Performs routine and standardized tests in blood center and transfusion services

14. _____ Uses equipment that produces sound waves, resulting in images of internal structures

15. _____ Uses the nuclear properties of radioactive and stable nuclides to make diagnostic evaluations of the anatomic or physiologic conditions of the body

16. _____ Prepares the operating room by selecting and opening sterile supplies

17. _____ Uses purposeful activity and interventions to achieve functional outcomes to maximize the independence and maintenance of health

18. _____ Performs tests to detect and diagnose various diseases and works closely with pathologists

19. _____ Provides medical care to patients who have suffered an injury or illness outside the hospital setting

20. _____ Formulates strategic, functional, and user requirements related to the processing of health data

j. Kinesiotherapist
k. Occupational therapist
l. Orthoptist
m. Physician assistant
n. Surgical technologist
o. Respiratory therapist
p. Athletic trainer
q. Medical technologist
r. Emergency medical technician
s. Health information specialist
t. Nuclear medicine technologist

CASE STUDY

Read the case study and answer the questions that follow.

Rebecca is a new employee at the Blackburn Clinic. She recently graduated from an accredited medical assisting school and completed her externship in a family practice clinic. She enjoys the variety of patients who come to the office, and she respects the physicians for their dedication to the art and science of medicine. The physicians with whom Rebecca works are strong proponents of continuing education, and they want Rebecca to attend no less than two seminars each year. Research the history of family practices and answer these questions:

1. What types of patients are seen in family practice clinics?

_____
_____
_____

2. What educational background does the physician need to become a family practitioner?

_____
_____
_____

3. What are some of the more common illnesses that present in a family clinic?

4. What are the goals of the American Association of Family Practitioners?

Workplace Applications

Read the following information and complete the exercises.

1. Visit a local hospital and introduce yourself to five medical professionals. Make an appointment to interview them and find out their job duties and their professional backgrounds. Write a thank-you note to each person after the interview.

2. Interview an office manager at a family practice. Ask about the positive and negative aspects of working with a variety of patients each day.

Internet Activities

1. Choose one of the early medical pioneers discussed in this chapter and research him or her using the Internet. After conducting the research, write a report and present the person to the class. Be creative with the presentation, using PowerPoint or some type of audiovisual equipment.

2. Research the history of a particular illness. Prepare a short report on that illness and present it to the class.

3 The Medical Assisting Profession

VOCABULARY REVIEW

Fill in the blanks with the correct vocabulary terms from this chapter.

1. Sandra should consider both the _____ and the _____ as she considers the various positions offered to her on graduation from her medical assisting training.

2. Robert is anxious to learn _____, because he would like to draw blood and possibly work in a local hospital laboratory.

3. The Wray Clinic recently began to offer _____ _____ to the employees, which gives them a part of the profits the clinic earns over the year.

4. It is important for graduates of medical assisting programs to gain _____ as soon as possible after graduation and to maintain it throughout their medical assisting career.

5. It is clear to Paula that there are many _____ to working as a medical assistant that make the profession worthwhile in ways other than compensation.

6. Alberta is interested in administrative medical assisting, because she is unsure whether she would enjoy performing _____ procedures.

7. Some high schools offer classes that allow students to explore the _____ _____ _____.

8. Both the American Association of Medical Assistants and the American Medical Technologists offer _____ _____ _____ for medical assistants.

9. _____ helps a team of medical assistants cover for one another in the event of illness or absence.

10. Medical assistants are the most _____ allied health professionals.

11. Some for-profit organizations offer _____ _____ after an employee has worked there for a specific period.

12. Bethany is looking forward to her _____ in a family practice clinic next month.

SKILLS AND CONCEPTS

Part I: The Medical Assisting Profession

1. Name the two major areas of medical assisting practice.

2. List five administrative duties a medical assistant might perform.

_____
_____
_____
_____
_____

3. List five clinical duties a medical assistant might perform.

_____
_____
_____
_____
_____

4. Provide an example of cross-training.

_____

5. Explain why hiring a medical assistant without any formal training often is more expensive.

_____
_____

6. Explain in your own words the history of medical assisting as a profession.

_____
_____

Part II: Professional Appearance

Determine which of the following normally would be part of the medical assistant's professional appearance. Place a check mark in the box marked "yes" or "no" to indicate whether that item would be acceptable in today's medical facilities.

	Yes	No	
1.	❏	❏	Hoop earrings
2.	❏	❏	Clear nail polish
3.	❏	❏	White uniforms
4.	❏	❏	Red nail polish
5.	❏	❏	One ear piercing
6.	❏	❏	Scrub tops
7.	❏	❏	Facial piercings
8.	❏	❏	Tennis or running shoes
9.	❏	❏	Excessive jewelry
10.	❏	❏	Tongue rings
11.	❏	❏	Lab coats
12.	❏	❏	Heavy eye makeup
13.	❏	❏	Street clothes with a lab coat
14.	❏	❏	Jeans

Part III: Externships and Internships

Explain briefly the solution you would choose for the following situations that might occur during an externship or internship. Discuss and compare answers during class.

1. Anna notices that her supervisor at the externship frequently arrives late and leaves work early. The physician asks Anna casually one day if the supervisor is helpful and cordial to her. What should Anna say about the supervisor?

2. One of Dr. Hammersly's patients, Brock Anderson, is extremely attractive, and Suzanne, the extern at the clinic, would like to get to know him better. When working with Brock's chart, Suzanne notices his home telephone number. She considers writing it down and contacting Brock after her externship is completed. Would this be acceptable behavior?

3. On a very stressful day, Georgia assists a drug representative in placing drug samples in the storage area. She has battled a headache for most of the day. One of the drugs left behind is a mild painkiller called Ultram. Georgia has taken Ultram before for her headaches and doesn't think the physician will mind if she takes one at work. Would this be appropriate?

4. Natasha was one of the most industrious medical assistant students in her class, always working hard and going the extra mile. When she begins her externship, she notices that the other assistants in the office are allowing her to do a large part of the work while they gossip and explore the Internet during working hours. How should Natasha handle this when her supervisor asks her how the externship is going?

5. Randy graduated from the same school Angela currently is attending for medical assisting training. The two meet during Angela's externship at the office where Randy works, and they quickly become friends. Randy would like to ask Angela, a single parent, to a company picnic the following weekend, after Angela finishes her externship. Would this be acceptable behavior?

6. Dr. Morton confides in Catrina, an extern, that he plans to fire Ashley, the medical assistant who books appointments for the clinic. He offers Catrina the job, which pays slightly more than she expected to make just out of school. The office is located very close to Catrina's apartment. Later in the week, Ashley and Catrina go to lunch together, and Ashley mentions that she is about to buy a new car. Should Catrina steer her away from such a major purchase, knowing that she is about to be fired?

7. Bailee, an extern, is shocked to see one of the other medical assistants, Kristen, take $20 from the petty cash drawer and put it in her purse. When the physician asks about the petty cash balance, Kristen mentions that she gave a Girl Scout troop a $20 donation. What should Bailee do?

___

8. Dr. Schilling storms into the clinic and calls a meeting. Taylor, an extern who has been at the clinic for 1 week, attends the meeting with the two other medical assistants in the office. When the physician insists that one of the three of them took a vial of Demerol from the drug cabinet, the two medical assistants look at Taylor. If Taylor is not guilty, how should she handle this situation professionally?

___

Part IV: Professional Organizations

Fill in the blanks with the correct word choice.

1. Gail uses the CMA credential after her name, which stands for _____ _____ _____.

2. The CMA examination is offered by which organization? _____

3. Patty uses the RMA credential after her name, which stands for _____ _____ _____.

4. The RMA examination is offered by which organization? _____

5. Two agencies that accredit medical assisting programs are the _____ and the _____.

6. Explain the purpose of CEUs.

___

7. Do both the AAMA and the AMT either require CEUs or offer them as an option for recertification?

___

8. Explain the mission of the AAMA.

___

9. Explain the mission of the AMT.

___

16

Chapter 3 The Medical Assisting Profession

Part V: Short Essay Questions

Answer the following questions using complete sentences.

1. List several personal attributes a student should display during his or her externship.

2. Explain why continuing education is critical to the success of the medical assistant.

3. What are some of the subjects that will be included in most medical assistant training programs?

CASE STUDY

Read the case study and answer the questions that follow.

Maryanne entered a medical assisting training program in June, and by mid-July she was struggling to do homework, take care of her infant son, and work part-time. She loves her classes but feels overwhelmed by the amount of work school requires. At times she thinks about quitting school, but she also realizes that a job as a medical assistant will be more rewarding than her current part-time job. Maryanne wants a position that she can be proud to hold. One of her instructors suggested that she make plans for the situations that could prompt her to give up her schooling.

1. How can Maryanne make plans for situations that might go wrong throughout her time in school?

2. What types of situations could present problems for her?

3. How can Maryanne budget her time effectively so that she is able to meet all her responsibilities?

Workplace Applications

Write a reasonable dress code policy for a fictional medical office. Include regulations for both male and female employees. Be specific about jewelry (e.g., nose rings, piercings, and so on), fingernail length, clean shoes, and all other aspects of an acceptable dress code.

Internet Activities

1. Research the requirements for taking both the CMA and RMA examinations. Request or download an application to become a member of the American Association of Medical Assistants and the American Medical Technologists. Obtain a money order for the application fee and send the fees with your application. Answer the following questions:

    What CMA examination date is closest to your graduation? _____

    What is the fee for the CMA examination? _____

    How much are the initial dues for joining the AAMA based on your state of residence? _____

    How much are annual dues for the AAMA based on your state of residence? _____

    What local chapter is closest to you? When and where are the meetings held?

    _____

    _____

    What RMA examination date is closest to your graduation? _____

    What is the fee for the RMA examination? _____

    How much are the initial dues for joining the AMT? _____

    How much are annual dues for the AMT? _____

    What local chapter is closest to you? When and where are the meetings held?

    _____

    _____

2. Research the medical assistant's scope of practice and write a report on this subject. Present the report to the class.

3. Research the requirements of other certifications that you might be interested in obtaining. Which would you like to work toward, if any? Secure applications for those additional certifications.

4 Professional Behavior in the Workplace

VOCABULARY REVIEW

Fill in the blanks with the correct vocabulary terms from this chapter.

1. Dr. Babinski struggles with _____, often putting off doing tasks that should be completed.
2. Anna has worked as a medical assistant for almost 30 years, and her professionalism and compassion are above _____.
3. Susan Bessler is a CMA who has supervised externships for almost 10 years; she expects students to display _____ when performing their duties at her clinic.
4. _____ is one of the most important attributes that medical assistants should display as they go about their duties.
5. James has learned that he must use _____ when dealing with the patients in the clinic, being careful not to reveal any confidential information to an unauthorized third party.
6. Roberta _____ the notes from the last staff meeting to all employees.
7. A few of the _____ that the professional medical assistant should show include loyalty, initiative, and courtesy.
8. Because Julia has been dishonest about her reasons for missing work, her _____ has been called into question.
9. Kristen has a pleasant _____ when working with patients.
10. Medical assistants receive pay that is usually _____ with their experience and training.
11. Jessica holds drawings for small gifts at her staff meetings, which helps to raise employee _____.
12. Gene evokes a professional _____ when talking with patients that encourages them to place their trust in him.
13. Medical assistants must take _____ when they are performing both externship and job duties.
14. _____ is a cause for immediate dismissal from employment.
15. The phrase "office politics" has a negative _____.

SKILLS AND CONCEPTS

Part I: Short Answer Questions

Briefly answer the following questions.

1. List the eight characteristics of the professional medical assistant.

   a. _____

   b. _____

   c. _____

   d. _____

   e. _____

f. _____

g. _____

h. _____

2. List five obstructions to professionalism.

   a. _____

   b. _____

   c. _____

   d. _____

   e. _____

3. Define teamwork in your own words.

   _____
   _____
   _____
   _____

Part II: Practicing Professional Behavior

Answer the following questions.

1. Karen has developed a friendship with Angela, who has a wonderful personality but does not always do her share in the family practice clinic where they work together. Dr. Rabinowitz tells Karen that Angela is going to be terminated on Friday, and she asks Karen to take over some of Angela's duties until a replacement is found. How can Karen demonstrate loyalty to her employer in this situation? To her friend, Angela?

   _____
   _____
   _____
   _____

2. Martin Smith is a patient who always disrupts the clinic. He constantly complains about everything from the moment he enters until the moment he leaves. Karen is at the desk when he arrives to check out and pay his bill. When she tells him that he has a previous balance from a claim that his insurance did not pay, he argues that Karen filed the claim incorrectly. Karen is not in charge of filing insurance claims and did not handle any part of the claim in question. How can she be courteous to this patient?

   _____
   _____
   _____
   _____

3. Karen works in the office laboratory. She is often asked questions about insurance and billing that she must refer to other personnel. How should Karen efficiently request information or assistance for the patient from other office personnel?

   _____
   _____
   _____
   _____

4. Karen and her fiancé ended their relationship last week. How can she deal with personal stressors while she is in the workplace?

5. A patient needs to be scheduled for an outpatient endoscopic examination. When Karen gives the instruction sheet to the patient, she suspects from his reaction that the patient is unable to read. How can Karen professionally handle this situation without causing embarrassment to the patient?

6. Which of the characteristics of professionalism is your greatest strength? Explain why.

7. Which of the five obstructions to professionalism will be most difficult for you to overcome? Explain why.

8. Explain the difference between drug abuse and drug addiction.

9. List the four criteria of substance abuse.

   a. _____
   b. _____
   c. _____
   d. _____

10. List the seven criteria that determine abuse if three are met within a 12-month period.

   a. _____
   b. _____
   c. _____
   d. _____
   e. _____
   f. _____
   g. _____

CASE STUDY

Read the case study and answer the questions that follow.

Aaron is a new medical assistant in Dr. Royce's family practice. He was an exceptional student, and he consistently performed well on his externship, receiving commendations from the externship office manager as well as a written recommendation from the physician. One month after he started his job, Bethany asked him to make a bank deposit for her, usually a duty that she performs daily. Bethany told him she was leaving the bank deposit in Aaron's bottom left drawer at his desk. When Aaron looked for the deposit at the end of the day, it was not anywhere in his desk; he looked in every drawer and even took the drawers out to make sure it had not fallen behind them. All the employees looked for the deposit, which was not found. No one was able to reach Bethany on the phone. The next morning when Aaron opened his left bottom desk drawer, the deposit bag was there, but it was empty. Bethany had already reported to the physician that the deposit had not been made. The physician calls Aaron to his office to discuss the situation.

1. What do you think happened?

   _____
   _____
   _____

2. How can you deal with employees who are determined to cause problems for others in the clinic?

   _____
   _____
   _____

3. How can situations such as this be proven effectively when one is unsure about exactly what happened?

   _____
   _____
   _____

WORKPLACE APPLICATIONS

Professionalism is a word used often with regard to medical personnel. What does professionalism mean? Write a report on the meaning of professionalism, highlighting a person you believe is the epitome of professionalism in the medical field. This person could be an instructor, a physician, or some other healthcare worker whom you have come to know. Be specific about the ways professionalism is apparent in this individual's actions and speech.

INTERNET ACTIVITIES

1. Find four articles on medical professionalism. What seems to be the primary issues in attempting to maintain professionalism in medical facilities?

2. What are some ways medical professionalism is taught in medical schools? Do these methods apply to medical assistants?

5 Interpersonal Skills and Human Behavior

VOCABULARY REVIEW

Fill in the blanks with the correct vocabulary terms from this chapter.

1. Jill commented that the new office policies are confusing and _____.
2. Giving a patient an injection against his or her will could be considered _____.
3. Shane's remark was insulting and _____.
4. Whitney _____ denied leaving the narcotics cabinet unlocked.
5. With the increasing number of lawsuits, medical personnel can conclude that our society is quite _____.
6. Angry employees who are being terminated might turn _____ in a short time.
7. The notion that large individuals are lazy is an example of a(n) _____.
8. Sayed uses positive _____ while training a new employee.
9. Rahima demonstrates _____ when she attempts to get her way in every situation.
10. Paula has learned that she uses _____ _____ when she feels threatened by her supervisor.
11. Karen felt intense _____ when her grandmother died.
12. _____ helps Angela make sure she understands exactly what a patient meant.
13. Roberto eventually was terminated for using _____ with several of the patients in the clinic.
14. Bobbie attended a seminar last week and learned about _____, which included the study of the spatial separation that individuals naturally maintain.
15. Sue Ann definitely felt out of her _____ _____ when she was asked to be a guest speaker at a regional AAMA meeting.
16. Mrs. Robinson is able to _____ her words quite distinctly.
17. Dr. Kirkham warned that no employee should speak to the _____ about any of his celebrity patients.
18. Rodman has a(n) _____ _____ at work, because he speaks so little English.
19. It is important to consider the patient's _____ of the staff, clinic, and physician.
20. Dr. Rockwell took Julia off phone duty because the high _____ of her voice was disconcerting to many patients.

SKILLS AND CONCEPTS

Part I: Open-Ended and Closed-Ended Questions

Label the following questions or statements as either open ended (O) or closed ended (C).

1. _____ Are you taking blood pressure medication?
2. _____ Are you allergic to aspirin?
3. _____ Would you tell me about your past surgeries?
4. _____ Do you have asthma?
5. _____ What types of attempts have you made to stop smoking?
6. _____ Explain what you feel when your migraines begin.
7. _____ Do you have hospitalization insurance?
8. _____ Do you want a morning or afternoon appointment?
9. _____ How are you feeling today?
10. _____ What type of trouble do you have when swallowing pills?

Part II: Defense Mechanisms

Match the following defense mechanisms with the appropriate statements.

1. _____ "Everyone forgets to clock in from lunch once in a while. Why am I being singled out and written up?"
2. _____ "I refuse to believe that I'm HIV positive. I've only had sex with two people in the past 5 years."
3. _____ "I would do a better job at work, but I can't do everything in 1 day like I'm expected to."
4. _____ "I know that the office manager is angry with me because I've been late, and I should talk to her, but I just can't deal with that stress right now."
5. _____ "Why are you attacking me about not filling out the narcotics log? You certainly aren't the perfect medical assistant!"
6. _____ "I know my blood sugar is high, and I have tried to avoid sugar, but at least I'm doing my exercises twice a week."
7. _____ "Dr. Roberts only yells at me because he's stressed about his patient load."
8. _____ "It doesn't matter what I do to please my family. They hate me anyway, and there's nothing I can do about it."
9. _____ "I have enough on my mind and don't need my co-workers complaining that I'm not doing my share of the work!"
10. _____ "I can't bear to go to Memorial Park for our office picnic, because that's where my ex-husband told me he wanted a divorce."
11. _____ "Sure she looks good, if you like people from the 60s!"

a. Verbal aggression
b. Projection
c. Sarcasm
d. Compensation
e. Physical avoidance
f. Regression
g. Apathy
h. Rationalization
i. Displacement
j. Repression
k. Denial

Part III: Barriers to Communication

Determine which of the five barriers to communication applies in each example given.

1. Cylinda has lived in the South all her life, and when Bruce came to work at the office, his brusque attitude made her feel defensive. She was so offended by his manner of speaking that she began to avoid him in the hallways and during breaks. He constantly spoke of how much more he'd been paid in New York and stressed the efficiency of the clinic where he formerly worked. Cylinda considers him a typical Northerner, and her dislike of him is based largely on the fact that he is different from her and most of the people she knows.

2. Aretha dreads the days that Rahima Bathkar comes to the office. She is a pleasant patient, but Aretha cannot understand her well and feels as if she is not providing Rahima with the care she deserves. She is always worried that she is missing some information the physician needs to know to diagnose and treat the patient properly. Aretha takes extra time with Rahima, but she is concerned, because there is no one to interpret for Rahima when she cannot find the right word in her broken English.

3. Allan and Rebecca Poe are an elderly couple who visit the clinic twice a month for Rebecca's diabetes. Rebecca is blind in one eye and cannot read easily. Allan has vision problems as well, so the staff must read to them any documents they are required to sign to ensure that they understand the information.

4. Tommy Lightman approached the office manager because he was concerned about the manner in which Sarah spoke to him in the office. He expressed that Sarah was quite short with him last Tuesday and seemed very distracted as she talked with him in the examination room before the physician came in to treat him. He also said that the physician seemed to spend less time with him that day than usual. Tommy was concerned that he was not wanted in the clinic and wanted to have his records sent to another physician. The office manager checks the appointment book and realizes that Tommy was in the office last Tuesday at 11 o'clock, which was the exact time that another patient was being transported to the hospital because of heart failure.

5. Teresa has a difficult time dealing with Orlando Guiterrez. He comes for appointments twice a month and is trying desperately to lose weight. He currently weighs 435 pounds. He is a pleasant person, but Teresa has been raised to believe that those who are overweight are lazy individuals. She tries to avoid caring for him when he visits the clinic.

Part IV: Dealing with Barriers to Communication

Reread the scenarios in the previous section and explain how each situation could be professionally handled by the medical assistant using good communications skills.

1. How can Cylinda develop a positive working relationship with Bruce?

2. What can Aretha do to improve communication with Rahima?

3. How can the medical assistant make Rebecca Poe feel more comfortable with her disability in the physician's office?

4. What can Sarah and the office manager do to change Tommy's perception about the incident that happened during his last office visit?

5. What does Teresa need to do personally to deal with patients she doesn't care for who visit the clinic?

Part V: Communication During Difficult Times
Read the following descriptions and suggest effective ways to communicate with the patient. Identify whether the patient is probably experiencing anger, shock, grief, or a combination of these emotions.

1. Joanna Taylor has just been brought to the physician's office after learning that her 16-year-old son was killed in a car accident. She is not responding to questions.

2. Lafonda Williams has come to the physician's office because of injuries she sustained when her estranged husband assaulted her.

3. Jackson Holland is seeing the physician today for antidepressants because of work-related stress, as well as difficulty dealing with the death of his elderly mother.

4. James Ackard comes to the physician's office for treatment of a work-related injury.

Part VI: Death and Dying
List the stages of grief in proper order.

1. _____
2. _____
3. _____
4. _____
5. _____

Part VII: Resolving Conflict

1. List three ways to resolve conflict.

   a. _____

   b. _____

   c. _____

2. How would the medical assistant professionally resolve a conflict with a co-worker?

   _____

   _____

   _____

3. How would the medical assistant professionally resolve a conflict with a supervisor?

   _____

   _____

   _____

Part VIII: Boundaries

1. Define self-boundaries.

   _____

   _____

   _____

2. List the four steps of setting boundaries at work.

   a. _____

   b. _____

   c. _____

   d. _____

Part IX: Communicating with People of Other Cultures

1. If a non–English-speaking patient comes to the office without an interpreter, what should the medical assistant do?

   _____

   _____

   _____

2. How can the medical assistant put a patient at ease who seems nervous about an office visit or a procedure?

   _____

   _____

   _____

3. Why should the medical assistant avoid the phrase "I know how you feel"?

   _____

   _____

   _____

Part X: Maslow's Hierarchy of Needs

Draw and label the Hierarchy of Needs as shown in Figure 5-7 in the text.

Part XI: The Process of Communication

Draw and label the transactional communication model as shown in Figure 5-4 in the text.

CASE STUDY

Read the case study and answer the questions that follow.

Janet has tried for months to reach Mr. Robinson, a cancer patient who comes to the clinic every 3 weeks. He does not have any family in the area, and he feels that no one is interested in him or the problems he faces. He is estranged from both of his daughters, whom he has told to stay out of his life. They have not seen or spoken to him in more than 10 years. Each visit, Mr. Robinson complains about how worthless his family is and how they have all deserted him in his time of need. However, Janet knows from reviewing the chart that Mr. Robinson was insistent that his daughters stay out of his life.

1. How involved should Janet get in this patient's life?

_____

_____

_____

2. How can she deal with Mr. Robinson's attitude during his office visits?

_____

_____

_____

3. Does Janet or the physician have the right to contact the daughters and discuss Mr. Robinson's condition with them?

WORKPLACE APPLICATIONS

Solicit 10 volunteers to come to the classroom and role-play patients and co-workers. Develop several personalities by writing a synopsis of the chief complaints and general personality traits. Allow each student to experience each "patient" or "co-worker" and react to them using professional interpersonal behavior and good human relations skills. Discuss the activity in class and talk about what this role-play activity can teach medical assisting students.

INTERNET ACTIVITIES

Use the Internet to answer the following questions.

1. How many different career fields do human relations and interpersonal skills affect?

2. What is organizational behavior?

3. How are human relations and interpersonal skills practiced in classrooms?

Write a classroom policy that stresses positive interpersonal skills and human relations. Share this policy with the class.

6 Medicine and Ethics

VOCABULARY REVIEW

Fill in the blanks with the correct vocabulary terms from this chapter.

1. Melissa believes that one of her roles as a medical assistant is to be a patient _____, supporting both the patient and family members during illnesses.
2. Ben has conflicting views about _____ and is unsure as to whether he would want the option to die with dignity if he had an incurable, debilitating disease.
3. Jill understands that the _____ of her actions while she is at work could affect whether a patient complies with the physician's instructions.
4. _____ allows the medical assistant to consider his or her personal feelings about various ethical issues before being faced with those decisions while working with actual patients.
5. _____ or handicapped patients need special understanding and patience from those who are employed in medical facilities.
6. Bianca is an infertile patient who is participating in _____ _____ to research a new drug that may help her to conceive a child.
7. The members of the Council on Ethical and Judicial Affairs issue _____ about medical situations, similar to the way that the Supreme Court justices consider matters that are brought before the court.
8. _____ is a devotion to the truth.
9. Kristy considers being friendly toward the patients in the clinic as her _____ and a vital part of her job performance.
10. When a person has breached an ethical standard, _____ may be necessary to atone for the action.

SKILLS AND CONCEPTS

Part I: Making Ethical Decisions

List the five steps of ethical decision making.

1. _____
2. _____
3. _____
4. _____
5. _____

For the following scenarios, determine the type of ethical problem presented, the agent or agents, the course of action, and the outcome. Although these situations may present more than one ethical problem, choose only one possibility for each exercise.

Two sisters have arrived at a medical facility to discuss with the attending physician the course of action they should take regarding their dying father. Mr. Roberts, the patient, is no longer responsive. Cassandra wants to continue all possible medical treatment to keep her father alive. Janet insists that her father would not want his life prolonged by artificial means. Mr. Roberts did not give either sister a power of attorney, and he did not leave a written record of his wishes on this issue.

1. Type of ethical problem

   _____

2. Agent or agents

   _____

3. Course of action (Suggest one.)

   _____

4. Outcome (Suggest one.)

   _____

5. How can the medical assistant refrain from inflicting his or her own opinions on patients?

   _____

   _____

   _____

Dr. Patrick is the chief of staff at a regional medical center. His specialty is oncology, and the hospital is considering the construction of a cancer center as part of a multimillion-dollar project. One of Dr. Patrick's partners, Dr. Adams, is vehemently opposed to the project because of the cost to the local taxpayers who support the hospital. Dr. Adams has threatened to leave the practice unless Dr. Patrick votes against the project. Dr. Patrick wants the center to be built, but he also realizes that if Dr. Adams leaves, the practice will suffer a drastic loss of income.

1. Type of ethical problem

   _____

2. Agent or agents

   _____

3. Course of action (Suggest one.)

   _____

4. Outcome (Suggest one.)

   _____

5. How would you handle an ethical decision that has an equal number of pros and cons?

   _____

   _____

   _____

Part II: Types of Ethical Problems

Identify the type of ethical problem that each diagram represents.

1.

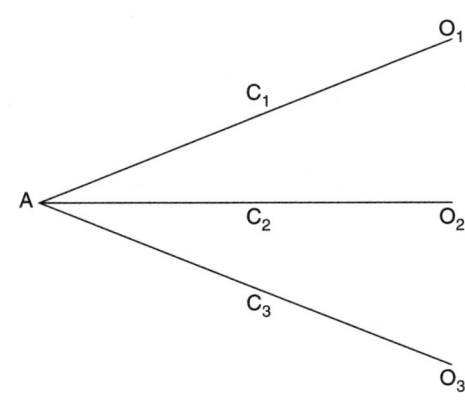

2.

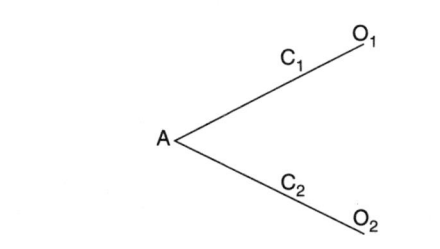

3.

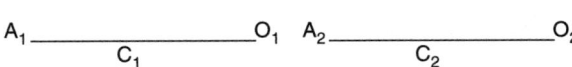

4.

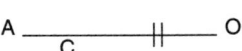

Part III: Opinions on Medicoethical Issues

Write your personal opinion regarding the following medicoethical issues. After writing your opinion, consider differing opinions by writing a brief opposing argument.

1. Abortion

_____
_____
_____

2. Abortion: opposing opinion

_____
_____
_____

3. Stem cell research

___

4. Stem cell research: opposing opinion

___

5. Human cloning

___

6. Human cloning: opposing opinion

___

7. Genetic counseling

___

8. Genetic counseling: opposing opinion

___

9. Physician-assisted suicide

___

10. Physician-assisted suicide: opposing opinion

___

Part IV: Ethics and the Medical Assistant

1. Describe the behavior of an ethical medical assistant in your own words.

   _____

   _____

   _____

   _____

Part V: Rights and Duties

Identify the following as a right, a duty, or neither.

1. Healthcare services for all Americans

   right   duty   neither

2. Owning a gun when licensed

   right   duty   neither

3. Providing care to an elderly parent

   right   duty   neither

4. Nondiscrimination

   right   duty   neither

5. Life

   right   duty   neither

6. Are there times when a right or duty in the preceding list is invalid or could be argued to be so? Explain your answer.

   _____

   _____

   _____

Part VI: Confidentiality

1. List several physical places within the physician's office where confidentiality could be breached.

   _____

   _____

   _____

2. What are the usual consequences of breach of patient confidentiality?

   _____

   _____

   _____

3. Explain why confidentiality is critical in the medical environment.

   _____

   _____

   _____

CASE STUDIES

Read the case studies and answer the questions that follow.

1. Robert is a patient who has tested positive for the human immunodeficiency virus (HIV). His employer invites the local blood bank to come to the workplace every 6 months and conduct a blood drive. Robert has declined to donate in the past because of his HIV status, but he often feels pressured by co-workers to give blood. None of them is aware that he is HIV positive. How do blood banks handle this situation today? Does Robert have alternatives that will resolve the situation? Explain your answer.

_____

_____

_____

2. Cameron works for Dr. Christian, and she works hard to earn the trust of the patients. Mrs. Rainer confides to Cameron that she has been smoking, against Dr. Christian's advice, and she asks Cameron not to tell the physician. How should Cameron handle this situation? What should she tell the patient?

_____

_____

_____

WORKPLACE APPLICATIONS

Stepping into the medical environment, where confidentiality is so important, may be a difficult adjustment for some new medical assistants. In any medical facility, you must think before speaking. At times, discussion of patients and their conditions will not be appropriate. How can you change your way of thinking and be constantly aware of the constraints that patient confidentiality places on discussion of patient information?

INTERNET ACTIVITIES

1. Peruse the Web site for the Health Insurance Portability and Accountability Act (HIPAA) and download the quick fact sheets. Study this information to gain a basic knowledge of HIPAA guidelines before studying the law in more detail in Chapter 16.

2. Discuss ethics in the classroom. How do medical assisting students perform ethically while completing their education? Research this issue on the Internet and talk about it in class.

3. Read the preamble and the nine principles of medical ethics posted on the American Medical Association's Web site. Discuss each principle. What changes would you make to these principles? Are they applicable to the situations that arise in the medical world today?

7 Medicine and Law

VOCABULARY REVIEW

Fill in the blanks with the correct vocabulary terms from this chapter.

1. Dr. Parker insists that a medical assistant be present during all of his patient examinations in order to avoid any _____ of wrongdoing or abuse.

2. Many physician offices require patients to sign a(n) _____ agreement, which means disagreements may be settled by a qualified third party.

3. If a person contributes to a patient's poor condition, he or she may be charged with _____.

4. Dr. Samantha Beddingfield was called to court to discuss her knowledge of malpractice cases as a(n) _____.

5. When a patient offers his or her arm to have blood drawn, he or she has _____ consent.

6. A doctor of _____ studies the law.

7. Dr. Cartwright failed to follow the care of a hospital patient to whom he was assigned and may be guilty of _____ and/or _____.

8. Civil cases must be proved by a(n) _____ of the _____.

9. Criminal cases must be proved by _____ _____.

10. Roger Askew is bringing a case against a physician in the death of his wife during surgery, making him the _____ in the case.

11. Something put into one's own words is _____.

12. A court must have _____ over a case before it can hear the arguments and make a judgment.

13. If Alisha writes down comments that are untrue and inflammatory about another person, she might be accused of _____.

14. City court is often called _____ court.

15. City regulations are often called city _____.

16. If either side in a lawsuit is unhappy with the results, in most cases the decision can be _____.

17. Vince suffered the loss of use of his arm after surgery, loss of wages by being rendered unable to work, and loss of his ability to earn a living. These losses are called _____ in court.

18. The constitutional guarantee that legal proceedings will be fair is called _____.

19. Judge Roberts has 12 cases on the _____ for the day.

20. The person who stands accused of a crime in court is called the _____.

21. The person who stands accused in a civil trial is called the _____.

22. Alyssa may be held _____ for damaging her boyfriend's car.

23. An intentional attempt to injure another person is called _____.

24. The unlawful use of force or violence against another person is called _____.
25. A(n) _____ is a major crime, such as rape or murder.
26. Consent that is detailed and usually in writing is called _____ consent.
27. Judge Conlin uses previous cases as models to determine his decisions on current cases. The previous cases are called _____.
28. Barbara Harris was served a(n) _____, which required her to appear in court.
29. The document requiring that records be produced in court is called a(n) _____ _____.
30. The final decision of the judge or jury is called the _____.

SKILLS AND CONCEPTS

Part I: Classifications of Law

1. The three basic categories of criminal law discussed in this chapter are:
   a. _____
   b. _____
   c. _____

2. The three basic categories of civil law discussed in this chapter are:
   a. _____
   b. _____
   c. _____

3. A law that is minor in nature and usually a breach of municipal regulations is called a(n) _____.
4. Civil law involves cases that are brought to court by _____.
5. Criminal law involves a crime against the _____ or _____.
6. Medical professional liability falls under what category of civil law? _____

Part II: Anatomy of a Medical Professional Liability Lawsuit

1. List the four elements of a valid, legal contract.
   a. _____
   b. _____
   c. _____
   d. _____

2. List the three steps in the creation of the physician-patient relationship.
   a. _____
   b. _____
   c. _____

3. What must a letter of withdrawal of care state?

   a. _____

   b. _____

   c. _____

4. How should a letter of withdrawal be mailed? _____

5. Does the letter of withdrawal have to explain to the patient the reason the physician chose to withdraw from care of the patient? Explain your answer.

   _____

   _____

   _____

6. Explain what is meant by having jurisdiction over a case.

   _____

   _____

   _____

7. What is the ultimate appellate court in the United States?

   _____

8. Explain the difference between a deposition and an interrogatory.

   _____

   _____

   _____

9. List three of the five ways to determine whether a subpoena is valid.

   a. _____

   b. _____

   c. _____

10. Briefly explain how a person called to testify in court should dress.

    _____

    _____

    _____

11. What is a defendant in a civil trial often called? _____

Part III: Medical Professional Liability and Negligence

Find the words in the list in the following puzzle.

```
Y S R Z S T F P E M Z S T D B P X K F Q W U T F
M R K O F U N H C H A F C B M N G J K M M T E U
Y R O T U B I R T N O C T F E W X L A B J D Y O
M R U T T P A A Q M S N B I L E V U Y K I W Y S
S D E L A N O I S S E F O R P G S G J L U G S R
B E C N A S A E F L A M O I Y V P G H K W P E G
V N N K Y B N J M A B X H H T R E P X E I Z W S
T I A Q F Y E E U U E A T I U A I M B S Q H O U
B C S A P H G N P W H A K D D O G S E P H F R B
T I A I H I L E O M Z H E I M V B E J M N B K M
S D E R E L I C T I O N A C Z M F G L J E F F Z
C E F F O F G N G Q T C N V F Q K A T L D G S S
K M S R U R E A S O N A B L E X E M P L A R Y S
B W I C I D N S W Z G Q G D V E D A T L I R N N
K X M V E Z C A C S U V N I I V H D T O M R R T
R D F C L O E E A P O N D K T X I J W K L M K I
Q K E K H U D F W D W G S K I I Y R U D E W U S
L D R P X Z F N P A Z R B V N F L P Y P X V M I
L Y Y S O J S O P L D G Q U U V G P E F R U J P
A V P J X X J N C L W U I S P S N N I P A V F T
D B W T R U V R V C Z Q D X O W U F E Q S T W Z
```

Act	Duty	Nonfeasance
Allegation	Exemplary	Professional
Compensatory	Expert	Prudent
Contributory	Litigation	Punitive
Damages	Malfeasance	Reasonable
Decedent	Misfeasance	
Dereliction	Negligence	

Part IV: Fill in the Blanks

Fill in the blanks with the correct answers.

1. The formal action of a legislative body is called a(n) _____.
2. The performance of an act that is wholly wrongful and unlawful is _____.
3. The agency that regulates safety in the workplace is _____.
4. A law enacted by the legislative branch of a government is called a(n) _____.
5. Failure to perform an act that should have been performed is _____.
6. A solemn declaration made by a witness under oath in response to interrogation by a lawyer is called _____.
7. The pretense of curing disease is called _____.
8. The improper performance of a legal act is _____.
9. Something that is easily understood or recognized by the mind is called a(n) _____.
10. An authoritative decree or direction usually set forth by a municipal regulation is called a(n) _____.
11. The law that promotes accuracy in medical laboratories is _____.

Part V: Inside the Courtroom

Circle T or F to indicate whether the statement is true or false.

1. T F Lying under oath constitutes perjury.
2. T F Arriving late to the courtroom is acceptable if the witness has a good excuse.
3. T F Attorneys usually discover new information when questioning their clients in the courtroom.
4. T F A sustained objection means that the judge disagrees with the objection and will allow the question to stand.
5. T F It is not necessary to use "ma'am" or "sir" in the courtroom when addressing the judge.
6. T F If a question is confusing to a witness, he or she should ask the attorney to restate or repeat the question.
7. T F Discovery is pretrial disclosure of pertinent facts or documents pertaining to a case.
8. T F Arbitration is a cost-saving alternative to trial.

Part VI: The Four Ds of Negligence and Damages

1. A patient was given the wrong medication. No adverse effects occurred. Which of the four Ds is missing? Why does this affect the possibility of a lawsuit?

   _____
   _____
   _____

2. A car accident occurs at an intersection outside a physician's office during normal business hours. Do the physician and staff have a duty to provide direct care for the injured? Why or why not?

   _____
   _____
   _____

3. A patient is treated for low back pain caused by a fall at the local mall. The patient sues the physician, because the pain is unresolved. Which of the four Ds would be the most difficult for the patient's attorney to prove? Why?

_____
_____
_____

4. A medical assistant mislabeled a vial of blood that was sent to an outside laboratory. Because of this mistake, a child was given the wrong diagnosis and later died. The child's family sued the medical assistant, the physician, and the hospital that owned the practice. The child's family was awarded $4 million. What type of damages is this?

_____
_____
_____

5. A female patient was awarded punitive damages after a physician sexually molested her during her annual pelvic examination. What are punitive damages designed to do? Do you think punitive damages should be limited to a specific amount of money?

_____
_____
_____

CASE STUDY

Read the case study and answer the questions that follow.

A 10-year-old girl was brought to a physician's office with a complaint of a headache after gymnastics practice in mid-August. The clinic was a freestanding, minor emergency center and not the child's regular physician's office. The girl and the adult who had brought her to the clinic, her aunt, both denied that she had been in any type of accident and stated that her only complaint was the headache and being tired and hot. The aunt mentioned that the girl also seemed a bit disoriented during the drive to the clinic. The girl didn't recall having been at gymnastics practice less than an hour earlier. The child told the physician that she had been a gymnast for 6 years and that she really liked her coach.

The outside temperature had reached 101° F that day. The physician examined the patient and suggested that she be taken home to rest and rehydrate. No prescriptions were written, and the girl left the clinic. Two hours later, she could not be roused from sleep; her aunt immediately took her to the emergency department (ED) at the closest hospital. The girl's mother met them at the hospital just in time to be told that the girl had slipped into a coma. The ED physician suspected that the girl had experienced heat stroke. The aunt was shocked and mentioned that she had taken the girl to a clinic earlier; she questioned why this diagnosis has not been considered at that time. The girl's mother immediately called the clinic and berated the physician for putting her child in a coma.

What went wrong in this case? Who is responsible for the child's condition? Is this a "good" malpractice case?

_____
_____
_____
_____
_____
_____
_____

WORKPLACE APPLICATIONS

Research the laws that apply to medical clinics in your state. If possible, interview an office manager about the laws that apply to local clinics and ask what challenges arise in trying to comply with them. Share what you learn with the class.

INTERNET ACTIVITIES

1. Use the Internet to find the place in your area where a small claims case would be filed. Obtain the paperwork necessary to file a claim. Create a fictional case and complete the paperwork as if you plan to file it in court.

2. Research mediators in your area using the Internet. Find the name and contact information for at least three. With your instructor's permission, contact a mediator and ask the individual to speak to the class.

3. Research medical malpractice attorneys in your area using the Internet. Find the name and contact information for at least three. With your instructor's permission, invite the attorney to speak to the class on how medical assistants can help prevent medical malpractice claims.

8 Computer Concepts

VOCABULARY REVIEW

Fill in the blanks with the correct vocabulary terms from this chapter.

1. Jacob uses a(n) _____ _____ to write data onto a blank compact disk and stores the CD as a backup for the clinic's blank forms.

2. To assist with patient diagnosis, Dr. Matthews uses software that is equipped with a type of _____ _____.

3. The smallest unit of information inside the computer is called a(n) _____.

4. Olivia installed new _____ _____ on the office computers that will allow patients to check in without the assistance of a receptionist.

5. Ethan has asked that all the computer users in the clinic clear the computer _____ periodically so that Web sites stored there will be erased and the system will run faster.

6. The office manager asked Samantha to print a(n) _____ _____ of the minutes of the meeting for each person attending.

7. Daniel likes to change the _____ in the different sections of the clinic's patients' newsletter to make it more readable and attractive.

8. A picture that represents a program or an object on the computer is called a(n) _____.

9. Information entered into and used by the computer is called _____.

10. Tyler is responsible for the operation of the clinic's _____, which manages shared network resources.

11. Information that is processed by the computer and transmitted to a monitor or printer is called _____.

12. Christian was able to easily connect a(n) _____ to his home computer, which allows information to be transmitted over telephone lines and enables him to connect to the Internet.

13. Any type of storage of files used to prevent their loss in the event of hard drive failure is called _____.

14. The _____ tracks all patient information, including addresses, phone numbers, and details about insurance coverage.

15. Megan purchased a(n) _____ _____ to backup the patient database and archive computer files.

16. A personal _____ assistant is a handheld computer that can perform many functions.

17. The initial part of a URL listing is called a(n) _____ _____.

SKILLS AND CONCEPTS

Part I: Matching Exercises
Match the following terms with their definitions.

1. _____ Approximately 1 billion bytes   A. Terabyte
2. _____ Approximately 1 trillion bytes   B. Bit
3. _____ 8 bits   C. Megabyte
4. _____ Binary digits   D. Byte
5. _____ Approximately 1,024 bytes   E. Kilobyte
6. _____ Approximately 1 million bytes   F. Gigabyte

Part II: Input, Output, and Storage Devices
Label each of the following as an input, output, or storage device.

	Device			
1.	Mouse	Input	Output	Storage
2.	Keyboard	Input	Output	Storage
3.	Printer	Input	Output	Storage
4.	Scanner	Input	Output	Storage
5.	Speakers	Input	Output	Storage
6.	CD-ROM	Input	Output	Storage
7.	Zip drive	Input	Output	Storage
8.	Touch screen	Input	Output	Storage
9.	Floppy disk	Input	Output	Storage
10.	Flash drive	Input	Output	Storage

Part III: Parts of the Computer
Provide the name of the computer part described below.

1. Central unit of the computer that contains the logic circuitry and carries out the instructions of the computer's programs

   _____

2. Main circuit board of the computer

   _____

3. Devices inserted into a computer that give it added capabilities

   _____

4. Device used to display computer-generated information

   _____

5. Magnetic disk inside the computer that can hold several hundred gigabytes of information and is used to store the application software that runs on the computer

   _____

6. Device used to take information from one CD-ROM and write it to another CD-ROM

   _____

7. Device over which data can be transmitted via telephone lines or other media, such as coaxial cable

8. Allows music or MIDI files to be heard from the computer

9. Software installed on a computer to allow a hardware device to function

Part IV: The Computer as a Co-Worker
List seven ways computers assist workers in medical offices.

1. _____
2. _____
3. _____
4. _____
5. _____
6. _____
7. _____

Part V: Basic Computer Functions
Describe how the following functions are performed on the computer.

1. Open a document

2. Save a document

3. Rename a document

4. Cut and paste text

5. Copy text

6. Exit a program

7. Turn the computer on

_____

_____

8. Turn the computer off

_____

_____

Part VI: Short Answer Questions

1. The three elements that differentiate microprocessors are:

   a. _____

   b. _____

   c. _____

2. Explain peripheral devices and give one example of a peripheral device.

   _____

   _____

3. What is the function of a browser?

   _____

   _____

4. Define computer networking.

   _____

   _____

5. Why is computer security so important in today's medical office?

   _____

   _____

Part VII: File Formats and Printer Types

Match the following terms with their definitions.

1. _____ Inexpensive printer that provides a moderate-quality hard copy

2. _____ File format that supports color and often is used for scanned images

3. _____ Bitmapped graphics compiled by a graphics image set in rows or columns of dots

4. _____ Printer output similar to that of a photocopier; capable of complex graphics

5. _____ File format in which characters are represented by their ASCII codes

6. _____ File type commonly used for photographs

a. .doc
b. .gif
c. Laser
d. .jpeg
e. .bmp
f. Dot matrix

7. _____ File type that combines ASCII codes with special commands that distinguish variations

8. _____ File usually created by a word processor for various documents, including letters and forms

9. _____ Printer that uses a heating element that is energized during the printing process

10. _____ Type of printer that serves as a scanner, fax, and copier

g. .txt
h. Ink jet
i. .rtf
j. Multifunctional

CASE STUDY

Read the case study and answer the questions that follow.

Brooke Comis works for Dr. Tomms as a clinical medical assistant. She is a former office computer specialist who worked in the computer field for 12 years before she entered medical assisting school. She changed career fields because of the work prospects in technology and acted on her dream to enter the medical field. Unfortunately, she is the only person in the office who is knowledgeable about computers, the Internet, and networking. Whenever a computer is not functioning correctly or a problem occurs with the network, Dr. Tomms asks Brooke to fix it. When he decided to buy new computers, he expected Brooke to assemble all of them and set up a new network. Brooke gets more and more irate each time she is asked to perform these duties, because she is not compensated other than her normal hourly pay. She knows that if Dr. Tomms paid someone to do this work, it would cost him more than her monthly salary. Brooke is not certain how to handle this situation. What should she do first? How should she approach the physician? Should she refuse to perform computer work? What could happen if she refuses?

WORKPLACE APPLICATIONS

Assume that you have been selected to order a new computer system for the physician. The clinic's personnel include three physicians, six administrative personnel, and four clinical assistants, plus you, the office manager. Describe the minimum equipment needed. Consider printers, Internet access, scanners, and wireless needs. Investigate computers using the Internet and prepare a folder with photos and/or specifications that detail the equipment you have selected.

INTERNET ACTIVITIES

Use the Internet to locate a company that sells computers in your geographic area. Explore the site. Find a computer that you might consider purchasing, then answer the following questions.

1. How much RAM and ROM does the system have?

2. What is the clock speed?

3. What is the baud rate of the modem?

4. What software, if any, comes with the system?

5. What is the total cost before taxes are applied?

9 Telephone Techniques

VOCABULARY REVIEW

Fill in the blanks with the correct vocabulary terms from this chapter.

1. Taylor Medical USA sells durable medical equipment and supplies to the public, so the company is considered to be a(n) _____.

2. Julie is careful of her _____, because she wants her voice to be clear and effective when she is speaking on the telephone.

3. Cassie's voice has a nice _____, which is a change in pitch or loudness when speaking.

4. Dr. LeGrand wants to _____ her relationships with patients of different cultures so that she can understand their needs.

5. The office manager cautions the medical assistants to avoid _____, because most patients do not understand complicated medical terms.

6. The highness or lowness of sound is called its _____.

7. Laura _____ will be at work on time and will stay until the last patient leaves.

8. When speaking on the phone or in public, Dr. Conn knows that he should avoid _____ speech to keep the listeners interested and enthusiastic about what he has to say.

9. The medical assistants at Wray Medical and Surgical Clinic are proficient at _____.

10. Being placed on hold for an extended time becomes quite _____.

11. The utterance of articulate, clear sounds is _____.

12. It is pleasant to hear a person speak with _____.

13. Dr. Beard ordered the laboratory tests _____ so that the results would be reported to him immediately.

14. Mackenzie has learned to be _____ when she speaks with patients on the phone so that she maintains a good relationship with them.

15. Dr. Lightfoot prefers that the receptionist _____ all his calls so that he can concentrate on the patients in the office during their examinations.

SKILLS AND CONCEPTS

Part I: Answering Incoming Calls and Taking Phone Messages

Read the following incoming calls. Then use the telephone message forms to take an accurate message for each caller. The calls in quotations are taken from voice mail. Determine who should receive the message; three questions to ask the patient when the call is returned; and what actions need to be taken for proper follow-through. Although you are not required to list questions that are clinical in nature, you may include clinical questions if you like.

Staff Members at Dr. Julie Beard's Office

Physician	Dr. Julie Beard
Office Manager	Julia Carpenter
Clinical Medical Assistant	Trina Martinez
Clinical Medical Assistant	Dean Howell
Scheduling Assistant	Stephanie Dickson
Receptionist	Ginny Holloway
Insurance Biller and Medical Records	Gloria Richardson

1. "Hello, this is Peter Young. I saw Dr. Beard on Monday about a rash on my forearms. This thing isn't getting any better, and the cream she prescribed for me isn't helping the itching, and it's very uncomfortable. Is there anything else we can do to help it? My number is 972-555-9873." The message was received at 8:30 AM on Thursday, February 3.

   Who should receive this message?

   _____

   Questions to ask the patient when returning this call:

   a. _____
   b. _____
   c. _____

   What action should be taken after speaking with the patient?

   _____
   _____
   _____

2. Gerald Morris calls Dr. Beard's office to ask whether his insurance has paid for his last office visit. He is an established patient and has worked as a city police officer for more than 10 years. After asking to place Mr. Morris on hold, you pull up his account on the computer. No insurance payment has been credited to his account, and a note indicates that his insurance was not in effect at the time of his office visit. Mr. Morris asks you to check with the insurance company and call him back, because he is concerned about resolving this issue. His phone number is 972-555-8824. This message was taken at 3:45 PM on September 4.

   Who should receive this message?

   _____

   Questions to ask the patient when returning this call:

   a. _____
   b. _____
   c. _____

What action should be taken after speaking to the patient?

_____
_____
_____

3. "Hello, this is Savannah Yarborough. I visited with your receptionist earlier today, and she indicated that one of the medical assistants has resigned and you will have a position available in a few weeks. I am very interested in interviewing and presenting myself as a candidate for the job. I am a certified medical assistant with 6 years' experience. Please give me a call at your convenience. My telephone number is 817-555-9902. I look forward to speaking with you and perhaps scheduling an interview." This message was taken at 1:30 PM on May 1.

Who should receive this message?

_____

Questions to ask when returning this call:

a. _____

b. _____

c. _____

What action should be taken after speaking to Ms. Yarborough?

_____
_____
_____

4. Mr. Juan Ross called today at 10:15 AM to get his prescription for Ambien refilled. His pharmacy is Wolfe Drug, and the drugstore phone number is 214-555-4523. He is allergic to penicillin. Mr. Ross's phone number is 214-555-2377. Mr. Ross's message was received on July 23.

Who should receive this message?

_____

Questions to ask the patient when returning his call:

a. _____

b. _____

c. _____

What action should be taken after speaking to the patient?

_____
_____
_____

5. Mr. Benjamin Adams called to speak to the office manager to express his dissatisfaction with the times he was offered for an appointment. His job is strict about attendance, and he cannot leave work until 4 PM. He has requested appointment times after 4 PM, but the scheduling assistant tells him that he cannot have an appointment any later than 4 PM. Mr. Adams is concerned that he will not be able to be at the clinic at that exact time, and he is frustrated that the clinic is not more responsive to his needs. He called at 2:15 PM on March 14. His phone number at work is 972-555-6343, and his cell phone number is 214-555-8080.

Who should receive this message?

_____

Questions to ask the patient when returning the call:

a. _____

b. _____

c. _____

What action should be taken after speaking to the patient?

_____

_____

_____

6. "This is Ms. Garrett from Blue Cross/Blue Shield, and it's 10 AM on June 5. I am calling to discuss employee benefits for the coming year with the office manager. BCBS provides insurance coverage for your clinic employees. Would you please have the office manager return my call when she has a few moments to talk? My number is 800-555-0024, extension 415. Thank you!"

Who should receive this message?

_____

Questions to ask when returning the call:

a. _____

b. _____

c. _____

What action should be taken after speaking to Ms. Garrett?

_____

_____

_____

7. "This is Sarah at Cline Meador Lab with a stat lab report. It's 9:35 AM on November 16. The patient's name is Laura Williamson, and her WBC count is 18,000. Please notify Dr. Beard immediately. The lab phone number is 800-555-3333, and my extension is 255. If she has any questions, please have her give me a call. Thanks."

Who should receive this message?

_____

Questions to ask or information to verify when returning the call:

a. _____

b. _____

c. _____

What action should be taken after speaking to Sarah?

_____

_____

_____

8. Judy Jordan has migraine headaches and occasionally takes hydrocodone to relieve the pain. Dr. Beard leaves the office for the weekend at noon on Friday, and office policy dictates that she is not to be paged except in emergencies. Patients with routine or lesser health issues are to be instructed either to make an appointment to come in and see the physician or to go to the emergency department. Ms. Jordan calls at 4:45 PM on Friday afternoon, March 9, after Dr. Beard has left the office. She requests that the staff authorize a refill for her pain medicine and insists on speaking to the office manager, who is in a meeting. Ms. Jordan's phone number is 214-555-9822.

Who should receive this message?

_____

Questions to ask or information to verify when returning the call:

a. _____

b. _____

c. _____

What action should be taken in this situation?

_____
_____
_____

9. Gary Burritt is moving out of state, so he calls the office because he needs a copy of his medical records. Dr. Beard prefers to send medical records directly to the receiving physician. Mr. Burritt's phone number is 512-555-6679. Today's date is December 20, and this message was received at 11:45 AM.

Who should receive this message?

_____

Questions to ask or information to verify when returning the call:

a. _____

b. _____

c. _____

What action should be taken in this situation?

_____
_____
_____

10. Allan Jenkins is calling from the cleaning service to let the office manager know what supplies he needs. He leaves a message stating that the office needs window cleaner, paper towels, liquid cleanser, and floor cleaner. He says that the office manager does not have to call him back, but the service will be cleaning again on Friday evening and will need the supplies at that time. This message was received on Wednesday, April 7 at 8:10 AM. The caller leaves his phone number, 903-555-2378, in case the office manager has questions.

Who should receive this message?

_____

What action should be taken in this situation?

_____
_____
_____

11. "Hello. My name is Christina Cawtel, and I was referred to your office by Dr. Preston for evaluation of an ovarian cyst. Today is Wednesday, October 4, and it is 8 AM. I would like to make an appointment for early next week if possible. My phone number is 817-555-9325. Oh, and by the way, I need to know if you are a provider for Aetna, because my company just changed to their managed care plan. I probably need to have a mammogram, too, and I want to see if you will order it before I come in for the appointment. Thanks."

    Who should receive this message?

    _____

    Questions to ask or information to verify when returning the call:

    a. _____

    b. _____

    c. _____

    What action should be taken in this situation?

    _____
    _____
    _____

12. "My name is Janeen Shaw and I am Dr. Beard's patient. It is just before 2 PM, and I am trying to reach you as soon as you open your office after lunch. I am having a hard time breathing, and I have stomach pains. I am hurting all over my upper body, on my chest, my arms, my neck, just everywhere. I'm sweating, and I'm very nauseated. I'm 45, and I'm almost never ill. I wanted to find out if I can come in for an appointment today. Please call me back as soon as possible. My phone number is 601-555-3423. Thank you. Please call as soon as you can. I really feel awful."

    Who should receive this message?

    _____

    Questions to ask or information to verify when returning the call:

    a. _____

    b. _____

    c. _____

    What action should be taken in this situation?

    _____
    _____
    _____

Part II: Handling Difficult Calls

Briefly explain how the following callers and types of calls should be handled.

1. Angry callers

    _____
    _____
    _____

2. Sales calls

    _____
    _____
    _____

3. Emergency calls

4. Unauthorized inquiry calls

5. Callers with complaints

Part III: Using a Telephone Directory

Using your local telephone directory or internet directory, find the following telephone numbers for your city or community.

1. Nonemergency number for the police department

2. General information number for the nearest airport

3. Local tax office

4. American Red Cross office

5. Acute care hospital

6. Mental health and mental retardation center

7. Meals on Wheels

8. American Cancer Society

Part IV: Answering the Telephone

Use the local telephone directory or internet directory to find telephone numbers for the following medical specialty offices in your area. Call these offices to determine how they answer the telephone. Explain the purpose of your call to the staff member who answers the phone and record the phone greeting they use in the space provided below. Alternatively, write an original phone greeting for each of these medical specialty offices.

1. Ophthalmologist

   _____

2. Oncologist

   _____

3. General practitioner

   _____

4. Chiropractor

   _____

5. Cosmetic surgeon

   _____

6. Dermatologist

   _____

Part V: Short Answer Questions

Fill in the blank with the correct answer.

1. Selecting which calls will be forwarded to the physician immediately is a process called _____.

2. A study by Harvard University claims that the physician's _____ of voice has a direct link to medical professional liability claims.

3. The medical assistant should not eat, drink, or _____ while answering the office telephone.

4. The mouthpiece of the telephone handset should be held _____ inch(es) from the lips.

5. The medical assistant must maintain patient _____ at all times, even when on the telephone.

6. Telephone calls should be answered by the _____ ring.

7. Unsatisfactory progress reports from patients should be directed to the _____.

8. _____ calls help the physician communicate with family members in different parts of the country.

9. Medical offices should have a set of clearly written _____ that can be read to the caller who requests the information.

Part VI: Time Zones

Determine the correct times.

1. When it is 3 PM in Dallas, Texas, it is _____ in Los Angeles, California.

2. When it is 2 PM in Washington state, it is _____ in New York City.

3. When it is 5 PM in Las Cruces, New Mexico, it is _____ in Flint, Michigan.

4. When it is 4 PM in Augusta, Maine, it is _____ in Columbia, South Carolina.

5. When it is 11 AM in Biloxi, Mississippi, it is _____ in Chicago, Illinois.

Part VII: Telephone Technique

1. List five questions that might be asked of a patient who calls with an emergency situation:

   a. _____

   b. _____

   c. _____

   d. _____

   e. _____

2. The phrase that often calms an angry patient is _____ _____ _____ _____.

3. Explain the procedure for transferring a phone call.

   _____

   _____

   _____

4. What should the medical assistant do if a caller refuses to identify himself or herself?

   _____

   _____

   _____

5. List the seven components of a proper telephone message.

   a. _____

   b. _____

   c. _____

   d. _____

   e. _____

   f. _____

   g. _____

CASE STUDY

Read the case study and answer the questions that follow.

Denise has been the receptionist for a moderately large clinic for the past 3 months. She replaced Dorothy, who retired. Denise has been overwhelmed by the number of calls to the clinic, and the office manager has spoken to her twice about missing calls. Denise insists that she is constantly on the phone answering and transferring calls. She is beginning to lose faith in herself, but as she considers why she is failing at her job, she realizes that two new physicians have joined the practice since Dorothy left, and numerous calls come to the clinic for those two physicians. Denise wants to suggest to the office manager that perhaps the time has come for a second receptionist, but she is unsure how to broach the subject. How can Denise begin her conversation with the office manager? What should she not do or say?

_____

_____

_____

_____

WORKPLACE APPLICATIONS

Contact a clinic office manager and ask whether he or she would allow you to shadow the office receptionist for a day. Take note of the types of calls that come into the clinic and how they are handled. Discuss the results of the visit with the class.

INTERNET ACTIVITIES

1. Investigate telephone techniques and skills on the Internet and bring three tips to class. Share these with your classmates.

2. After researching information on the Internet, write a report that explains why the telephone is so important in making a good first impression.

3. Research the way telephones actually work. Prepare a brief report for the class.

4. Research the way Internet connections are made through phone systems. Prepare a brief report for the class.

10 Scheduling Appointments

VOCABULARY REVIEW

Fill in the blank with the correct vocabulary term from this chapter.

1. Angela arranged for a short time _____ between Dr. Patrick's speaking engagement and his first afternoon appointment so that he would have time for lunch.

2. Gayle gained _____ in computers by taking Saturday classes on the newest software.

3. A(n) _____ noise came from the autoclave when it was turned on this morning, so Pamela called service personnel to repair the machine.

4. Olivia realized that she needed to take a(n) _____ medical terminology course before she could register for anatomy and physiology.

5. All the medical assistants in the facility know that a(n) _____ _____ must be noted in the medical record, as well as the appointment book.

6. Before using an appointment book, establish the _____ by marking all times the physician is unavailable, so that patients will not be scheduled during those times.

7. A patient from a neighboring clinic caused a(n) _____ in the hallway as he left, because he disagreed with a billing statement.

8. _____ _____ are those who have been seen as patients in the clinic more than once.

9. The _____ among the staff at Dr. Wykowski's office has become strained since the office manager was terminated.

10. Cooperation and willingness to help other staff members is a(n) _____ part of the success of a practice.

11. The payment of benefits to the physician for services rendered is called _____.

12. A(n) _____ is a predeveloped page layout used to make new pages with a similar design, pattern, or style.

SKILLS AND CONCEPTS

Part I: Appointment Reminder Cards

Practice completing appointment reminder cards on the forms provided.

1. Gayle Jackson has an appointment for August 23, 20XX, at 3 PM with Dr. Lupez.

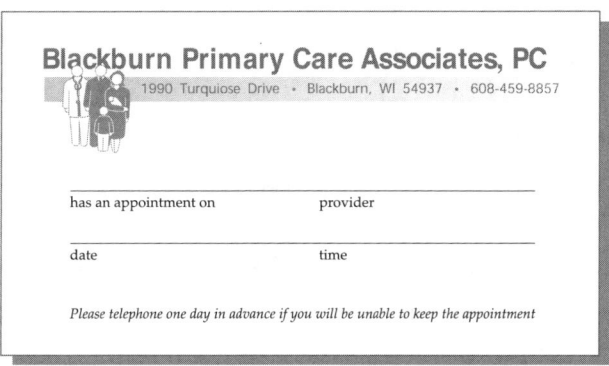

2. Debra Odom has an appointment for May 1, 20XX, at 9 AM with Dr. Hughes.

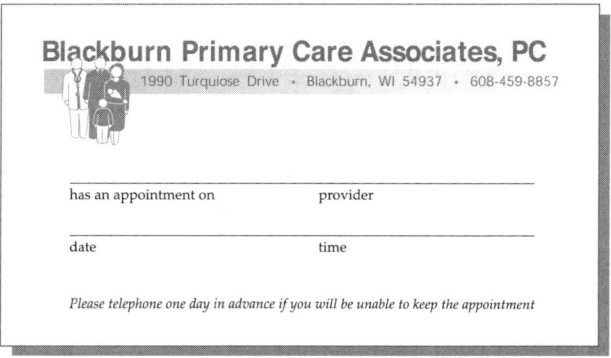

3. Katrina Shaw has an appointment for June 13, 20XX, at 11:45 AM with Dr. Hughes.

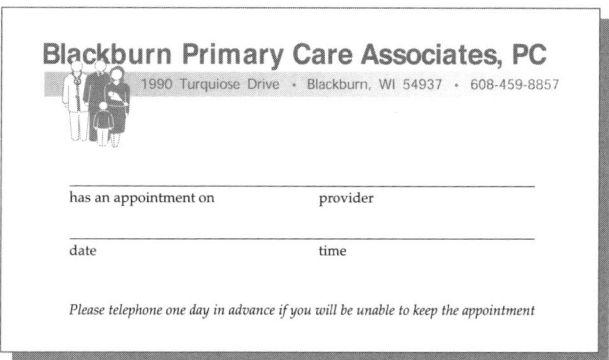

4. Joni Perry has an appointment for September 12, 20XX, at 2:40 PM with Dr. Lawler.

Blackburn Primary Care Associates, PC
1990 Turquoise Drive • Blackburn, WI 54937 • 608-459-8857

_____   _____
has an appointment on   provider
_____   _____
date   time

Please telephone one day in advance if you will be unable to keep the appointment

5. Savannah York has an appointment for December 15, 20XX, at 4:30 PM with Dr. Lupez.

Blackburn Primary Care Associates, PC
1990 Turquoise Drive • Blackburn, WI 54937 • 608-459-8857

_____   _____
has an appointment on   provider
_____   _____
date   time

Please telephone one day in advance if you will be unable to keep the appointment

Part II: Guides for Scheduling

1. What three items must be considered when scheduling appointments?

    a. _____

    b. _____

    c. _____

2. Why is patient need an important consideration when planning the services the clinic will offer?

    _____

    _____

3. How can the medical assistant handle a physician who habitually spends more than the allotted time with patients?

    _____

    _____

4. List one advantage and one disadvantage to using an appointment book for scheduling.

    Advantage _____

    Disadvantage _____

5. List one advantage and one disadvantage to using a computer for scheduling.

    Advantage _____

    Disadvantage _____

6. Explain why the time length of appointments is important.

7. Define a template and explain its use with regard to appointment scheduling.

8. What is a repeating appointment?

9. What is the difference between an emergency appointment and an urgent appointment?

10. Explain why an emergency call should never be placed on hold.

Part III: Advance Preparation and Establishing a Matrix

Prepare Appointment Page 1 (See Work Product 10-1 on p. 47 of the Procedures Checklists) according to the following directions.

1. The date is Monday, October 13, 20XX.
2. Dr. Lawler and Dr. Hughes have hospital rounds from 8 to 9 AM.
3. Dr. Lupez sees patients from 8 AM to noon and then has a medical conference.
4. Lunch is from noon until 2 PM.
5. Dr. Lawler has a 4 PM meeting at the hospital.
6. Dr. Hughes and Dr. Lawler both prefer a break from 3:15 to 3:30 PM to catch up on telephone calls and other duties.

Part IV: Scheduling Appointments

Prepare Appointment Page 2 (See Work Product 10-2 on p. 49 of the Procedures Checklists) according to the following directions. Appointments can be scheduled for subsequent days in these exercises.

1. The date is Tuesday, October 14, 20XX.
2. Lunch is from noon until 2 PM.
3. Dr. Lawler will be out Tuesday afternoon.
4. Dr. Hughes is out of town speaking at a conference.
5. Tracey and Keith Jones would like an appointment with Dr. Lawler right before lunch. Both are new patient physical examinations, and they would like to come to the office at the same time so that they can also discuss family planning.
6. John Edgar, Lydia Perry, and June Trayner are established patients who need follow-up appointments with Dr. Lupez.

7. Wayne Harris needs a new patient appointment with Dr. Lawler as early as possible.

8. Lucy Fraser needs an appointment with Dr. Lawler or Dr. Hughes and has to make the appointment after 3:30 PM, because she picks up her children from school.

9. Asa Nordholm, Carrie Jones, and Seicho Ando need follow-up appointments with Dr. Lawler.

10. Talia Perez called and is having trouble with her new blood pressure medication. The soonest she can get off work and come to the clinic is 2:15 PM.

11. Paula Nolen needs an allergy shot in the morning.

12. Amy Wainwright needs a well-woman examination and can come to the clinic any time before 3 PM.

13. Pam Billingsley wants to come to the clinic in the later afternoon for a return check about her migraine headaches.

14. Adam Angsley needs an appointment with Dr. Lawler in the afternoon.

Prepare Appointment Page 3 (See Work Product 10-3 on p. 51 of the Procedures Checklists) according to the following directions. Appointments can be scheduled for subsequent days in these exercises.

1. The date is Wednesday, October 15, 20XX.

2. All of the physicians are in the office today.

3. Lunch is from noon until 2 PM.

4. Dr. Lawler has three rechecks today, with Ella Jones, Fred Linstra, and Mary Higgins.

5. Winston Hill is an established patient coming in for an annual physical with Dr. Lawler. His neighbor can drive him to the clinic for a 2 PM appointment.

6. Elnar Rosen, an established patient, needs a physical with Dr. Hughes at around 10:15 AM.

7. A staff meeting is scheduled for 9 AM.

8. A representative from Allied Medical Supply is demonstrating a self-scheduling computer program at 4:30 PM for all staff members.

9. Bob Jones needs a morning appointment with Dr. Lupez.

10. Talia Perez is extremely nauseated and needs to return to the clinic today.

11. Robin Tower is a new patient who wants to see Dr. Lawler or Dr. Hughes.

12. Audrey Rhodes is a new patient who wants to see Dr. Lawler.

13. Victor Garner is a follow-up patient whom Dr. Lupez saw last week in the hospital. He is new to the clinic.

14. Charlie Robinson missed his appointment today at 11 AM with Dr. Hughes.

15. Peter Blake calls to see if he can be seen by one of the physicians at 11:15 AM.

Prepare Appointment Page 4 (See Work Product 10-4 on p. 53 of the Procedures Checklists) according to the following directions. Appointments can be scheduled for subsequent days in these exercises.

1. The date is Thursday, October 16, 20XX.

2. Dr. Hughes is not in the office, because his daughter is having a baby.

3. Lunch is from noon until 2 PM.

4. All patients must be seen in the morning because the clinic is closed on Thursday afternoons.

5. Cassie LeGrand is coming to the clinic as a new patient to see Dr. Lupez.

6. Cassandra LeBrock is coming to the clinic as an established patient to see Dr. Lupez.

7. Raymond Smith wants to make an appointment at 1:45 pm with Dr. Lawler.

8. Benjamin Charles requests an appointment with Dr. Lupez at 3:45 PM.

Prepare Appointment Page 5 (See Work Product 10-5 on p. 55 of the Procedures Checklists) according to the following directions.

1. The date is Friday, October 17, 20XX.

2. Dr. Lupez is the only provider in the office today.

3. Lunch is from noon until 2 PM.

4. Cassie LeGrand returns today for laboratory work and to consult with Dr. Lupez for surgery.

5. Bruce Wells is scheduled for a follow-up appointment at 10:15 AM.

6. Ronald Trayhan calls to make an appointment with Dr. Lupez for 2:30 PM.

7. Dr. Hughes calls to ask Dr. Lupez to see one of his young patients, Barbara Scott, at 3 PM for a high fever.

8. Stanley Allred calls for an appointment to see Dr. Lupez at 3 PM.

Part V: Types of Scheduling
Briefly describe each type of scheduling, and list one advantage and one disadvantage of each.

1. Scheduled appointments

___

2. Open office hours

___

3. Flexible office hours

___

4. Wave scheduling

___

5. Modified wave scheduling

___

6. Double booking

___

7. Grouping procedures

_____

_____

8. Advance booking

_____

_____

Part VI: Special Circumstances

1. How can the medical assistant deal with patients who are consistently late for appointments?

_____

_____

2. How does the medical assistant handle a patient who arrives at the clinic to see the physician but does not have an appointment?

_____

_____

Part VII: Verifying Appointments

1. Write a brief script that could be used to verify patient appointments and that does not violate patient privacy.

_____

_____

_____

_____

Part VIII: Scheduling Inpatient and Outpatient Admissions and Procedures

Complete the referral forms in Work Products 10-6 to 10-9 on pp. 57-64 of the Procedures Checklists for the following patients. Create fictional demographic information.

1. Cassie LeGrand is to report to Mercy Hospital for excision of a nasal polyp on Tuesday, October 24, 20XX. Dr. Lupez is her attending physician. Surgery is scheduled for Tuesday at 2 PM. She will need blood work that morning. The procedure is considered outpatient, and Cassie will go home later that day if she does well. ICD code: 471.0 (Work Product 10-6).

2. Bob Jones arrives at Presbyterian Hospital to have a magnetic resonance imaging (MRI) scan on his right knee on Friday, November 2, 20XX. He needs an early morning appointment. ICD code: 715.8 (Work Product 10-7).

3. Lucille Saxton is to be admitted to the hospital for surgery for a bowel obstruction. Her surgery date is June 14, 20XX, and she must be admitted a day in advance for laboratory work and a chest x-ray examination. ICD code: 560.9 (Work Product 10-8).

4. Pam Burton needs to be admitted for several tests because of recurrent irritable bowel syndrome. She will be in the hospital for at least 3 days and should check in on July 23, 20XX, in the afternoon so that she will have taken nothing by mouth (NPO) before the blood tests are performed and x-ray films are taken the following morning. ICD Code: 564.1 (Work Product 10-9).

CASE STUDY

Read the case study and answer the questions that follow.

Janie Haynes consistently arrives at the clinic 15 to 45 minutes late. She always has a "good" excuse, but she could make her appointments on time if she had better time management skills. The office manager has mentioned to Paula, the receptionist, that Janie is to be scheduled at 4:45 PM and if she is late, she will not be seen by the physician. Paula books Janie's next three appointments at that time, and Janie actually arrives early. However, on the fourth appointment, Janie arrives at 5:50 PM, and Paula knows it is her responsibility to tell Janie she cannot see the physician. How does Paula handle this task? Is more than one option available?

WORKPLACE APPLICATIONS

Choose five clinics and call the receptionist at each. Tell the receptionist that you are studying scheduling in medical assisting school and are interested in the scheduling method that clinic uses. Tally the results each classmate obtains, then graph or chart the results for the class on one document. Discuss the frequency of the various methods of scheduling.

INTERNET ACTIVITIES

1. Research scheduling software on the Internet and select a software package that would be functional for a physician's office. Gather information about the features and benefits and present the information to the class.

2. Research information about the different types of scheduling and how effective they are in physicians' offices. Determine the type of scheduling best suited to a family practice clinic. Present the ideas to the class.

3. Research self-scheduling software and determine the advantages and disadvantages of allowing patients to schedule appointments on the Internet. Present the information to the class or write an informative report about your findings.

11 Patient Reception and Processing

VOCABULARY REVIEW

Fill in the blanks with the correct vocabulary terms from this chapter.

1. Thomas noticed that the staff had _____ their supplies of gauze pads, so he ordered a case using the medical supplier's online system.

2. Jerri _____ the 1-inch syringes so that Thomas would know to order more of them for the clinic.

3. Dr. Raleigh installed a(n) _____ system so that he could speak to the medical assistants both in the front and the back offices from the examination rooms.

4. Medical assistants must be aware of the _____ patients have of the office staff and take steps to ensure it is a positive one.

5. Susan filed the laboratory reports in _____ order.

6. _____ information includes the patient's address, insurance information, and e-mail address.

7. Any _____ offered to a patient should be within the physician's orders, so make sure a beverage with sugar is not offered to a diabetic.

8. Angela uses _____ devices to help her remember the duties to complete before leaving the office.

9. Employees prefer to work in an office with a(n) _____ environment.

10. Dr. Lawson has a(n) _____ desire to serve his patients and promote wellness.

11. A secondary use of health information that cannot be reasonably prevented is called a(an) _____.

12. Medical assistants may find it helpful to write a patient's name using _____ spelling to remember its pronunciation.

SKILLS AND CONCEPTS

Part I: The Office Mission Statement

1. Create a mission statement for a fictional family practice.

_____

_____

_____

_____

_____

Part II: The Reception Area

1. Why is the first impression of the physician's office so important to patients?

2. List five items that might be found in the patient reception area.

   a.
   b.
   c.
   d.
   e.

3. If a computer is provided in the reception area, what cautionary measure should be taken to ensure patient privacy?

4. Describe the ideal receptionist for a physician's office.

Part III: Registration Procedures

1. List six items of demographic information found on a patient information sheet.

   a.
   b.
   c.
   d.
   e.
   f.

Part IV: Consideration for the Patient's Time

1. Why might a crowded waiting room be a sign of inefficiency rather than the physician's popularity?

2. Delays longer than _____ minutes should be explained to patients, and they should be allowed to reschedule if they want to do so.

3. No more than _____ or _____ patients should be waiting in the reception area at any given time.

4. What feelings do patients often experience when waiting in the physician's office?

_____

_____

_____

Part V: Patient Confidentiality

1. How can the medical assistant help prevent a breach of patient confidentiality by the placement of charts in wall holders?

_____

_____

_____

_____

2. How can the medical assistant help prevent a breach of patient confidentiality while using sign-in sheets?

_____

_____

_____

_____

3. Provide two examples of incidental disclosure.

   a. _____

   b. _____

4. Why would some offices limit the number of people who can accompany a patient into the exam room?

_____

_____

_____

5. Should the medical assistant ever discipline a disruptive child in the medical office? Why or why not?

_____

_____

_____

_____

6. How do glass partitions help keep patient information confidential? Are they useful in today's medical offices? Why or why not?

_____

_____

_____

_____

Part VI: Patient Checkout

Write a verbal response to the following patients in the checkout process.

1. Suzanne Anton is ready to leave the clinic, and she owes a co-pay of $25 plus a past due balance of $10 that her insurance did not pay. She questions the $10 balance.

___

2. Randy Stephens is leaving the clinic but is angry about his visit with the physician, who insists that he lose 40 pounds. He reluctantly pays his co-pay. He needs to schedule a follow-up appointment for 1 month, during which time the physician wants him to have lost 5 pounds by following a strict diet.

___

3. Alfreda Williams has come to the clinic for a checkup. She is being treated by the physician for colon cancer, and she usually is cheerful, despite her prognosis. Today she seems distressed and hesitates before paying her bill of $65.

___

Part VII: The End of the Day

1. Paige is preparing for the next work day. What are some tasks that will help her prepare for tomorrow's patients?

___

2. List several routine tasks for closing an office.

___

3. How can the medical assistant gain confidence in asking for payments and co-payments?

___

Part VIII: Evaluating Reception Areas

Visit several reception areas in physician's offices, hospitals, and/or clinics. Take note of the appearance and amenities in these facilities. Rate each reception area on a scale of 1 to 10. Total the figures to determine the "best" reception area.

AREA	Locations				
Cleanliness					
Color scheme					
Seating					
Lighting					
Comfort					
Amenities					
Noise level					
Total					

CASE STUDY

Read the case study and answer the questions that follow.

Jill is the receptionist for Dr. Boles and Dr. Bailey, who are psychiatrists. Each week Sara Ables comes to her appointments but brings her two small children, Joey and Julie, ages 8 and 6 years, respectively. When Sara goes back for her appointment, the children are almost uncontrollable in the reception area. Although there are never more than two patients waiting, the kids are a serious disruption in the clinic. When Jill mentioned the problem to Dr. Boles, he said that Sara really needed the sessions and that Jill should try to work with Sara on this issue. What can Jill do to remedy the situation?

_____

_____

_____

_____

WORKPLACE APPLICATIONS

Design a registration form for a fictional clinic that includes all information necessary for a new patient. Be creative with logos and fonts. Make the form attractive and easy to understand.

INTERNET ACTIVITIES

1. Search for innovations in patient reception on the Internet, including computers that allow patients to check themselves in for appointments. Present information on one of the systems to the class.

2. Find examples of office mission statements online. Compare them and write a brief report about the contents of the various statements.

3. Research the Americans with Disabilities Act. Determine what accommodations must be made in reception areas to comply with this law. Present the information to the class.

12 Office Environment and Daily Operations

VOCABULARY REVIEW

Fill in the blanks with the correct vocabulary terms from this chapter.

1. Julia noticed some _____ in the inventory when comparing last month's totals with the current month's totals.

2. Rhonda prefers that all _____ _____ be initialed by the person who checks in the package.

3. Dr. Hughes is _____ when dealing with conflicts within the office by talking with staff members and looking for ways to compromise.

4. Kayla enjoys developing a(n) _____ for office expenditures each fiscal year.

5. Items on _____ frustrate the office manager because of the follow-up required to make sure the item eventually arrives at the clinic.

6. When Douglas neglected to pay the supply bill by the due date, he _____ late charges and increased the total due by 2%.

7. Elaine, the office manager, was able to _____ a confrontation with the patient who complained about the bill by addressing his concerns in a cordial way.

8. By _____ Web sites she uses frequently, Ann is able to find medical suppliers and research the best prices quickly.

9. Dr. Tarago received a(an) _____ for speaking at the regional medical society meeting.

10. Physicians are constantly concerned about their _____ when budgeting and planning salary increases.

11. Julia knew that there were _____ circumstances involved with the patient statements being sent late during August.

12. September begins the _____ _____ for the clinic.

13. Dr. Hughes finally agreed to the _____ of his medical transcription.

14. Dr. Tarago gave Kayla a(n) _____ before she left to attend the medical assistant convention.

SKILLS AND CONCEPTS

Part I: Opening the Office

1. List six duties that should be completed before patients start to arrive.

   a. _____
   b. _____
   c. _____
   d. _____
   e. _____
   f. _____

2. What parts of the medical record should be checked to see whether additional forms need to be added before a patient arrives for an office visit?

3. Explain the precautions that should be taken with prescription pads.

4. Why is patient traffic flow an important consideration in the office environment?

Part II: The Office Environment

1. List 10 expenses the physician's office incurs on a month-to-month basis.

   a. _____
   b. _____
   c. _____
   d. _____
   e. _____
   f. _____
   g. _____
   h. _____
   i. _____
   j. _____

2. List six tasks the medical assistant can do between patients or during slower periods.

   a. _____
   b. _____
   c. _____
   d. _____
   e. _____
   f. _____

3. Explain the purpose of white noise.

4. List three things related to the office environment that the medical assistant can do to help the physician save money.

   a. _____

   b. _____

   c. _____

5. Explain why the number of individuals with keys and alarm codes should be limited in the medical office.

   _____

   _____

   _____

Part III: Medical Waste and Regular Waste

Note whether each of the following items should be classified as medical waste or regular waste.

1. Gauze used to stop bleeding after venipuncture

   _____

2. Tissues used in the reception room to clean eyeglasses

   _____

3. Blood tubes containing blood that has already been tested

   _____

4. Used syringes

   _____

5. Paper towels used to clean a mirror in a restroom used by patients

   _____

Part IV: The Office Policy and Procedures Manual

1. Why is the office policy and procedures manual important?

   _____

   _____

   _____

2. List five sections that might be found in an office policy and procedures manual.

   a. _____

   b. _____

   c. _____

   d. _____

   e. _____

Part V: Equipment Inventory

Complete an inventory of either administrative or clinical equipment at the school using the form in Work Product 12-1 on p. 93 of the Procedures Checklists. Give the form to the instructor when finished.

Part VI: Supply Inventory

Complete an inventory of either administrative or clinical supplies at the school using the form in Work Product 12-2 on p. 95 of the Procedures Checklists. Give the form to the instructor when finished.

Part VII: Purchase Orders

Complete two purchase orders using an office supply catalog, newspaper ad, or the Internet. Complete one purchase order for supplies (things that are used up on a routine basis); complete the other for equipment (things that are reusable and usually of value).

Name _____

Date _____

PURCHASE ORDER　　　　　　　　　　　　　　　　　　　　　No. 1554

Bill to:

Blackburn Primary Care Associates PC
1990 Turquoise Drive
Blackburn, WI 54937

Ship to:

Blackburn Primary Care Associates, PC
1990 Turquoise Drive
Blackburn, WI 54937

Vendor: _____

Terms: _____

ORDER #	DESCRIPTION	QTY.	COLOR	SIZE	UNIT PRICE	TOTAL PRICE
					SUBTOTAL	
					TAX	
					SHIPPING	
					TOTAL	

Name _____

Date _____

PURCHASE ORDER		No. 1554
Bill to:		**Ship to:**
Blackburn Primary Care Associates PC 1990 Turquoise Drive Blackburn, WI 54937		Blackburn Primary Care Associates, PC 1990 Turquoise Drive Blackburn, WI 54937

Vendor: _____
_____
_____

Terms: _____

ORDER #	DESCRIPTION	QTY.	COLOR	SIZE	UNIT PRICE	TOTAL PRICE
					SUBTOTAL	
					TAX	
					SHIPPING	
					TOTAL	

Part VIII: Maintenance Logs

Use the form in Work Product 12-3 on p. 97 of the Procedures Checklists to compile a log of the administrative equipment in your classroom. Follow the example given on the first line. Give the form to the instructor when you are finished.

Part IX: Travel Expense Reports

Complete a travel expense report using the form in Work Product 12-4 on p. 99 of the Procedures Checklists. Use the following information on the report. Allowed meal amounts are breakfast $10.00, lunch $18, and dinner $27.00. Figure the total for each expense category, the total expenses for the trip, and the amount to be reimbursed to the employee, if any.

Advance:
$200 cash

Expenses/Receipts:
Two hotel nights at the Regency Inn (May 2 & 3, 2010). Cost: $110.00 per night. Tax Rate: 8.25%
Cab from airport to hotel (May 2, 2010): $22.00 plus 18% tip.
Cab from hotel to airport (May 4, 2010): $22.00 plus 18% tip.
Breakfast: Free each day at the hotel buffet

Lunch: Figure all tips at 18%
   May 2—$12.56
   May 3—$16.24
   May 4—$10.54
Dinner: Figure all tips at 18%
   May 2—$18.35
   May 3—$22.34
Phone: Calls to office
   May 2—$2.13
   May 3—$3.43

A manual with examples of forms for the medical office was purchased at the seminar for $38.00. The seminar cost was paid several months in advance.

Part X: Emergency Preparedness

Using the Internet, find at least five agencies in your region that provide emergency preparedness. Present a brief report to the class on each agency and the services it provides. Complete Work Product 12-5 (on p. 101 of the Procedures Checklists) according to instructor specifications.

CASE STUDY

Read the case study and answer the questions that follow.

Dianna had worked at the Family Clinic for 6 years in the front office. When a new medical assistant, Kiran, was hired to work the phones and schedule appointments, Dianna noticed that she was not following the office policy and caused several problems with the schedule. Some patients were very late in seeing the physician; this was unusual for the office, so complaints were made. Dianna volunteered to work with Kiran to help her schedule according to policy. She noticed that Kiran accessed the Internet and her e-mail frequently, but that did not seem to detract from setting appointments. Kiran promised to perform according to office policy, but after 3 weeks, the problems continued.

1. What should happen in this situation?

2. Why is the scheduler such an important position in the facility?

Workplace Applications

1. Set up an interview with an office manager and discuss the cost of running a medical practice from month to month. Discuss the biggest expenses that the physician pays each month. Report what you discover to the class.

2. Discuss emergency preparedness for the medical office and determine with a team of classmates the logical contents of an emergency preparedness plan for a physician's office. Outline a plan and present it to the class.

Internet Activities

1. Find three medical suppliers on the Internet and compare their prices for each of the following items. Use local suppliers if information is available online about their products.

Item	Suppliers	Price #1	Price #2	Price #3
1 case of 4 × 4 gauze pads				
1 gallon of isopropyl alcohol				
1 case of table paper				

2. Research medical office layout designs on the Internet and design an office. Include a color scheme and floor plan. Present the design to the class using a computer presentation, poster, or handouts.

3. Research three local medical facilities on the Internet, looking for information such as company reports, financial information, company profiles, news, and current affairs. Write a report on one of the facilities to share with the class.

4. Research information on fire extinguishers, including their operation and the types for different uses. Prepare a report on the findings.

13 Written Communications and Mail Processing

VOCABULARY REVIEW

Fill in the blanks with the correct vocabulary terms from this chapter.

1. Roberta has a(n) _____ tone in her voice when she speaks to the office staff, and this has caused friction between her and the employees.

2. Most of the mail the Blackburn Clinic sends is classified as _____ mail, which means it is sent within the boundaries of the United States.

3. Savannah asked Noble to _____ a memo among all of the employees.

4. Dr. Lupez suggested that the clinic sell or donate all of the _____ computer equipment once the new system arrived and was installed.

5. Jaci sometimes gets confused about subject and predicate _____ when she is writing.

6. Mrs. Abernathy reminded the students to make the margins _____ to the left when writing memorandums.

7. Dr. Lawler asked Roberta to order new stationery and specifically requested that the _____ be of a high quality.

8. All the staff members enjoyed having Alicia as an intern because of her _____ personality with the patients.

9. The physicians considered rearranging the drug sample shelves _____ according to type of drug.

10. Dr. Hughes's _____ remark was out of character, and Suzanne was certain that he was simply stressed over a patient.

11. Ellen forgot to measure the _____ of a package before taking it to the post office to mail.

12. Jacqueline has a talent for writing _____ documents that are easy to understand.

13. Angela was _____ the newsletter yesterday afternoon.

SKILLS AND CONCEPTS

Part I: Correspondence and Envelopes

Label the parts of the letter in the figure below, and write in the number of lines required between each section.

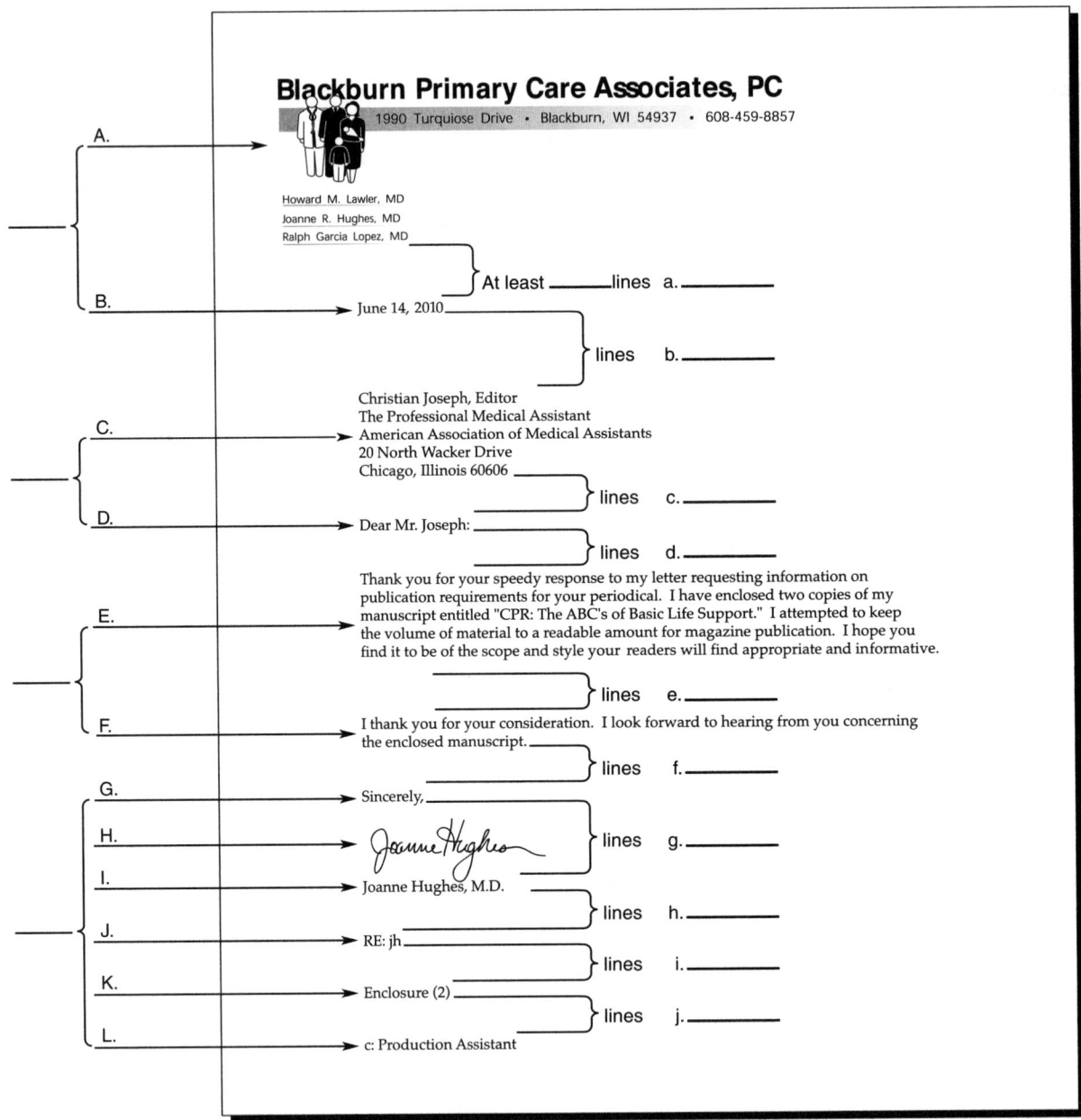

Complete Work Product 13-1 on p. 111 of the Procedures Checklists by writing the following addresses correctly according to OCR guidelines on the envelopes provided.

1. doctor john smith m.d. 301 west hughes street chicago illinois 54321

2. cindy johnson, physical therapist 1467 east green street suite 409b bayfield georgia 12345

3. jose kelley memorial lane number 321 west columbia florida 97654

Part II: Short Answers

1. What is a watermark?

2. Why is a portfolio useful in the medical office?

3. Explain how a ream of paper is determined.

4. List several pieces of equipment used for written communications.

5. List some of the supplies used for written correspondence.

6. What is standard letter-size paper?

7. List the four parts of a letter.

   a. _____

   b. _____

   c. _____

   d. _____

8. Name three items that should be on a continuation page.

   a. _____

   b. _____

   c. _____

9. What is the difference between registered and certified mail?

   _____

   _____

   _____

10. Name and briefly define the parts of speech.

    a. _____

    b. _____

    c. _____

    d. _____

    e. _____

    f. _____

    g. _____

    h. _____

11. List the four types of letter styles and the differences between each one.

    a. _____
       _____

    b. _____
       _____

    c. _____
       _____

    d. _____
       _____

12. List three things to do before answering a business letter.

    a. _____

    b. _____

    c. _____

Part III: Letters and Memos

Using the letterhead form in Work Products 13-2 and 13-4 (See pp. 113 and 117 in the Procedures Checklists), the memo form in Work Products 13-3 and 13-5 (see pp. 115 and 119 in the Procedures Checklists), and the fax form in Work Product 13-6, complete the following activities. Write the documents using one of the four letter styles discussed in the chapter. If allowed by the instructor, use templates for added creativity and customization.

A. Initiating Correspondence—Complete Work Product 13-2.

Write a letter from Dr. Hughes to the president of the American Medical Association suggesting a topic for the next national convention. In the letter, indicate Dr. Hughes's interest in presenting the topic.

B. Initiating a Memo—Complete Work Product 13-3.

Write a memo to all employees, making a change in office policy. The new policy should state that the new budget for continuing education per employee will change from $300 annually to $500 annually. Be sure to set an effective date.

C. Responding to Correspondence—Complete Work Product 13-4.

Respond to an invitation to speak at a local Rotary Club meeting on the subject "Health, Wellness, and Eating Well."

D. Responding to a Memo—Complete Work Product 13-5.

Respond to a memo from a supervisor who wants an update on the progress made toward arranging the drug sample area into categories as directed by the physician. Make sure to include an estimated date of completion for the project.

E. Initiating a Fax—Complete Work Product 13-6 on p. 121 of the Procedures Checklists.

Design a cover sheet for a fax message using the form in Work Product 13-6 or a template. On the cover sheet, indicate that test results for a patient are attached. Be certain to address the issue of patient confidentiality.

WORD FIND

Find the words in the list in the following puzzle. Be sure you know the definition of each word in the list in relation to written communications and mail processing.

```
Z F C T Y L H U I X C I M C N D L I T T X J O Z Q A E M M A G Q Y L Y C L Y M Z
P D D P H I L H A L Z A W D D E W R Y V C C O X H Z L X U K D N F F Z Q B A J Q
P V K Y U N F R A Y V A T V F W G C R O G J J O T L M L D R I F C J J C R Y N B
R N H P S T J U E C E X R E M Y H P N M S S J G I L T V N O A M I I L G I T J G
E T D C O E Y Q O K Z B C X G Q B T H R Z F W O J E C O A F B I P D I N N P U W
V U C Q V R J Y K R P E B U B O I E T A N I M E S S I D R S E R B N A N Y N Y C
S A K F C N W W W E W R L V W N R R N K Y J P C A N X X O K Z S D F L A G A T Z
D H Q U N A T K R W P Z C A U B J I Y X E E T C J H H B M W X G A U V N F J A Q
H J N P C T B H Z B B B Z A R P L U C J F R H Q O H Z X E H F V S B Q X Y J W R
M P V A W I F X I K J I T O N X P T K A D G R Z N D A X M Z Y Y W G S W L Q Q K
O P E S D O O G W M D I Z N L Y S I K H L J H Y O B E V I J Z L U I G I H Y O K
J R K U P N L H Z R O D L Z N P L Z W U O L W R A T Q Q V R C Q Q A C Y B B O H
E M C J H A P U L N R M E N X P O I B U K V Y L B I A N N G U T Z H T Z E F V I
R G G Q I L B X X F I K S F Q W J L O L V J W O R H X O C E D G P P P Y L H W D
X Z X Z E G A Z B C H B M Y O I R Q F N B Z X I Z H I U J H K P Z J N M U E A P
V W S L R K A Z G P W F E F J F E K C Y B P J W M T G C F J C F A K R O E V Z J
T H K V L I Z C Q U V H H E C N U B I O L Y G I A Y S X U J W Q A P V O M Y R C
E N C L O S U R E O U Z C X I E C C X I F F Q T J D V K T Z I F Y Y Y A Z V R C
B W F U H K B V Q K D N W A T A H P M W J T U X B O L N U Z F F J T Q A W M A L
E K E I N M W V T C E L A M S C Y G V B D L L C W B C T Z I W J S I I W X B O J
E L E G F B C G I D C L E M E U T N R O A X X C T Y F M Z J R W O Q G I Z M Q N
Q B Q X U V R W N U P F S K M L A J P S T L A Y Z G Q L R Y M D E U E Y M G B N
X M W T O P C O R H M O I G O T O P E N I N G U T E T X H F D K Z R J X W Z O I
A R K M R N P S B U E B R K D W R O Z M E R X R X U U K P B W Q V A L Z X R D B
J M N V P S I S K S V O U T U B V K B F R G T U L P T V V T T G R P G I H P D J
K V Z L E Q A X G Q V K J Q F C B F D V H K B Y R R J W N F F E H A S L J D Q D
C U L R U I S Y R X V N L H F O B J I J O F E O F G B V E W M M L L Y C E X S S
X J R T N W N I V Y I W L S T Q L A C F E D O M N U H G W X V L E L T I Y G L H
H O U F W W I E P N G Z T Q T R O I J R J F S I U Q I J B F U R J X I L U F Y N
C D K U X R E P K U L K L K K P I I O G R K D E L E A I C C X E M Q O E T Z N C
A P M C N U D L R Y C R Y O G L I G L E Z A F G G A D M M Z O M A B P T X I Q N
K M H G I P Q O U I G P B F L B V R A S E Q M Y I A A A Q V E R G I Y T Z X V H
Q C D X M S Z O Z N C N C L T S J D C H B T O S S W S Y K K V E P O L E V N E F
C O M P L I M E N T A R Y N R O R B I S D S F O M O Z S F V D A E X H R R G W X
H E E B V U T H T R S L G X X T U E X V T U S W O W Y H E E R R P U E I J M M Q
I L I G D J V B X I I E M M O Z W L U L L S U N F N Q X E M O J R M X O H E R Z
H R R W I R T J R N L I A M E J P L W S G S O T E J X Z D R I X A R O S G D B V
I C A R P A G C M S E K Z C X V K Y H I B U J P I S G B G A A U H T U B B X E O
X N B F I G A T L I T F K B R I R S U V C G I D Q O U Q M C D C Q Z Q I G V L I
I P I H Q B T M V C L C J U A D C J L X F D W O R S R V X Y G L L T A U K V X D
```

Chapter 13 Written Communications and Mail Processing

Body	Enclosure	Memorandum
Categorically	Envelope	Messages
Complimentary	Girth	Opening
Continuation	Heading	Portfolio
Correspondence	International	Postscripts
Disseminate	Intrinsic	Proofread
Domestic	Letter	Salutation
Email	Margin	ZIP code

CASE STUDY

Read the case study and answer the questions that follow.

Barbara recently graduated as a medical assistant and obtained employment at a local physician's office. She and the office manager have seemed to be at odds since Barbara redesigned several forms that had been in use at the clinic but had been copied over and over again and looked quite unprofessional. Barbara did not ask permission to redo the forms; she was attempting to help and to make a good impression. Since that incident, the office manager has given Barbara two written reprimands for minor issues.

1. What should Barbara do?

2. How could she have prevented this situation from the beginning?

3. Is the office manager at fault?

WORKPLACE APPLICATIONS

Collect several documents from various healthcare facilities. Compare the quality of the documents. Do they make a good first impression? Are they clearly copies that have been made over and over again? Grade the documents and revise those that are graded below a B so that they present a positive, professional image of the facility.

INTERNET ACTIVITIES

1. Compare the services offered by companies such as FedEx, UPS, DHL, and the USPS. Determine the lowest cost for sending an overnight letter or package.

2. Research reference books that would be valuable to the medical assistant's library. Find and compare costs and make a list of several books that would be useful in the physician's office.

3. Go to the Microsoft Office home page and look for templates. Download several of the business templates and customize them for the Blackburn Primary Care Associates.

14 The Paper Medical Record

VOCABULARY REVIEW

Fill in the blank with the correct vocabulary term from this chapter.

1. Veronica prefers a(n) _____ filing system, in which combinations of letters and numbers are used to identify a file.

2. Julia prefers a(n) _____ filing system, in which the letters of the alphabet are used to identify a file.

3. Paula Ann feels that only a(n) _____ filing system provides patient confidentiality.

4. Dr. Banford uses a _____ file to help him remember that a certain action must be taken on a certain date.

5. Teresa wants to _____ the current software library with programs for making brochures and designing Web sites.

6. The clinic physician records _____ information when questioning patients about their illness.

7. The clinic physician records _____ information when examining the patient.

8. When Mira files documents into medical records, she lays one report on top of another, with the most recent on top; this filing method is called _____.

9. The office manager is particular about the _____ under which documents are filed, because she wants to be able to access information quickly.

10. Dr. Lawler scheduled an appointment with his accountant to discuss the _____ of the office financial records.

11. Georgina avoids _____ by taking care of issues and documents as they are presented to her rather than setting them aside for later.

12. Naomi has a _____ interest in the success of the new hospital, because she owns shares in its stock.

13. The medical assistant must never remove entries in a patient's record by _____.

14. Dr. Lupez's _____ _____ was irritable bowel syndrome, not colon cancer.

15. Jose read the memo about the new medical records _____ schedule with interest, because his job includes filing.

SKILLS AND CONCEPTS

Part I: Filing Medical Records
Place the following names in the correct order for filing in the right column.

1. Cassidy Kay Hale   1. _____

2. Candace Cassidy LeGrand   2. _____

3. Taylor Ann Jackson   3. _____

4. Anton Douglas Conn   4. _____

5. Mitchel Michael Gibson   5. _____

6. Lorienda Gaye Robison   6. _____

7. LaNelle Elva Crumley   7. _____
8. Allison Gaile Yarbrough   8. _____
9. Sarah Kay Haile   9. _____
10. Marie Gracelia Stuart   10. _____
11. Karry Madge Chapmann   11. _____
12. Randi Ann Perez   12. _____
13. Cecelia Gayle Raglan   13. _____
14. Sarah Sue Ragland   14. _____
15. Riley Americus Belk   15. _____
16. Starr Ellen Beall   16. _____
17. Mitchell Thomas Gibson   17. _____
18. George Scott Turner   18. _____
19. Winston Roger Murchison   19. _____
20. Sara Suzelle Montgomery   20. _____
21. Tamika Noelle Frazier   21. _____
22. Alisa Jordan Williams   22. _____
23. Alisha Dawn Chapman   23. _____
24. Bentley James Adams   24. _____
25. Montana Skye Kizer   25. _____
26. Dakota Marie LaRose   26. _____
27. Robbie Sue Metzger   27. _____
28. Thomas Charles Bruin   28. _____
29. Percevial "Butch" Adams   29. _____
30. Carlos Perez Santos   30. _____

Part II: Subjective and Objective Information

Note whether the following information is usually subjective or objective.

1. Patient's address _____
2. Yellowed eyes _____
3. Patient's e-mail address _____
4. Insurance information _____
5. Elevated blood pressure _____
6. Bloated stomach _____
7. Complaint of headache _____
8. Weight of 143 pounds _____
9. Bruises on upper arms _____
10. Patient's phone number _____

Part III: Short Answers

1. List four reasons medical records are kept.

   a. _____

   b. _____

   c. _____

   d. _____

2. Explain the concept of the ownership of medical records.

   _____

   _____

   _____

3. Why might color-coded files be more efficient than an alphabetic filing system?

   _____

   _____

   _____

4. What are the two major types of patient records found in a medical office?

   a. _____

   b. _____

5. What type of form should be completed if a patient no longer wants to allow his or her medical records to be released to a person or an organization?

   _____

   _____

   _____

Part IV: Releasing Medical Records

Complete an Authorization to Release Medical Records form using your name as the patient.

```
                    RECORDS RELEASE AUTHORIZATION

    TO _____
                              Doctor or Hospital

       _____
                                   Address

    I HEREBY AUTHORIZE AND REQUEST YOU TO RELEASE TO:




    ALL RECORDS IN YOUR POSSESION CONCERNING _____

    _____ILLNESS AND/OR

    TREATMENT DURING THE PERIOD FROM _____ TO _____.
    NAME _____ TEL. _____
    ADDRESS_____
    SIGNATURE _____ DATE _____
                    (If relative, state relationship)
    WITNESS _____ DATE _____
               25-8104 © 1973 BIBBERO SYSTEMS, INC., PETALUMA,, CA.
```

Part V: Changing or Correcting Medical Records

Correct the following medical record entries as noted, as it would be done in a medical chart. Then rewrite the entry correctly on the line provided.

1. The correct date of the appointment below was October 12, 20XX.

    10-21-20XX   Patient did not arrive for scheduled appointment. *P. Smith, RMA*

    _____

2. The patient stated that the chest pain began 2 weeks ago.

    1-31-20XX   Patient complained of chest pain for the last 2 months. No pain noted in arms. No nausea. Desires ECG and blood work to check for heart problems. *R. Smithee, CMA(AAMA)*

    _____

    _____

3. The correct date for the last refill was 3-20-20XX.

   4-22-20XX   Patient requested that Rx for Vicodin be refilled. Last refill was 4-20-20XX. Dr. Lawton refused refill and requested patient schedule follow-up appointment. *S. Ragland, RMA*

   What additional follow-up might be needed in this situation?

4. Mr. Eric Robertson cancelled his surgical follow-up appointment today for the third time.

5. Angela Adams called to report that she was not feeling any better since her office visit on Monday. She wants the doctor to call in a refill for her antibiotics. The chart says that she was to return to the clinic on Thursday if she was not feeling better. Today is Monday, and she says she cannot come in to the clinic this week.

6. Mary Elizabeth Smith called the physician's office to report redness around an injection site. She was in the office 3 hours ago and received an injection of penicillin. She says she also is itching quite a bit around the site and is having trouble breathing. The doctor has left the office for the day.

Part VI: Filing Procedures

1. List and explain the five basic filing steps.

   a.

   b.

   c.

d. _____

e. _____

CASE STUDY

Read the information below and answer the questions.

The Blackburn Clinic is considering the purchase of new filing equipment. They currently use an open-shelf method, with the patient's names in alphabetic order. They would like to change to an alphanumeric system.

1. What must they consider before making this change?

   _____

2. How would the office implement this change so that it causes the least disruption to the patients and staff?

   _____

WORKPLACE APPLICATIONS

Visit three medical offices and determine the type of filing system each uses. Ask the receptionist about the pros and cons of each system. Share this information with the class.

INTERNET ACTIVITIES

1. Research paper-based filing systems on the Internet and determine which system you would choose for a medical office. Cite three reasons for your choice.

2. Look for special paper-based, color-coding systems on the Internet. How might these be used in a physician's office?

3. Look for filing tips on the Internet. Which of these tips might help you file faster and more efficiently in the medical office?

15 The Electronic Medical Record

VOCABULARY REVIEW

Fill in the blanks with the correct vocabulary terms from this chapter.

1. Jennifer explained that a(n) _____ of electronic health information usually included documents from two or more different health facilities.

2. The electronic record that originates from one facility is called the electronic _____ record.

3. The electronic record that originates from more than one facility is called the electronic _____ record.

4. Behavior that is generally or widely accepted is called _____.

5. A system that is capable of interacting with another system is said to be _____.

6. A(n) _____-based medical record is used in combination with a paper-based record to optimize patient care.

7. Medical _____ refers to the study of medical computing.

8. Any of a set of physical properties, the values of which determine characteristics or behavior, is its _____.

SKILLS AND CONCEPTS

Part I: Electronic Medical Records

1. List three of the five requirements listed in President George W. Bush's order establishing the goal of having electronic medical records for most Americans by 2014.

    a. _____

    b. _____

    c. _____

2. List five advantages of the EMR system.

    a. _____

    b. _____

    c. _____

d. _____

e. _____

3. List five disadvantages of the EMR system.

   a. _____

   b. _____

   c. _____

   d. _____

   e. _____

Part II: EMR Capabilities

1. What is the approximate cost of implementing an EMR system for a typical physician's office with one physician?

   _____

2. Briefly describe three capabilities of an EMR system. Why do you think each capability will enhance patient care?

   a. _____

   b. _____

   c. _____

Part III: The Patient and the EMR

1. Discuss how you would talk with a patient who has expressed legitimate fears about having health information in electronic form. Explain what you would say to the patient and how you would reassure the individual.

   _____

Part IV: Nonverbal Communication and the EMR

1. List several things to remember when in the exam room with the patient and the electronic device that houses the EMR system. Specifically, what should you, as the medical assistant, do to put the patient at ease?

   _____
   _____
   _____
   _____
   _____
   _____
   _____
   _____

Part V: Nationwide Health Information Network (NHIN)

1. Briefly explain the purpose of the Nationwide Health Information Network.

   _____
   _____
   _____
   _____

2. List two goals of the Nationwide Health Information Network.

   a. _____
   _____

   b. _____
   _____

3. What are some of the governmental agencies you think will be a part of the effort to meet the goals of the Executive Order of 2006?

   _____
   _____
   _____
   _____
   _____
   _____
   _____
   _____

Part VI: Backup Systems for the EMR

1. List three backup systems for an EMR system in a physician's office.

   a. _____
   _____

   b. _____
   _____

c. _____

CASE STUDY

Read the information below and answer the questions.

Dr. Adkins and Dr. Brooks want to expand their office to make sure they can take advantage of cutting-edge technology. Their goal is to use electronic equipment to perform as much of the work as possible so that all staff members can keep caring for the patients in the forefront of their minds. Dr. Adkins is fairly satisfied with the system the clinic has now. However, the medical assistant, Dr. Brooks, a "technology geek," wants the newest, greatest, and best electronics in his clinic. The office manager gives Sloan, the medical assistant, the opportunity to research electronic medical records systems to determine which are considered the best of the best.

Research what is available in your local and regional areas, make a brief report about the availabilities, and present it to the class.

1. What new possibilities did you discover in your research?

2. Why do you think many physicians are slow to adopt new technology?

3. As a medical assistant, what type of technology would make your duties easier?

WORKPLACE APPLICATIONS

Determine whether a local physician's office that uses an EMR system would allow the class to visit, perhaps on an afternoon when patients are not in the clinic. Take a list of at least five questions about using an EMR system. Observe how the system works and watch to see if the employees seem to have more or less of a workload. Watch the interaction of the employees with each other and ask whether they think the system is more of a help or a hindrance as they go about their duties.

INTERNET ACTIVITIES

1. Research the cost of an EMR system on the Internet. Find a low, moderate, and high cost system. Compare the features of each and share your information with the class.

2. Find a company that sells EMR systems. Ask a salesperson to present information to your class. Ask whether he or she can demonstrate the capabilities of the system.

3. Search for blogs used by medical assistants and look for those who have EMR systems in their clinics. What types of problems do they discuss? Are they promoting any specific systems that seem to work well?

16 Health Information Management

VOCABULARY REVIEW

Fill in the blanks with the correct vocabulary terms from this chapter.

1. Dr. Charles received a memo from Smith-Park Hospital that reminded him to _____ several of the medical records.
2. Janie records any _____ _____ that happens to a patient while he or she is in the hospital.
3. Chris asked if there was a way to _____ outgoing e-mail messages so that they could not be altered before reaching their destination.
4. Anne knows that medical facilities must meet certain _____ to maintain accreditation.
5. After reviewing several hundred files, Alex was concerned about the _____ information in several patient records.
6. Betty reminded Joanne to be careful not to _____ numbers or letters when entering information into the computer.
7. The _____ _____ office in a healthcare facility is concerned with providing the best and most efficient care possible to the patients.
8. Dr. Hughes knew that penicillin was a(n) _____ for Kathleen Schultz, so he ordered a different antibiotic.
9. The new user manual has several _____, which must be corrected.
10. The medical assistant should never attempt to _____ the regulations that apply to medical records.
11. An injury caused by medical management rather than the underlying condition of the patient is called a(n) _____ event.
12. A _____ _____ is a medical error that is corrected before it affects the patient.

SKILLS AND CONCEPTS

Part I: Short Answers

1. Define health information management in lay terms.

   _____

   _____

   _____

2. List five ways in which healthcare data are used.

   a. _____
   b. _____
   c. _____
   d. _____
   e. _____

3. Explain what is meant by the underuse of medical services.

4. Explain what is meant by the overuse of medical services.

5. List five of the statistics collected by the NCHS.
   a.
   b.
   c.
   d.
   e.

Part II: Characteristics of High-Quality Health Data

Determine which of the nine characteristics of high-quality health data is involved in the following scenarios. Use each quality only once, and choose the one that best represents the facts presented in the scenario.

1. Janeen is concerned because the computer system did not upload the entries made the previous day.

2. Suzanne found a notation inside the medical record that a patient was allergic to sulfa drugs, but she noticed that the sticker on the outside of the record was marked NKA.

3. Sabrina brought a chart to the physician's attention in which he had written to prescribe 200 mg of Imitrex to a patient. Sabrina had heard the physician tell the patient that he was prescribing 100 mg. The physician corrected the error before writing the prescription.

4. Steven was unfamiliar with an abbreviation used in the medical record. He asked the office manager about the abbreviation, and she explained its use in the physician's office. In previous facilities, Steve had seen the same abbreviation used a different way.

5. After an employee was terminated, Chris changed applicable passwords so that the individual could no longer access the system.

6. Patricia researched the HIPAA Web site to make certain she understood a portion of the privacy law.

7. The new patient database allows several staff members to access data at the same time.

8. Joshua was reprimanded for not filing laboratory reports on a daily basis and for allowing the documents to stack up over several days.

9. Dr. Adams realized that some information entered into the patient database was not being used for treatment purposes, so he sent a memo to the staff and confirmed that the information no longer needed to be collected.

Part III: Acknowledging and Disclosing Medical Errors

1. Number the following events in the order they would be performed in the event of a medical error at the physician's office.

    a. _____ Offer a sincere apology when talking to the patient.

    b. _____ Call the patient and ask him or her to come to the office.

    c. _____ Give the patient the opportunity to ask questions.

    d. _____ Tell the physician about the error.

    e. _____ Complete an incident report and document the error in the chart.

    f. _____ Document the discussion of the error with the patient.

    g. _____ Meet with the patient in a private area where there will be no interruptions.

    h. _____ Allow the physician to explain the error to the patient.

Part IV: Medical Errors

1. Define an adverse event.

2. Define a sentinel event.

3. Define a near miss.

4. List five reasons a physician might be hesitant to disclose a medical error to the patient.

    a. _____

    b. _____

    c. _____

    d. _____

    e. _____

5. Who should be told about an error first?

Part V: Incident Reports

A medical assistant gives an injection of penicillin to a patient who reported an allergy to amoxicillin. The patient complains of itching and experiences shortness of breath and wheezing while sitting in the treatment room. The physician gives the patient epinephrine and observes him for 30 minutes, during which time the itching, shortness of breath, and wheezing fully resolves. Complete an incident report for this sentinel event.

Incident Report
Do Not File in Medical Records

Confidential and privileged health care quality improvement information prepared in anticipation of litigation

Name: _____ Employee ☐ Patient ☐ Visitor ☐

Attending physician: _____
MR # _____ SS # _____
D.O.B. ___/___/___   Sex: M[ ] F[ ]
Admission date: ___/___/___
Primary diagnosis: _____

Facility name: _____
Site (if applicable): _____
City: _____
Facility ID#: _____
State: _____
Phone #: _____

SECTION I: General Information

General Identification (circle one)
001 Inpatient
002 Outpatient
003 Nonpatient
004 Equipment only

Location (circle one):
005 Bathroom/toilet
006 Beauty shop
007 Cafeteria/dining room
008 Corridor/hall
009 During transport
010 Emergency department
011 Exterior grounds
012 ICU/SCU/CCU
013 Labor/delivery/birthing
014 Nursery
015 Outpatient clinic
016 Patient room
017 Radiology
018 Recovery room
019 Recreation area
020 Rehab
021 Shower room
022 Surgical suite
023 Treatment/exam room

Treatment Rendered (circle one)
024 Emergency room
025 First aid
026 None
026 Transfer to other facility
027 X-ray

SECTION II: Nature of Incident (Circle all that apply):

001 Adverse outcome after surgery or anesthetic
002 Anaphylactic shock
003 Anoxic event
004 Apgar score of 5 or less
005 Aspiration
006 Assault or altercation/combative event
007 Blood or IV variance
008 Blood/body fluid exposure
009 Code/arrest
010 Damage/loss of organ
011 Death
012 Dental-related complication
013 Dissatisfaction/noncompliance*
014 Equipment operation*
015 Fall with injury*
016 Fall without injury*
017 Handling of and/or exposure to hazardous waste
018 Informed consent issue
019 Injury to other
020 Injury to self
021 Loss of limb
022 Loss of vision
023 Medication variance*
024 Needle puncture/sharp injury
025 Paralysis
026 Patient-to-patient altercation
027 Perinatal complication*
028 Poisoning
029 Suspected nonstaff-to-patient abuse
030 Suspected staff-to-patient abuse
031 Thermal burn
032 Treatment/procedure issue
033 Ulcer: nosocomial stage III/IV

* Complete appropriate area in Section III

SECTION III: Type of Incident

If death, circle all that apply:
001 After medical equipment failure
002 After power equipment failure or damage
003 During surgery or postanesthesia
004 Within 24 hours of admission to facility
005 Within 1 week of fall in facility
006 Within 24 hours of medication error

Blood/IV Variance Issues (circle all that apply):
007 Additive
008 Administration consent
009 Contraindications/allergies
010 Equipment malfunction
011 Infusion rate
012 Labeling issue
013 Reaction
014 Solution/blood type
015 Transcription
016 Patient identification
017 Allergic/adverse reaction
018 Infiltration
019 Phlebitis

Dissatisfaction/Noncompliance (circle all that apply):
020 AMA
021 Elopement
022 Irate or angry (either family or patient)
023 Left without service
024 Noncompliant patient
025 Refused prescribed treatment

Falls (circle all that apply):*
001 Assisted fall
002 Found on floor
003 From bed
004 From chair
005 From commode/toilet
006 From exam table
007 From stretcher
008 From wheelchair
009 Patient states—unwitnessed
010 Unassisted fall
011 While ambulating
012 Witnessed fall

Medication Variance Issues (circle all that apply):
013 Contraindication/allergies
014 Delay in dispensing
015 Incorrect dose
016 Expired drug
017 Medication identification
018 Narcotic log variance
019 Not ordered
020 Ordered, not given
021 Patient identification
022 Reaction
023 Route
024 Rx incorrectly dispensed
025 Time of dose
026 Transcription

* For any marks in this field, Section V must be completed

Part VI: Confidentiality Statement

Evaluate the confidentiality statement for Diamonte Hospital below. Revise the statement to make it appropriate for a medical practice setting. Use proofreader marks to indicate your proposed changes in the confidentiality statement. Rewrite the completed, revised statement on the letterhead form on the next page.

DIAMONTE HOSPITAL

Diamonte, Arizona 89104 • TEL. 602-484-9991

CONFIDENTIALITY STATEMENT

I, _____ , understand that in the course of my activities/business at or for Diamonte Hospital, I am required to have access to and am involved in the viewing, reviewing, and/or processing of patient care data and/or health information.

I understand that I am obligated by State Law, Federal Law, and Diamonte Hospital to maintain the confidentiality of these data and information at all times.

I understand that a violation of these confidentiality considerations may result in punitive legal action against me.

I certify by my signature below that this Confidentiality Statement has been explained to me, and I agree to the principles contained herein as a condition of my activity/business at or for Diamonte Hospital.

_____
Signature/date

_____
Witness/date

Blackburn Primary Care Associates
1990 Turquoise Drive
Blackburn, WI 54937
(555) 555-1234

CASE STUDY

Read the case study and answer the questions that follow.

Alberto discovered that three people accessed the medical records of a player on the local professional football team who had been brought to the physician's office for follow-up on injuries sustained in a car accident. He realizes that the information accessed involved the results of the player's blood alcohol level.

1. What should Alberto do?

2. What type of penalty, if any, is appropriate for those who accessed the information?

WORKPLACE APPLICATIONS

Determine how total quality management ideas can be worked into the mission statement for a physician's office. Write a mission statement that stresses quality management. How does quality management affect patients in a medical office?

INTERNET ACTIVITIES

1. Explore the NCHS website. Investigate one of the issues in the Vital Statistics area. Use information found there to write a report about any area of interest and present it to the class.

2. Explore the Joint Commission (formerly JCAHO) Web site. Peruse the sections of the site that refer to standards, patient safety, and sentinel events. Choose a fact and write a brief report.

3. Research total quality management on the Internet and write a two-page report on how quality management can improve efficiency in a physician's office.

17 Privacy in the Physician's Office

VOCABULARY REVIEW

Fill in the blanks with the correct vocabulary terms from this chapter.

1. Dr. Lawton is considered a healthcare _____, because he provides services and treatments to patients.

2. The _____ against Dr. Rosales was one of his former patients, Risa Jackson, who believed that his staff had violated her privacy.

3. Byron knows that he is not allowed to _____ any information about a patient without a release from the patient for that information.

4. Sarah could _____ from what the patient said that he was nervous about his upcoming surgery.

5. STAT Medical Billing provides services to the Blackburn Clinic, so the company is considered a(n) _____ _____.

6. Julia has difficulty understanding the _____ in which many federal documents and regulations are written.

7. Janease knew that she could _____ two employees from guilt, because they were both at lunch when the incident happened.

8. The _____ on the privacy statement was hard for a layperson to understand, so Annette decided to rewrite the document.

9. Roberta was assigned to be the temporary _____ _____ at the clinic while Maritza was on maternity leave.

10. The Office of _____ _____ investigates breaches of laws that pertain to HHS.

11. The Office of _____ _____ enforces privacy standards.

12. Dr. Hughes had to prove _____ _____ in that he made every attempt to notify the patient before mailing test results to her home.

13. The _____ _____ _____ _____ in a patient's record is private and must not be shared without a release from the patient.

14. Health information that is transmitted in electronic form is called _____ _____ _____.

15. The patient's information that pertains to his or her health is called _____ _____ _____.

SKILLS AND CONCEPTS

Part I: The Health Insurance Portability and Accountability Act

1. 1. List six benefits provided by the HIPAA Privacy Rule to patients and/or providers.

    a. _____

    b. _____

    c. _____

111

Chapter 17 Privacy in the Physician's Office

d. _____

   e. _____

   f. _____

2. Briefly explain the Title I provision of HIPAA.

   _____
   _____

3. Briefly explain the Title II provision of HIPAA.

   _____
   _____

4. List six rights HIPAA gives to patients.

   a. _____

   b. _____

   c. _____

   d. _____

   e. _____

   f. _____

5. List six items of information a Notice of Privacy Policies must include.

   a. _____

   b. _____

   c. _____

   d. _____

   e. _____

   f. _____

Part II: Patients' Rights under HIPAA

Determine which right under HIPAA applies to each of the following scenarios. Use each right only once.

1. Susan Enlow discovered that her date of birth was incorrect when she requested her medical records from the Blackburn Clinic. She was moving to another city and wanted to take the records with her to her new provider. Susan surmised that the error might have been the reason her insurance company rejected several claims. She contacted the Blackburn Clinic in writing and asked them to correct the error and then to determine whether any claims were outstanding that might need to be resubmitted to her insurance carrier.

   Right to _____

2. Keiran requested that the clinic send a copy of his most recent physical examination and laboratory results to Dr. Ballard, who was seeing him about a long-standing problem with his knees.

   Right to _____

3. Louie requested that all communication from the physician's office be sent to his office address, because he was in the midst of a tense divorce.

   Right to _____

4. The Blackburn Clinic gives a copy of its Notice of Privacy Policy to all patients and makes sure a signature is obtained or a note is attached to prove that the policy was offered to the patient.

   Right to _____

5. A few days after seeing Dr. Reynolds, Rita received an e-mail from a company that offered multivitamins. Dr. Reynolds had suggested that she begin taking multivitamins and mentioned that a friend sold a vitamin drink that she might be interested in trying. Rita did not give permission for release of her e-mail address at the visit. She called the clinic and asked whether her e-mail address had been distributed to anyone outside the clinic.

   Right to _____

6. Suyen made a written request to the Blackburn Clinic that no information about her treatment for drug dependency be released to anyone without her specific written permission.

   Right to _____

Part III: Incidental Disclosures

Determine which of the following situations could be classified as an incidental disclosure.

	Situation	Incidental Disclosure	
		Yes	No
1.	Ms. Allen, a patient waiting in the x-ray department of a large clinic, overhears Dr. Smith mention that another patient has been diagnosed with testicular cancer, but she does not hear the patient's name during the discussion.		
2.	Bob Mitchell, a patient at Mercy Hospital, overhears a physician telling his roommate that he needs surgery for carpal tunnel syndrome.		
3.	As Zaria passes the nurses' station at a local hospital, she hears the nurses talking about the patient in room 2114. They mention that he has been diagnosed with terminal cancer. Zaria knows the patient's family and hears that the diagnosis has not been given to them yet.		
4.	Paula Stanley signs in at the front desk of the medical clinic and notices that her college professor signed in to see the physician 30 minutes ago.		

Part IV: Notice of Privacy Practices

Read the Notice of Privacy Practices in Figure 17-1 of the textbook. Based on the information in that policy, answer the following questions.

1. Can the patient obtain a copy of his or her medical record?

   ❑ Yes   ❑ No

2. Can the patient request that certain information in his or her medical record not be released to certain persons or organizations?

   ❑ Yes   ❑ No

3. Can the patient have a copy of the Notice of Privacy Practices?

   ❑ Yes   ❑ No

4. Can the clinic use the information in the patient's medical record to compile statistics about certain diseases treated by the practice without additional permission from the patient?

   ❑ Yes   ❑ No

5. Does the clinic have to honor all requests from the patient regarding the release of his or her protected health information?

   ❑ Yes   ❑ No

Part V: Privacy in the Physician's Office

Find the words on the list in the puzzle.

```
P R O V I D E R V E G H E Y T Y G O C O T V G P S P N O F J F R L N O I L D K C
L D I S Q A T Q R S P N Z T Z M B X W A E D B R R D I X Y B R U U E E N Y O K T
Z L A T N E D I C N I L N I O H L C I R U T B O D O H F K S Y T D G G T O H Y F
X L E N V C H L R I A S E T U Z S L B Q Z M T C S T M P C F N S I Y U A R H O U
K C J X P E L C F I F A P N F V L I K P Q E L Q R H E O O E A H O W J M L L Y C
V E W J B L D G T I P B L E K Z A Y N B C S B P C B W U M R Y T Z V N C T E K N
A O K J C N G N C R N W P Z I G H W D T D S M M T N G E G L U V I D D N Q B S L
J W A S Q G E T O D R I C N E D B U E G I E V F E B L Q W G Y S P D B G N Z Z E
K T R D M D T V C V R S Y C N J N D E G S W Y U P P D A K R H M L P Z M H O R T
T V B G I A I Q O V T R X Q U H H E A V C D X Q M R K V Y S R E Q Q I B N Q K V
O X W F W S P L J K C Y H R J E E C W I L N M I P A R P D K A K Z B S Q W D K X
E X N M I Y P N J F C I D K A E F N G Y O G F S P L J J R K Y L G Q V L O W A H
W O V O Y U K M D O O B M L J O A A G Q S I H A X G M O A V B D P J V W O F S N
C A N V V T H O T R F N T A T M O R P E U E U J V G P C P S I V U B S J A B Z I
F S N S W T I U M J E H W I S U K U T K R U M W I J V S L L J E Y I V L O R S B
W O A F J H D L U S I C R Z I F T S X W E O X X R F D F G F D C H T L M M Y X F
H S I B K P G T I N N A W M T G S N W C S W B A C S B T C O P N H E K Y A A Y E
Q K K H J K E C F B R L I W Z C X I S U Q R T B B A Z Q M G X E P Z Y Q H W O M
Z L F M N P V O W Y A R L P G M C R G C X S Y Z P S Z S Y H P G K W U H T M C M
K K F R C N R Q O P V T I S Q P Q B Z T Y H A K S U K A Y J A I E Q W E I S I A
Y F Z B J M U Q L O J P N I Q E P N V R B L I S O H C P H H L L Y X K V W G G S
F C M U A N S J I Q J R A U Z N B N U I Z Y E B E M Q K D Q K L S Q J U X F H E
T R A T N Y W V N P F F K A O W P L S M X G G J Y D T X U Y X I P Z R T Z C T O
W R I V U A F W H L K F W B N C Z I I X N W N H Y D M N M E M D W I X S D X F U
F O A B I R A Y F X C Z M B C Y C W N C U D N A P X T V E W N E U H B K Y R M M
N X I N E R H C I L W W C O M P L A I N A N T Y I K Z O S L S U V S L J R E J W
Q C K F S K P A C P X R D N Q C C D F D Z X G K E K R U L P A D J D O D G D Q W
P S N I S A K H R T J P V N P N H P F L H K Q R I K M A F H K V V D P P H P A O
C I R F E T C F J Q A Z P Q K C U L V G J Z O F C Z D B H S O D E A S A R R B Z
K J N D O L D T E H U M E F K W M D E A Y L T H L B S C X D F N F R V M C E Q E
V E J M X D G V I C B B U H S T K U M X P L B T N G V D O Y W X Y A P B J C M V
O H T F H W Y Z Y O B Z C D G R S Q X F E T A I C O S S A S S E N I S U B L Q H
W C E P M X X B I V N A N Z Z P V B G Q O P H P N Q W X R B G I E O Z P B U C B
L K L A V U Z N G X U D Q I Y I X G S L X V P E T J U O A J M N K V Q R Y D M A
V F F K A V R P F S T C X J C J L A N I Z D A J R E A K N U V X M Z K J V E R D
W S K F C X O A F Y E W S P C W N C D F I J P P J T Y Y F R B J Z W I F P M E V
Q B V Z Z V K Y E H D R R D V F N F R N I Y H H G W A F M J H M W X N I X I C F
P J Q U G M O P R Z R M M J K V Y V Z P L D X V G Q T H F U E N C N F A V C V Q
C G M G M O L X I Y U T I L B T A L A F U X R U Y X J S E O Q F A D R G B F K J
R J Y C W A V G L M Y P I G P Z L Q Q I C Q B I U V S W A Y J E I G Z B W M E E
```

Accountability
Business associate
Complainant
Confidential
Disclosures
Divulge
Due diligence
Entity
Implement
Incidental
Infer
Insurance
Legalese
Preclude
Prevalent
Privacy
Protected health information
Provider
Provisions
Transaction
Verbiage

CASE STUDY

Read the case study and answer the questions that follow.

Morgan was given a copy of the Privacy Law and told to write the Notice of Privacy Practices for their clinic. After she began reading the law, she became somewhat discouraged because of the legalese and the slow pace at which she had to read to make sure she comprehended the message and requirements. She decided to attend a private training seminar on HIPAA compliance and found the instructor to be very knowledgeable.

1. How can such seminars be beneficial to the practice?

___

2. How can the medical assistant determine whether a seminar is worth attending?

___

Research seminars in your area and request information about them. Compare data with the information collected by the rest of the class.

WORKPLACE APPLICATIONS

Determine what certifications are available that relate to HIPAA. What are the requirements for obtaining these special certifications? Why might these be beneficial for the medical assistant? Is there a particular certification you are interested in obtaining?

INTERNET ACTIVITIES

1. Research the HIPAA Web site and find information about complaints. Then write an office policy for patients that details how to make a complaint if the patient thinks that his or her privacy has been violated.

2. Find the exact Public Law number that details the Health Insurance Portability and Accountability Act.

3. Research and write a report on HIPAA's Security Standard.

4. Find five additional links, other than the HIPAA Web site, that provide useful information on HIPAA compliance.

5. Determine misleading marketing ploys that sometimes are used in promoting HIPAA training.

6. Research programs that provide a specialized certificate in HIPAA proficiency.

18 Basics of Diagnostic Coding

VOCABULARY REVIEW

Fill in the blanks with the correct vocabulary terms from this chapter.

1. In medical coding, assessment and diagnostic statement are synonymous with _____.
2. _____ is any contact between a patient and a provider of service.
3. The _____ is the physician's determination of what is or may be wrong with the patient based on the findings from the H&P.
4. The abbreviation "CC" is a statement in the patient's own words that describes why the person sought medical attention. The letters "CC" stand for _____ _____ _____.
5. _____ is the signs and symptoms of a disease.
6. The _____ lists conditions, injuries, and diseases in alphabetical order by main terms, modifying terms, and subterms.
7. Services that support patient diagnoses (e.g., laboratory or radiology services) are known as _____.
8. In the context of the ICD-9-CM, the word *and* should always be interpreted as _____.
    a. and
    b. and/or
    c. or
9. _____ are broad sections of the ICD-9-CM coding manual grouped by disease or illness.
10. _____ is used when one or more codes are necessary to identify a given condition.
11. Converting verbal or written descriptions into numeric and alphanumeric designations is called _____.
12. _____ is the abbreviations, punctuation, symbols, instructional notations, and related entities that provide guidance to the medical assistant or coder in selecting an accurate and specific code.
13. The determination of the nature of a disease, injury, or congenital defect is a(an) _____
14. The _____ is the information about the diagnosis or diagnoses of the patient which have been extracted from the medical documentation.
15. The cause of the disorder; a claim may be classified according to _____.
16. _____ terms are always written in italics, and the word _____ is often enclosed in a box to draw particular attention to these instructions.
17. H&P or HPE is an acronym for _____ _____ _____.
18. _____ is the current system for classifying disease to facilitate collection of uniform and comparable health information, for statistical purposes, and for indexing medical records for data storage and retrieval.
19. _____ is the initial identification of the condition or complaint the patient expresses in the outpatient medical setting.
20. The term _____ must always be followed and is found in the Alphabetic Index, volumes 2 and 3; it is a direction given to a coder to look in another place.

21. _____ is a direction given to the coder to look elsewhere if the main term or subterm (or subterms) for that entry are not sufficient for coding the information.

22. _____ is a direction given to the coder to see a specific category (three-digit code). This must always be followed.

23. SOAP notes are a system of charting that includes the following four things:

_____

_____

_____

_____

24. The term _____ appears only in volume 1 in those subdivisions in which the user should add further information by means of an additional code to give more complete picture of the diagnosis.

25. In the context of the ICD-9-CM, the terms _____, _____, and _____ dictate that both parts of the title be present in the statement of the diagnosis in order to assign the particular code.

SKILLS AND CONCEPTS

Part I: Getting to Know ICD-9-CM Coding

1. The use of ICD-9-CM codes is important for several reasons. Circle the letters of the ones that do NOT apply:

    a. Standardizing a system of diagnostic coding accepted and understood by all parties in the reimbursement cycle

    b. Creating a more convenient method of data storage and retrieval

    c. Assisting in the maximization of reimbursement

    d. Lengthening the claims processing time

    e. Facilitating and measuring regulatory compliance by use of guidelines and other instructions

    f. Assisting in measuring the appropriateness and timeliness of medical care

2. Fill in the blanks in the paragraph below:

    The ICD-9-CM code is located in volume 1, the Tabular Index, of the ICD-9-CM coding manual. The code consists of a(n) _____ category code that represents a specific disease, illness, condition, or injury within a general disease category. For example, 250 is the disease classification, or category, for diabetes mellitus. Up to _____ additional digits can be used, which add further definition and specificity.

    These additional digits are the fourth digit, or _____; and the fifth digit, or _____, respectively.

3. The basic ICD-9-CM manual has three volumes. Fill in the blanks regarding these three volumes:

    _____ are used for diagnostic coding by hospitals, physicians, and all other providers of service.

    _____, also known as the Tabular Index, contains all of the diagnostic codes grouped into 17 chapters of disease and injury. _____ are broad sections of the ICD-9-CM coding manual grouped by disease or illness (e.g., Chapter 10 contains diagnostic codes for diseases of the genitourinary system).

    _____ is called the Alphabetic Index and is used in the same way an alphabetic index in any textbook is used, except that it refers the user back to the category codes in the Tabular Index rather than page numbers. _____ is used by hospitals to code procedures and services performed in the hospital environment. This volume is not used by most physician providers.

4. Match the following:

   _____ Section   a. Fourth digit

   _____ Category   b. Also called a *chapter*

   _____ Subcategory   c. Fifth digit

   _____ Subclassification   d. Also called a *classification*

5. The _____ _____ is used to describe whether any disease process or manifestation exists that was caused by the disease. _____

6. The _____ is used on occasions when the patient is not currently ill or to explain problems that influence a patient's current illness, condition, or injury. _____

7. The _____ is used to classify environmental or external causes of injury, poisoning, or other adverse effects on the body. _____

8. Match the following:

   _____ Morphology of Neoplasms   a. Appendix C

   _____ Glossary of Mental Disorders   b. Appendix A

   _____ Classification of Drugs   c. Appendix E

   _____ Classification of Industrial Accidents   d. Appendix B

   _____ List of Three-Digit Categories   e. Appendix D

9. The abbreviation _____ is the equivalent of "unspecified" and means that the diagnostic statement does not provide more specificity or definition.

10. The abbreviation _____ is to be used only when the coder lacks the information necessary to code the term to a more specific category. _____

11. Four basic forms of punctuation are used in the Tabular Index. Circle the letter of the one that is NOT one of those forms:

    a. Brackets

    b. Parentheses

    c. Question marks

    d. Braces

    e. Colon

12. Two other conventions found in both the Alphabetic Index and the Tabular Index are the use of _____ and _____ fonts.

13. _____ type is used for all codes and titles in the Tabular Index.

14. _____ type is used for exclusion notes and to identify any diagnosis that cannot be used as the primary diagnosis.

Instructional notations are notes included in the Tabular Index to provide additional guidance for selecting a specific diagnosis code. The following are the most common instructional notations. Fill in the blank with the appropriate term.

15. A notation indicating that under a category or other subdivision, separate terms can be found that will serve to further define, give examples of, or provide modifying adjectives and sites or conditions. _____

16. Terms that are enclosed within a box and are printed in italics. These notations indicate that some code classifications cannot be used with the code being selected. _____

17. Used to define terms and give coding instructions. They often are used to list the fifth-digit subclassification or subclassifications for certain categories. _____

18. The _____ instruction follows a main term and indicates that a different term should be referenced.

19. This notation is a variation of the SEE instruction. _____

20. The _____ instruction generally is found after a main term in the Alphabetic Index and directs the coder to another area with additional index entries that may be useful.

21. This note directs the use of codes that are not normally intended to be used as a principal diagnosis or are not to be sequenced before the underlying disease. _____

22. This word should be interpreted to mean *and* or *or*. _____

23. This word in the Alphabetic Index is sequenced immediately after a main term. It provides additional definition or specificity to the code description. _____

24. Match the following:

    _____ Main terms   a. Are always indented two additional spaces from the level of the preceding line
    _____ Modifying terms   b. Appear in bold print
    _____ Subterms   c. Are found in the Alphabetic Index indented below main terms
    _____ Modifiers   d. Are indented two spaces to the right under the main term

25. Three tables and one supplementary index are in the Alphabetic Index. The tables include the: _____, _____, and _____.

26. The supplementary index is the Index to _____ (E codes).

27. The _____ Table lists the types of hypertension and the manifestations and causes of hypertension.

28. _____ is defined as a type of hypertension in which the clinical course progresses rapidly to death.

29. _____ hypertension is a type that does not threaten a patient's health status significantly.

30. _____ hypertension is used only when no documentation is provided in the clinical record that the hypertension is malignant or benign.

31. The _____ Table lists neoplasms by anatomic location.

32. A benign neoplasm is a(n) _____.

Part II: Beginning the Encounter Process

1. Information pertinent to code selection is culled from a variety of medical documents. Circle the letter of the one that is NOT a part of the diagnostic statements:

    a. Encounter form

    b. Treatment notes

    c. Discharge summary

    d. Operative report

    e. Nurses' notes

    f. Radiology report

    g. Pathology report

    h. Laboratory report

2. The _____ generally is a preprinted form and is also the most common form used by the medical assistant to obtain the charges and diagnosis when performing charge and payment data entry and insurance billing.

3. _____ are the second most common medical document from which diagnostic information can be obtained.

4. The _____ begins with a statement in the patient's own words that describes the reason the person is seeking medical attention. This statement is called the _____ and is often abbreviated _____ in the History documentation in the medical record.

5. The _____ is used primarily for extracting procedure and diagnostic information for patients who were hospitalized rather than seen in the physician's office.

6. The _____ will also be used for extracting procedure and diagnostic information for patients who underwent surgery as an outpatient or inpatient.

7. _____, _____, _____ reports are not used to obtain diagnostic statements. Any findings from these reports must be documented in the treatment notes in the medical record to be used for diagnostic coding, charge entry, or insurance billing purposes.

8. A(n) _____ describes a disease, condition, or injury named after a person, such as Hodgkin's disease.

9. _____ are abbreviations of words that create a new word. For example, the _____ for gastroesophageal reflux disease is GERD. *GERD* and *gastroesophageal reflux disease* are both medical terms.

10. _____ are slightly different; abbreviations are "shorthand" for common medical terms.

11. _____ are words similar in meaning that can be used interchangeably.

12. A series of questions called a(n) _____ can assist the medical assistant in navigating the Alphabetic and Tabular Index while performing the steps for diagnostic coding. The _____ for the main text is designed to guide the selection of the appropriate ICD-9-CM diagnostic code

Part III: Coding Exercises

Code the following diagnoses to the highest level of specificity

1. The Smiths' newborn has a birthmark on his neck.

2. Mr. Epstein suffers from Bruck's disease.

3. Jenny developed bronchitis over spring break after inhaling gas fumes while sitting in a traffic jam.

4. Carolyn has experienced dumping syndrome periodically since her gastric bypass surgery.

5. Robert has experienced pain when he urinates for the past 3 weeks.

6. Julia has been nauseated for about a week but has not complained of vomiting.

7. Paul has trench foot, which is a condition of moist gangrene caused by freezing of wet skin.

8. Benjamin was given a health examination the night he entered prison to serve a life sentence.

9. Angela was classified as morbidly obese, so she qualified for gastric bypass surgery.

10. Joseph was diagnosed with academic underachievement disorder and sent for counseling.

11. Morgan Smith had an acute myocardial infarction, commonly referred to as a heart attack.

12. Jessica was placed in the neonatal ICU because she was diagnosed with transient tachypnea at birth.

13. Terri constantly struggles with her maxillary sinus, especially in the winter.

14. The physician told Roger that he had epididymitis, but it was not a result of a venereal disease.

15. Judy has experienced neck pain for 1 week, but she does not know why the pain began.

16. Kevin has suffered from low back pain for years.

17. Brad was bitten by a brown recluse spider.

18. The Abbotts' child died of sudden infant death syndrome.

19. Mitral stenosis was Mrs. Richland's final diagnosis.

20. Georgia went into anaphylactic shock after drinking milk.

21. Joey was taken to a psychologist because he was having recurrent nightmares.

22. Roger has benign essential hypertension.

23. Susan was having trouble breathing, and her physician told her that she had a nasopharyngeal polyp that needed to be removed.

24. Kristy's son, Christian, suffers with croup syndrome and has been hospitalized three times because of the disorder.

25. Ron saw Dr. Jarrett because of an anal fissure, which resulted from a nontraumatic tear of his anus.

26. Griffin saw Dr. Redford for treatment of a common head cold.

27. A tetanus toxoid vaccination was administered to a child who stepped on a rusty nail.

28. Mrs. Garrett developed a decubitus ulcer on her buttocks while she was a patient in a nursing home.

29. Paige has a migraine headache, and the physician did not mention intractable migraine in the medical record.

30. Pat has Graves' disease, and the physician did not mention thyrotoxic crisis or storm on the medical record.

31. Mary is in rehabilitation for episodic cocaine dependence.

32. Jonathan has been diagnosed with attention deficit disorder, without mention of hyperactivity.

33. Angelica has had chronic cystic mastitis for years.

34. Mr. Robertson had a TIA at home and was rushed to the hospital.

35. Ray noticed a ringing in his ears after working for 6 months on a construction site.

36. Raul has been diagnosed with iron-deficiency anemia, because he is not getting enough iron in his diet.

37. Camille has had recurrent earaches in the 2 years since her birth, and the physician diagnosed chronic purulent otitis media.

38. Sally's newborn was diagnosed with pyloric stenosis and required surgery.

39. Stephanie has a urinary tract infection, but the physician does not yet know what organism caused the illness.

40. Don has insomnia, which the physician thinks is a result of drug abuse.

41. Mabel Johnson has rheumatoid arthritis and takes daily medication to control the pain.

42. Cynthia has a plantar wart but does not want to have it removed yet.

43. Sebastian fractured his clavicle at the sternal end during a football game. The fracture was closed.

44. Peggy contracted herpes simplex with herpetic vulvovaginitis.

45. Eric noticed blood in his semen, and the physician diagnosed hematospermia.

46. Kayla had a sore throat and fever and was diagnosed with infectious mononucleosis.

47. Gerald has osteoarthritis in his shoulder region and is scheduled to begin physical therapy next week.

48. Tray has had three headaches, not diagnosed as migraines, in the past week.

49. Amanda was diagnosed with multiple sclerosis.

50. Jeffrey has a personal history of alcoholism.

51. Butch had four back surgeries and developed a continuous dependence on hydrocodone.

52. Jake went to an ophthalmologist to have a splinter removed from his cornea.

53. Tammy suffered from severe pain in the temporomandibular joint area.

54. Josephine was struck by lightning during a thunderstorm.

55. Barry's alcoholism has caused cirrhosis of the liver.

56. The Wickers' newborn had a skin condition called *cradle cap*.

57. Adam has been a paraplegic since a car wreck 2 years ago.

58. Hudson suffered a ruptured abdominal aneurysm and had emergency surgery.

59. Mr. Emmett had atherosclerosis of the extremities with gangrene just before his death.

60. The woman with Munchausen syndrome had three children who died before law enforcement grew suspicious.

61. Ginger experienced dermatitis as a result of using a tanning bed.

62. The Lewises' first child was born with Down syndrome.

63. Lee Anna has experienced painful menstruation during her last three cycles.

64. James had one testicle removed because of seminoma. The tumor was the primary site and incident of his cancer.

65. Jacqueline has uncontrolled diabetes mellitus type 2 with ketoacidosis.

66. Mrs. Julius died last week from congestive heart failure.

67. Gary saw the physician to follow up on his previous diagnosis of cardiomegaly.

68. Dr. Albertez thinks that Mr. Tidwell's Parkinson's disease was drug induced.

69. Jerry developed Kaposi's sarcoma during the final stages of AIDS. The sarcoma was present in his lymph nodes.

70. Sally developed a postoperative fever because of an infection (code infection only).

71. Terri attempted suicide by ingesting a handful of lithium.

72. Beaumont's divorce affected every aspect of his life.

73. Mr. Maxwell's physician knew that his patient would have to be hospitalized once he diagnosed diverticulitis of the colon with hemorrhaging. Mr. Maxwell, at age 95, could not risk staying at home and allowing the bleeding to continue.

74. Susan was stung by a jellyfish while swimming off the coast of Mexico.

75. Alaydra has tunnel vision, which makes it difficult to drive safely.

76. The escaped criminal was cornered by the police and shot because he raised his gun and pointed it at a policeman.

77. Riley has acute myocarditis and was admitted to the hospital.

78. Alisha underwent artificial insemination in an effort to have a child.

79. Jackie's baby was breech and was delivered using forceps.

80. Ordell has acute esophagitis and complained that he had been sick for 3 days.

81. Robert dislocated his shoulder while playing baseball. This was a closed anterior dislocation of the humerus.

82. Betty has allergic gastroenteritis.

83. Mrs. Ralphy was diagnosed with systemic lupus erythematosus.

84. Winston has synovitis of the knee.

85. Mrs. Radson had a skin condition known as bullous pemphigoid, in which blisters formed in patches all over her skin.

86. Osteomalacia made it impossible for Robbie to walk.

87. Henry has oral leukoplakia, which may have been caused by smoking a pipe.

88. Ricky was diagnosed with acute lymphocytic leukemia.

89. The Smithsons' 4-year-old daughter has Hurler's syndrome, which was diagnosed a few months after she was born.

90. Patricia has had uterine endometriosis for several years and may require a hysterectomy in the future.

CASE STUDY

Dr. Rogers saw Mrs. Arrant in the office this morning. Mrs. Arrant has been diagnosed in the past with congestive heart failure, diabetes mellitus type 2, and chronic myelocytic leukemia. She came to the clinic today complaining of chest pain, and she had a fever of 101.8° F. Code all these conditions. In what order would they be written on an encounter form?

WORKPLACE APPLICATIONS

Determine what certifications are available that relate to coding. What are the requirements for obtaining these special certifications? Why might these be beneficial for the medical assistant? Is there a particular certification you are interested in obtaining?

INTERNET ACTIVITIES

1. Research the AHIMA Web site and explore opportunities for a career in coding.

2. Locate a job description for a medical billing and coding specialist and determine the daily duties that coders perform in medical offices and/or large clinics.

3. Write a report on the importance of coding accurately. Share the information with the class.

4. Find five additional links other than the AHIMA Web site that provide useful information on billing and coding.

5. Research programs that provide a specialized certificate in billing and/or coding proficiency.

19 Basics of Procedural Coding

VOCABULARY REVIEW

Fill in the blanks with the correct vocabulary terms from this chapter.

1. The primary procedure or service code selected when performing insurance billing or statistical research is a category _____ code.

2. Jerri sometimes has difficulty with _____ codes, which designate procedures or services that are grouped together and paid for as one procedure or service.

3. Jules prepared a(n) _____ or summary of the diagnostic statements on Mr. Ford's medical record.

4. _____ are found at the beginning of each of the six sections of the CPT-4 manual, and Rebecca refers to them often when coding procedures.

5. Category _____ codes are for new or experimental procedures.

6. A procedure, service, or diagnosis named after a person is called a(n) _____.

7. Codes in which the components of a procedure are separated and reported separately are called _____ codes.

8. Code additions that explain circumstances that alter a provided service or provide additional clarification or detail are called _____.

9. The main divisions of the CPT-4 manual are called _____.

10. Abbreviations are also called _____.

CODING EXERCISES

Code the following procedures.

1. Dr. Smith visits Eula Fairbanks, a patient with dementia, in the nursing home for less than 30 minutes.

2. Jessica Lundy, a newborn, was admitted to the pediatric critical care unit after her birth, where Dr. Williams provided her initial care.

3. Because Lucille Westerman had multiple health problems, she was admitted for observation after a fainting spell. Dr. Adams took a comprehensive history and performed a thorough examination and then made medical decisions of high complexity regarding her care.

4. Dr. Wray saw Tammy Luttrell in the office as a new patient. He took a detailed history and performed a detailed examination and then made medical decisions of low complexity.

5. Sylvia Julius saw Dr. Bridges for her allergies. The physician took a problem-focused history, performed a problem-focused examination, and made straightforward decisions regarding her care.

6. Bonnie Sadler comes to the office to have blood work drawn for an obstetric panel. What is the code for the obstetric panel only?

7. The office charges Bonnie Sadler, a college student, for drawing a blood specimen. What is the code for venipuncture?

8. Terri Smithson had laparoscopic gastric bypass surgery involving the Roux-en-Y procedure.

9. Kim Errant had outpatient kidney imaging with vascular flow to make sure her kidneys were functioning normally.

10. Georgie Ebersol had blood drawn for a total bilirubin. Code the blood test only.

11. Roy Messing's urine was tested for total protein.

12. Jerry Orchard was tested for his blood alcohol level.

13. Andrea Adams has a bleeding disorder and has to undergo regular coagulation time tests. Her physician uses the Lee and White method.

14. Dr. Airheart sent Roberto's specimen to the microbiology laboratory to check for *Cryptosporidium* organisms.

15. The body was sent to the county medical examiner's office for a forensic autopsy, which was performed by Dr. Stein.

16. Jonathan Boyd was required to have a polio vaccination by his school. He received an oral dose.

17. Julia Anderson has a lithium level drawn to make certain that her dosage was accurate and appropriate.

18. Cynthia Hernandez was exposed to hepatitis, so her physician ordered an acute hepatitis panel.

19. Sam Livingston, a baby in the neonatal unit, had total bilirubin tests drawn each morning.

20. Susan's husband has blood drawn regularly to measure his quinidine levels.

21. Bobby had to undergo treatment of a clavicular fracture, without manipulation, after his injury during a football game.

22. Betty received anesthesia for the vaginal delivery of her child.

23. Anesthesia was provided to Ron Smith, a brain-dead patient whose organs were being harvested for donation.

24. Dr. Partridge participated in a complex, lengthy telephone call regarding a patient who was scheduled for multiple surgeries.

25. When Terri Anderson was involved in a major car accident, the emergency department physician took a comprehensive history, performed a thorough examination, and made highly complex decisions.

26. Tim Taylor is a new patient with a small cyst on his back. Dr. Young took a problem-focused history and performed a problem-focused examination and then made straightforward medical decisions.

27. Jim Angelo, an established patient, saw the physician for a minor cut on the back of his hand. The physician spent approximately 10 minutes with Jim.

28. Vera Carpenter was admitted to the hospital for diabetes mellitus, congestive heart failure, and an infection of unknown origin. Dr. Antonetti performed a consultation that took about an hour, including the time spent writing orders in her medical record.

29. Carla had a nasal polyp removed that was hindering her ability to breathe. The excision was a simple one and was performed in Dr. Wilson's office.

30. Darla's son, Andy, was examined for pinworms.

31. The police asked the laboratory technician to perform an arsenic test on a tube of blood.

32. An incision was made into the newborn's pyloric sphincter to allow food to travel through his digestive system.

33. Ben, a 6-year-old, had his tonsils and adenoids removed because of recurrent infections.

34. Edward had one testicle removed because of a growing tumor attached to it. An inguinal approach was used, and during the surgery, the physician explored the abdominal area to look for other growths.

35. Alex's mother insisted that she have her ears pierced by a physician so that the procedure would be as clean as possible.

36. Fonda was diagnosed with an abdominal ectopic pregnancy, which Dr. Tomlinson removed surgically.

37. The medical assistant performed a simple urinalysis, using a dipstick and a microscope to examine the specimen.

38. Wayne had blood drawn for a CBC with an automated WBC.

39. Paula had an inflammation somewhere inside her body, as evidenced by her sedimentation rate. The test was automated.

40. Jimmie's physician ordered computed tomography of his abdomen with contrast material.

41. Joan had a laparoscopic biopsy of her left ovary.

42. Craig had to undergo a direct repair of a ruptured aneurysm of the carotid artery, which was performed via a neck incision.

43. Emma was given a urine pregnancy test in the clinic before receiving x-ray examinations to diagnose her back disorder; a color comparison test kit was used.

44. Jennifer's child was tested for serum albumin.

45. Angela had a qualitative lactose test using a urine specimen.

46. Sarah was required to have a blood chemistry test for methadone by her probation officer.

47. The two children who had been lost in the woods were tested for Rocky Mountain spotted fever.

48. Marcus has a total T-cell count every month.

49. After her needle-stick injury, Felicia was tested for the hepatitis B surface antibody.

50. Dr. Torrid felt that Katrina might have the Epstein-Barr virus, so he tested for the early antigen.

51. Dr. Battson performed a chlamydia culture on the vaginal specimen.

52. Juan was given a test for herpes simplex type II.

53. Mr. Albertson was given a blood test for uric acid.

54. Derrick had a Western Blot test last week. The interpretation and report are due back to the physician by tomorrow.

55. Roy had a urine test for total protein.

56. The emergency physician ordered a lead test on the small child, thinking that she had perhaps ingested some paint chips.

57. Joy has monthly blood tests to evaluate her iron-binding capacity.

58. Andi was tested for chromium yesterday and has a return appointment next week.

59. All gastric bypass patients are required to have a basic metabolic panel before surgery is scheduled.

60. June had an obstetric panel run on her second appointment with the physician.

61. Royce had a chest x-ray film, single frontal view, to check for pneumonia.

62. Dr. True suspected that Joey had fractured his sternum, so he ordered an x-ray film that would show two views of the bone.

63. Jessalyn had an MRI scan of her spinal canal and its contents.

64. Dr. Tompkins visited a new patient at her home and spent about 20 minutes diagnosing and treating her for the flu.

65. Dr. Revy was on standby for about 20 minutes while the decision was made as to whether the patient would have a cesarean section.

66. Judge Jordan has his blood checked for potassium levels monthly.

67. Steven Pauly needs a chest x-ray examination, and the physician has requested four views.

68. Linda Ellis had a complete hip x-ray examination with two views, because her physician was considering hip replacement surgery.

69. Judy had blood drawn for determination of a theophylline level during her last office visit.

70. Joy had a closed treatment of a coccygeal fracture.

71. Mrs. Dickson went to see Dr. Donner for a complete radiologic examination of the scapula.

72. Bobbie returned to the physician's office to have a short leg walking cast applied after having worn a larger cast for 4 weeks.

73. Dr. Angell ordered a radiologic examination of Sylvia's mastoids, requesting two views.

74. Sammy had a uric acid test during his last office visit.

75. Peter asked his physician to repeat his CPK total, because it had been slightly high on his last visit.

76. Bryce has a digoxin level drawn every 3 months.

77. The pathologist prepared tissue for drug analysis.

78. Julie was quite dehydrated for a week, so her physician ran an electrolyte panel.

79. Frank asked the physician how a magnesium level related to his illness.

80. Joel's physician believed that Joel had adrenal insufficiency, so he ordered an ACTH stimulation panel.

81. All three children who lived in the condemned home were subjected to a quantitative carbon monoxide test.

82. When Ariel turned 50, her physician recommended that she have an occult blood test annually.

83. Most diabetics periodically have a blood glucose test performed at the physician's office in addition to the test strip checks that they perform at home.

84. Selenium can be detected with a blood test.

85. Sarah's infant returned to the physician's office to have a PKU test a few weeks after she was born.

86. Van Stephens had blood work done on Monday to check his triglyceride level.

87. Karry has been to the physician for several days in a row to have ovulation tests, which are done by visual color comparison.

88. Samuel's vitamin K test results were slightly below normal.

89. Dr. Grant runs a spun microhematocrit on each of his pregnant patients at every prenatal visit.

90. Trent had a serum folic acid test run this morning at his physician's office.

CASE STUDY

In the following text, highlight all procedures that need to be coded for billing purposes.

Roberta Sleether is a new patient who saw Dr. Morganstern. She complained of feeling tired all the time. She stated that she was exhausted even after a full 8 hours of sleep at night. Roberta said that she did not have much of an appetite and that she had been eating mostly salads and chicken, with a bowl of fruit as snacks. She is not overweight, and her blood pressure and other vital signs were normal. Dr. Morganstern decided to perform a CBC, an electrolyte panel, and a lipid panel. He also ordered a urinalysis, an iron-binding capacity, and a vitamin B_{12} test. The physician asked if she had noticed any blood in her urine or stool, and she denied blood in the urine but did mention she had several episodes of diarrhea. Dr. Morganstern added an occult blood test as well as a stool culture to check for pathogens. The physician placed Roberta on multivitamin therapy and told her to return in 1 week to discuss her laboratory test results. He spent approximately 30 minutes with Roberta, taking a detailed history, performing a detailed examination, and making low-complexity medical decisions. Roberta scheduled her appointment for the following week and left the clinic.

WORKPLACE APPLICATIONS

1. Select a medical specialty and research the procedure codes that would be commonly used in that practice.

2. Contact a practice and make an appointment to meet the person or persons who perform coding tasks. Discuss the challenges and rewards of the job. Prepare a report for the class based on the interview with the coders.

3. Design an encounter form for a fictional medical practice. Choose the specialty and make sure the codes chosen for the form are applicable to the specialty practice.

INTERNET ACTIVITIES

1. Research job postings on the Internet that relate to billing and coding.

2. Working in groups, prepare a report on the sections of the CPT-4 manual. Discuss the most common codes in each section.

3. Search for coding hints and tips online. Prepare a report for the class and discuss the tips and how to use them to code more effectively.

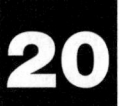
Basics of Health Insurance

VOCABULARY REVIEW

Fill in the blanks with the correct vocabulary terms from this chapter.

1. _____ is the maximum amount of money many third-party payers allow for a specific procedure or service.

2. A term used in managed care for an approved referral is _____.

3. An individual entitled to receive benefits from an insurance policy or program or from a government entitlement program offering healthcare benefits is considered the _____.

4. The amount payable by an insurance company for a monetary loss to an individual insured by that company, under each coverage, is known as _____.

5. This rule states that when an individual is covered by two insurance policies, the insurance plan of the policyholder whose birthday comes first in the calendar year (month and day, not year) becomes the primary insurance.

6. _____ is a payment method used by many managed care organizations in which a fixed amount of money is reimbursed to the provider for patients enrolled during a specific period of time, no matter what services were received or how many visits were made.

7. In the insurance business, companies that assume the risk of an insurance policy are considered the _____.

8. CHAMPUS is the acronym for _____.

9. The health benefits program run by the Department of Veterans Affairs (VA) that helps eligible beneficiaries pay the cost of specific healthcare services and supplies is (give full name and acronym) _____.

10. A(n) _____ provision frequently is found in medical insurance policies whereby the policyholder and the insurance company share the cost of covered losses in a specified ratio.

11. This type of plan reimburses the insured for expenses resulting from illness or injury according to a specific fee schedule as outlined in the insurance policy and on a fee-for-service basis. _____

12. A(n) _____ is the sum of money paid at the time of medical service; a form of co-insurance.

13. Typically met on a yearly or per-incident basis, this specific amount of money, a(n) _____, is what a patient must pay out of pocket before the insurance carrier begins paying.

14. _____ are the spouse, children, and sometimes domestic partner or other individuals designated by the insured who are covered under a healthcare plan.

15. This type of insurance provides periodic payments to replace income when an insured person is unable to work as a result of illness, injury, or disease. _____

16. The _____ is the date on which an insurance policy or plan takes effect so that benefits are payable.

17. _____ is a term that indicates whether a patient's insurance coverage is in effect and the patient is eligible for payment of insurance benefits.

18. The term for limitations on an insurance contract for which benefits are not payable is _____.

19. A letter or statement from the insurance carrier that describes what was paid, denied, or reduced in payment and that also contains information about amounts applied to the deductible, the patient's co-insurance, and the allowed amounts is called the _____ _____.

20. A letter or statement from Medicare describing what was paid, denied, or reduced in payment and that also contains information about amounts applied to the deductible, the patient's co-insurance, and the allowed amounts is called the _____ _____.

21. An established schedule of fees set for services performed by providers and paid by the patient is called _____.

22. A _____ _____ is an organization that contracts with the government to handle and mediate insurance claims from medical facilities, home health agencies, or providers of medical services or supplies.

23. Medicaid and Medicare are examples of _____ plans.
    a. local
    b. basic
    c. organizational
    d. government

24. Insurance written under a policy that covers a number of people under a single master contract issued to their employer or to an association with which they are affiliated would be considered a(n) _____ policy.

25. The _____ is the person responsible for paying a medical bill.

26. _____ _____ is protection in return for periodic premium payments that provides reimbursement of expenses resulting from illness or injury.

27. The Kassebaum-Kennedy Act, which was designed to improve portability and continuity of health insurance coverage; to combat waste, fraud, and abuse in health insurance and healthcare delivery; to promote the use of medical savings accounts; to improve access to long-term care services and coverage; to simplify the administration of health insurance; and to serve other purposes, is also called the (please provide the whole name and the acronym) _____
_____.

28. A(n) _____ is an organization that provides a wide range of comprehensive healthcare services for a specified group at a fixed periodic payment. These organizations may be sponsored by the government, medical schools, hospitals, employers, labor unions, consumer groups, insurance companies, and hospital-medical plans.

29. _____ _____ pay for all or a share of the cost of covered services, regardless of which physician, hospital, or other licensed _____ provider is used. Policyholders of these plans and their dependents choose when and where to get healthcare services.

30. What type of insurance policy is designed specifically for the use of one person (and his or her dependents) and is not associated with the amenities of a group policy (e.g., lower premiums)? _____ _____.

31. The individual or organization covered by an insurance policy according to the policy terms, and usually the individual or group that pays the premiums, is called the _____.

32. An umbrella term for all healthcare plans that provide healthcare in return for preset monthly payments and coordinated care through a defined network of primary care physicians and hospitals is _____.

33. Tax-deferred bank or savings accounts that are combined with a low-premium, high-deductible insurance policy and designed for individuals or families who choose to fund their own healthcare expenses and medical insurance are called _____.

34. Matching terms:

    _____ Medicaid   a. A federally sponsored health insurance program for those over age 65 and those under age 65 who are disabled
    _____ Medicare   b. A term sometimes applied to private insurance products that supplement Medicare insurance benefits
    _____ Medigap   c. A federal and state sponsored health insurance program for the medically indigent

35. A(n) _____ _____ is a physician or other healthcare provider who enters into a contract with a specific insurance company or program and by doing so agrees to abide by certain rules and regulations set forth by that particular third-party payer.

36. The person who pays a premium to an insurance company and in whose name the policy is written in exchange for the insurance protection provided by a policy of insurance is the _____.

37. _____ is a process required by some insurance carriers in which the provider obtains permission to perform certain procedures or services or to refer a patient to a specialist.

38. The periodic (monthly, quarterly, or annual) payment of a specific sum of money to an insurance company for which the insurer, in return, agrees to provide certain benefits is called a(n) _____.

39. The _____ is a general practice or nonspecialist provider or physician responsible for the care of a patient for some health maintenance organizations; also called a *gatekeeper*.

40. An insurance term used when a primary care provider wants to send a patient to a specialist: _____.

41. An explanation of benefits that comes from Medicaid is called a(an) _____ _____.

42. The fee schedule designed to provide national uniform payment of Medicare benefits after adjustment to reflect the differences in practice costs across geographic areas is called the _____.

43. A(n) _____ is a special provision or group of provisions that may be added to a policy to expand or limit the benefits otherwise payable. It may increase or reduce benefits, waive a condition or coverage, or in any other way amend the original contract.

44. A type of insurance plan funded by an organization with an employee base large enough to enable it to fund its own insurance program: _____.

45. When a patient or insured individual refers himself or herself to a specialist without requesting the referral from the primary provider, this is known as _____.

46. _____ _____ plans provide benefits in the form of certain surgical and medical services rendered rather than cash. This type of plan is not restricted to a fee schedule.

47. An organization that processes claims and performs other business-related functions for a health plan is a(n) _____.

48. Entities that make payment on an obligation or debt but are not parties of the contract that created the debt are known as _____.

49. A government-sponsored program under which authorized dependents of military personnel receive medical care; the program originally was called CHAMPUS but now is called _____.

50. A(n) _____ _____ is a review of individual cases by a committee to make sure services are medically necessary and to study how providers use medical care resources.

51. Insurance against liability imposed on certain employers to pay benefits and furnish care to employees who are injured and to pay benefits to dependents of employees killed in the course of or arising out of their employment is known as _____ _____.

FOR QUESTIONS 52-61: Read the following paragraph and then fill in the blanks.
The medical assistant's tasks related to health insurance processing are initiated when the patient encounters the provider, either by appointment, as a walk-in, or in the emergency department or hospital. To complete insurance billing and coding properly, the medical assistant must perform the following tasks.

52. Obtain information from the patient and insured, including _____, employment, and _____ data.

53. Verify the patient's _____ for insurance payment with the insurance carrier or carriers, as well as _____ available, exclusions, and whether _____ are needed to refer patients to specialists or to perform certain services or procedures, such as surgery or diagnostic tests.

54. Perform _____ and _____ coding and review the encounter form or charge ticket for completeness once the patient has been seen by the provider.

55. Calculate insurance _____ and co-insurance amounts and provide the patient with a statement showing the _____ expense, the amount owed by the patient.

56. Obtain _____ for referral of the patient to a specialist or for special services or procedures that require advance permission.

57. Complete an insurance claim form and submit it to the insurance company for _____ for services and procedures performed.

58. Post payments and adjustments on the patient ledger or account and examine the _____ (EOB), _____ (EOMB) or the _____ (RA) from the insurance company to identify what was paid, reduced, or denied.

59. Make adjustments to the account of the allowable amount, which is either written off (adjusted) or passed on to the patient for _____.

60. Bill the patient for any _____ _____, or, if there is a secondary insurance, complete the secondary insurance claim form and submit it to the insurance company.

61. _____ on any rejected or unpaid claims and any requests from the insurance carrier for more information about specific claims.

QUESTIONS 62-73: Match each type of insurance benefit with its description

62. _____ Hospitalization
63. _____ Surgical
64. _____ Basic medical
65. _____ Major medical
66. _____ Disability
67. _____ Dental care
68. _____ Vision care
69. _____ Medicare supplement

a. Pays expenses involved in care of the teeth and gums
b. Provides reimbursement for all or a percentage of the cost of refraction, lenses, and frames
c. Helps defray medical costs not covered by Medicare
d. Protects a person in the event of a certain type of accident, such as an airplane crash
e. Provides payment of a specified amount on the insured's death
f. Covers a continuum of broad-ranged maintenance and health services to chronically ill, disabled, or mentally retarded individuals
g. Pays all or part of a surgeon's and/or assistant surgeon's fees
h. Weekly or monthly cash benefits provided to employed policyholders who become unable to work as a result of an accident or illness

70. _____ Special risk insurance

71. _____ Liability insurance

72. _____ Life insurance

73. _____ Long-term care insurance

i. Pays all or part of a physician's fee for nonsurgical services, including hospital, home, and office visits

j. Provides protection against especially large medical bills resulting from catastrophic or prolonged illnesses

k. Pays the cost of all or part of the insured person's hospital room and board and specific hospital services

l. Often includes benefits for medical expenses payable to individuals who are injured in the insured person's home or in an automobile accident

74. List three advantages of the managed care concept.

75. List three disadvantages of the managed care concept.

76. List 10 items of information the medical assistant should obtain from the patient before calling the insurance company for preauthorization or precertification.

a. _____
b. _____
c. _____
d. _____
e. _____
f. _____
g. _____
h. _____
i. _____
j. _____

77. List two types of people who would qualify for Medicare.

78. List two types of people who would qualify for Medicaid.

79. The _____ _____ is the official daily publication for rules, proposed rules, and notices of federal agencies and organization, as well as Executive Orders and other presidential documents.

CASE STUDY

Survey all class members and determine the various types of insurance coverage the students have. Assign each student a different insurance company and have them call to verify benefits. Choose a medical procedure and have the students call and verify the amounts of coverage for that particular procedure. If students are uncomfortable exchanging health insurance information, allow them to verify and obtain amounts of coverage for their own insurance.

WORKPLACE APPLICATIONS

1. Working in small groups, obtain a quote for health insurance coverage for a small group. Use the Internet to research companies and choose three or four from which to obtain quotes.

2. Design a document that provides information on what should be placed in each box of the health insurance claim form. Place the document in a report cover with sheet protectors and turn it in for a special project grade.

3. Obtain encounter forms from several different physicians' offices. Use them to create mock patients, listing a diagnosis and several procedures. Complete an insurance claim form for each patient and encounter form. As an option, work in groups and present the patient to the class.

INTERNET ACTIVITIES

1. Research the various individual policies available. Obtain a quote for healthcare coverage from one company. Share the information with the class and compare the cost of individual policies with those of group policies. Discuss the differences.

2. Investigate medical savings accounts and determine how these accounts work, as well as how benefits for healthcare expenses are paid.

3. Conduct a survey of 25 physicians and ask them what insurance plans they see in the office most frequently. Research these companies on the Internet and determine their benefits and costs. Prepare a report that compares the five most frequently mentioned companies.

21 The Health Insurance Claim Form

VOCABULARY REVIEW

Fill in the blanks with the correct term from this chapter.

1. _____ is the transfer of the patient's legal right to collect benefits for medical expenses to the provider of those services, authorizing the payment to be sent directly to the provider.

2. The process of examining claims for accuracy and completeness before submitting the claims is called a(n) _____, which can be performed manually or electronically with computer billing software.

3. Often referred to when tracking medical services used by patients or researching claims, a(n) _____ _____ is the path left by a transaction when it has been completed.

4. _____ _____ are insurance claim forms that have been completed correctly and that can be processed and paid promptly if they meet the restrictions on covered services and blocks.

5. A centralized facility to which insurance claims are transmitted, a(n) _____ separates, checks, and redistributes claims electronically to various insurance carriers.

6. A method of electronic claims submission in which computer software allows a provider to submit an insurance claim directly to an insurance carrier for payment is called _____ _____.

7. _____ claims are claims that contain errors or omissions that must be corrected so that the claims can be resubmitted to an insurance carrier to obtain reimbursement.

8. _____ claims are claims that are submitted to insurance processing facilities using a computerized medium, such as direct data entry, direct wire, dial-in telephone digital fax, or personal computer download or upload.

9. The transfer of data back and forth between two or more entities using an electronic medium is called _____, or _____.

10. A(n) _____ _____ is a mark that is accepted as proof of approval of and/or responsibility for the content of an electronic document.

11. The number used by the Internal Revenue Service to identify a business or an individual functioning as a business entity for income tax reporting is known as a(n) _____ _____ number, or _____.

12. A claim that is missing information and is returned to the provider for correction and resubmission is called a(n) _____ _____ or sometimes an *invalid claim*.

13. _____ or _____ is the electronic scanning of printed blocks as images and the use of special software to recognize these images as ASCII text for uploading into a computer database.

14. The term for the acronym NPI is _____.

15. The term for the acronym PIN is _____.

16. The term for the acronym UPIN is _____.

17. Hard copies of insurance claims that have been completed and sent by surface mail are known as _____ _____.

18. Any company, individual, or group that provides medical, diagnostic, or treatment services to a patient is considered a(n) _____.

19. A number assigned to a provider by a carrier for use in the submission of claims is called a(n) _____ or _____.

20. _____ claims are claims that have been returned unpaid to the provider for clarification of questions and that must be corrected before resubmission.

21. The number assigned by fiscal intermediaries to identify providers on claims for services is the _____ or _____.

22. The universal claim form was developed by the Health Care Financing Administration (HCFA) (now known as the Centers for Medicare and Medicaid Services [CMS]) and approved by the American Medical Association (AMA) for use in submitting all government-sponsored claims. It now is also known as the _____.

23. A medical assistant may submit insurance claims to a third-party payer or an insurance carrier in one of two ways: _____ or _____.

24. Name two advantages of using hard copy (paper) claims.
    _____
    _____

25. Name two disadvantages of using hard copy (paper) claims.
    _____
    _____

26. List two benefits of the ICR scanning system.
    _____
    _____

27. A number of rules must be followed when completing the paper CMS-1500 form so that the insurance carrier can scan the claim. Give 10 examples of when a blank space should be used when completing a paper CMS-1500.
    a. _____
    b. _____
    c. _____
    d. _____
    e. _____
    f. _____
    g. _____
    h. _____
    i. _____
    j. _____

28. Now list the other six rules for completing the paper CMS-1500 form so that the insurance carrier can scan the claim.

    a. _____

    b. _____

    c. _____

    d. _____

    e. _____

    f. _____

29. The transaction and code set for the CMS-1500 electronic claims submission is called the _____.

30. Implementation Guides for each of the transaction and code sets requirements for electronic data submission can be obtained through the Center for Medicare and Medicaid Services (CMS). The data that can be submitted electronically include (list three):

    a. _____

    b. _____

    c. _____

31. List two ways electronic claims can be submitted.

    _____

    _____

32. Clearinghouses typically also provide additional services; list three of them.

    a. _____

    b. _____

    c. _____

33. Give one major advantage of electronic submission of insurance claims.

    _____

34. The first section of the patient registration form includes the patient information; list four items that are recorded in this section.

    a. _____

    b. _____

    c. _____

    d. _____

35. The patient registration form should be completed by the patient or the patient's guardian. The medical assistant should confirm the information by doing two things:

    a. _____

    b. _____

QUESTIONS 36-51:
Detail the 16 steps for gathering patient information and the other information required to complete an insurance claim form.

36. _____

37. _____

38. _____

39. _____

40. _____

41. _____

42. _____

43. _____

44. _____

45. _____

46. _____

47. _____

48. _____

49. _____

50. _____

51. _____

52. Once the patient's and the insured's demographic and insurance information has been collected, the next step is to verify the patient's eligibility and benefits. By what method or methods is this usually done?

_____

_____

_____

_____

53. If any diagnostic or therapeutic services or procedures are to be rendered by the provider that require preapproval, a(n) _____ must be done to obtain an authorization number.

54. A CMS-1500 claim form has _____ blocks, or items. The blocks are divided into _____ sections.

55. List the information contained in each section of a CMS-1500 claim form.

    Section 1 _____

    Section 2 _____

    Section 3 _____

56. The type of insurance the patient has is indicated in block _____.

57. Block 1a is used for what vital piece of information?

    _____

58. Block 2 should contain the patient's name. This is the person receiving treatment or supplies. In what order should the patient's name be entered? _____.

    a. First, middle initial, last

    b. Middle initial, last, first

    c. Last, first, middle initial

59. Block 3 contains what two pieces of information?

    _____

    _____

60. Block 4 contains _____; this is the person who owns the policy.

61. The patient's (permanent) address and phone numbered are entered in which block? _____.

    a. Block 5

    b. Block 5a

    c. Block 5b

62. Block 6 is Patient Relationship to Insured; explain what the following titles mean in this block.

    a. Self _____

    b. Spouse _____

    c. Child _____

    d. Other _____

63. The insured's address and telephone number are entered in block 7. How does the information in this block differ from that in block 5?

 _____

 _____

64. Block 8 is Patient's Status; to what specifically does this refer and why is this information important?

 _____

 _____

65. In Section 3, the Patient/Insured Section, which blocks are completed for the primary insurance and which blocks are completed only if a secondary insurance claim is being submitted?

 Primary insurance _____

 Secondary insurance _____

66. Block 12 contains which signature? _____

 a. Insured's or authorized person's signature

 b. Patient's or authorized person's signature

67. Block 13 contains which signature? _____

 a. Insured's or authorized person's signature

 b. Patient's or authorized person's signature

68. The name of the referring provider, ordering provider, or other source that referred or ordered the service or procedure on the claim is entered in block 17. Explain the difference between a referring physician and an ordering physician.

 _____

 _____

 _____

 _____

69. Block 21 contains an important piece of information; what is it?

 _____

 _____

70. When entering the appropriate diagnosis or ICD-9-CM code or codes, what is the maximum number of codes that should be used on one claim form?

 _____

71. What number is placed in block 26, and who assigns this number?

 _____

72. What information is provided in block 28? _____.

 a. Balance due

 b. Total charge

 c. Amount paid

73. What information is provided in block 29? _____.

   a. Amount paid
   b. Balance due
   c. Total charge

74. What information is provided in block 30? _____.

   a. Total charge
   b. Balance due
   c. Amount paid

75. Many guidelines for reviewing a claim must be followed prior to submission of the claim. List 10 of those guidelines.

   a. _____
   b. _____
   c. _____
   d. _____
   e. _____
   f. _____
   g. _____
   h. _____
   i. _____
   j. _____

76. The two main reasons for denial of payment are:

   _____
   _____

77. A clean claim is defined as _____
   _____.

78. A dirty (or dingy) claim is defined as _____
   _____.

79. A rejected claim is defined as _____
   _____.

SKILLS AND CONCEPTS

Part I: Completing Insurance Claim Forms

Complete a claim form using the patient information in each of the following scenarios. Use the claim forms in Work Products 21-1 through 21-5.

1. Complete Claim Form 1 (Work Product 21-1) using the following information.

Today's date: 9-29-20XX

Mr. Jackson, an established patient, has suffered from situational depression since his wife of 47 years died last winter. He has a history of congestive heart failure and intermittent high blood pressure. He comes to the office on July 23, 20XX, for treatment of his depression. Dr. Swakoski sees Mr. Jackson and counsels him about medication for his condition. He is with the patient for about 25 minutes. He gives Mr. Jackson a week's worth of samples of Cymbalta and writes a prescription for the drug that is refillable for 3 months. The charge for the office visit is $85. File this claim with BC/BS.

Donald W. Jackson (patient and insured)
77834 High Road Way
Los Angeles, CA 90010
818-665-0098 (home)
SS# 567-99-0067

Insurance: BC/BS and Medicare
ID# 567990067
Employer: Retired
DOB: 3-8-1940

Diagnosis: Depression, CHF, HTN
Procedures: Office visit
Account Number: JAD0067

Family Health Center
120 E. Northwest Highway
Los Angeles, CA 90010
818-624-0112
Federal Tax ID# 75-6102034

BC/BS
11001 Spring Way, Suite 200
Sacramento, CA 90012
800-443-0033

Theodore Swakoski, MD
NPI# 6170421616
BS Provider# 621604211

2. Complete Claim Form 2 (Work Product 21-2) using the following information.

Today's date: 9-29-20XX

Mr. Adams, an established, married patient, comes to the office because of an episode of bronchitis. He states that he has felt poorly for about 1 week and that he now is having trouble getting a full breath of air. He has had moderate pain on coughing and admits that the cough has kept him awake or has awakened him. He says he has bronchitis about once a year in the fall. Dr. Abbott sees Mr. Adams for about 15 minutes in the office. She prescribes an antibiotic, a cough syrup, and Hycodan. Dr. Abbott knows that Mr. Adams is also diabetic, so she draws blood for a glucose test to make sure the levels are normal. She suggests that Mr. Adams stay home from work for the 2 days leading into the weekend and return to work on Monday. Dr. Abbott asks whether Mr. Adams is still having trouble sleeping, as reported on his last office visit. He admits that he is still suffering from insomnia even apart from the bronchitis. Mr. Adams also admits that his marriage is failing, and he says that the stress may be contributing to the insomnia. Dr. Abbott gives him a prescription for Ambien CR along with the other prescriptions. Mr. Adams is to return to the clinic in 1 week if he is not feeling better. The charge for the office visit is $77, and the blood sugar test is $12. Mr. Adams pays his $20 co-pay.

Benjamin C. Adams
55180 Grand Avenue Parkway
Austin, Texas 78706
512-998-1354 (home)
SS# 445-74-8363

Insurance: Humana PPO
ID# 445748363
Employer: Texas Department of Public Safety
DOB: 7-2-1954

Diagnosis: Acute bronchitis; diabetes mellitus type II, controlled; insomnia
Procedures: Office visit, blood glucose test
Account Number: ADB8363

Family Medical Clinic
1216 E. Lamar Blvd.
Austin, Texas 78704
512-624-0112
Federal Tax ID# 75-8210612

Humana
PO Box 3031103
Chicago, IL 60068
800-611-1216

Barbara Abbott, MD
NPI 4712678920

3. Complete Claim Form 3 (Work Product 21-3) using the following information.

Today's date: 9-29-20XX

Ms. Snell comes to the office complaining of severe pain in the lower left quadrant. She states that the pain came on suddenly and that she has a history of ovarian cysts. Ms. Snell is clearly in severe pain, so Dr. Jackman gives her an injection of Toradol. Once the medication has taken effect, he performs a pelvic examination and determines that the most likely cause of her pain is a ruptured ovarian cyst. Dr. Jackman sends Ms. Snell to the hospital for an ultrasound examination and will see her in the emergency department later in the afternoon. Ms. Snell has no other significant health problems. Her office visit is $85, and the injection is $25. Dr. Jackman spent about 40 minutes with her.

Suanne L. Snell
4545 Rustic
Los Angeles, CA 90002
818-445-9970 (home)
SS# 665-76-5568

Insurance: Aetna HMO
ID# 665765568
Employer: Marriott Hotels International
DOB: 9-3-1964

Diagnosis: Ruptured ovarian cyst
Procedures: Office visit, injection
Account Number: SNS5568

Medical Surgical Clinic
4800 S. Broadway Blvd.
Los Angeles, CA 90012
818-261-1122
Federal Tax ID# 75-6120662

Aetna
PO Box 310661
Sacramento, CA 90121
800-996-8445

James Jackman, DO
NPI 8216740292

4. Complete Claim Form 4 (Work Product 21-4) using the information below.

Today's date: 9-29-20XX

Ms. Huntington, a single female, arrives at the clinic today as a new patient. She was referred to Dr. Tyler by Dr. William R. Curry, a friend of Dr. Tyler from medical school. Ms. Huntington has been diagnosed with systemic lupus erythematosus and periodically experiences a great deal of pain. She arranged to forward her medical records to Dr. Tyler several weeks ago, and she made today's appointment before her move to New Rochelle. Dr. Tyler has worked with numerous patients who have lupus and is understanding about their needs and the challenges they face in living a normal life. Ms. Huntington states that she needs to refill her medications, and Dr. Tyler reviews them with her, agreeing to refill her prescription Motrin (800 mg), Lortab (10 mg), and Phenergan suppositories (50 mg). Ms. Huntington says that she uses the Motrin almost every day but rarely uses the Lortab, although she prefers to keep a supply on hand for times when the disease strikes aggressively. She mentions that she has not had a well-woman examination in 2 years because of the sale of her home and the purchase of a new one in New Rochelle. Dr. Tyler performs the well-woman examination and writes Ms. Huntington an order for a mammogram. She also performs a breast examination, which is included in the well-woman examination. Dr. Tyler spends about 45 minutes with the patient. She asks Ms. Huntington to return in 3 months if she does not feel the need to do so before then. Ms. Huntington is charged $179 for the new patient office visit and $55 for the Pap smear and well-woman examination. She leaves with her prescriptions.

Celeste C. Huntington
554 Georgetown Way
New Rochelle, NY 10801
914-889-6675 (home)
SS# 433-99-2364

Insurance: United Health Care PPO
ID# 433992364
Employer: Loist and Earnest Law Firm
DOB: 9-3-1960

Diagnosis: Systemic lupus erythematosus
Procedures: Office visit, Pap smear
Account Number: HUC2364

New Rochelle Family Medicine
2002 Front Street, Suite 600
New Rochelle, NY 10800
914-661-0001
Federal Tax ID# 75-6234710

United Healthcare
PO Box 292928
New York, NY 10021
212-660-1100

Rene Tyler, MD
NPI 6779354390
William R. Curry, MD
NPI 4619907217

5. Complete Claim Form 5 (Work Product 21-5) using the following information.

Today's date: 9-29-20XX

Mrs. Saxton, a married female, has several health problems and is a frequent visitor to Dr. Handley's office. She is insured through her own policy with Unicare and also through her husband's policy with Assurant Health. She has Graves' disease, malignant HTN, bursitis of the right knee, and carpel tunnel syndrome. She arrives at the office today to have her blood pressure checked. In the waiting area, she develops mild chest pains, so the medical assistant brings her to the back office immediately and performs an ECG. Upon checking the strip, Dr. Handley believes that Mrs. Saxton may recently have had a mild heart attack, so he refers her to Dr. Stern, a cardiologist. The office sets up an immediate appointment for Mrs. Saxton, and she leaves the clinic with her husband with instructions to drive directly to Dr. Stern's office. They promise to do so. Mrs. Saxton is charged for the office visit ($165) and an ECG ($45). She is with Dr. Handley for approximately 50 minutes.

Patricia N. Saxton
13104 Highway 798 South
Tyler, TX 75701
903-882-4453 (home)
SS# 334-88-9907

Insurance: Unicare PPO
ID# 334889907
Employer: Self-employed
Husband: Levern R. Saxton
Employer: Kelly Tires
SS# 621-12-6701
ID# 621126701
DOB: 7-8-1953

Diagnosis: Malignant HTN, Graves' disease, bursitis, carpel tunnel syndrome
Procedures: Office visit, ECG
Account Number: SAP9907

South Tyler Health Clinic
120 E. West Street
Tyler, Texas 75703
903-566-1112
Federal Tax ID# 75-2162704

Unicare
12000 Walker Blvd., St. 100
Dallas, Texas 75225
800-921-0091

Wendle Handley, DO
NPI 5682103541

Assurant Health
PO Box 704
Dallas, Texas 75229
800-621-1000

Part II: Determining Diagnosis and Procedure Codes

Determine the proper diagnosis and procedure codes.

1. Diagnosis: Lou Gehrig's disease; hydrocodone dependence

    Diagnostic code(s) _____

    Procedure: Office visit, new patient (10 minutes)

    Procedure code(s) _____

2. Diagnosis: Generalized osteoarthritis in the upper arm

    Diagnostic code(s) _____

    Procedure: Office visit, established patient (10 minutes); basic metabolic panel; lipid panel

    Procedure code(s) _____

3. Diagnosis: Foreign body in the ear

    Diagnostic code(s) _____

    Procedure: Office visit, established patient (10 minutes)

    Procedure code(s) _____

4. Diagnosis: Burn over 40% of body surface because of car accident with another vehicle; passenger in the car

    Diagnostic code(s) _____

    Procedure: Hospital admission, new patient, physician spends approximately 50 minutes treating patient

    Procedure code(s) _____

5. Diagnosis: Rosacea

    Diagnostic code(s) _____

    Procedure: Office visit, established patient (15 minutes)

    Procedure code(s) _____

6. Diagnosis: Sunburn, third degree

    Diagnostic code(s) _____

    Procedure: Office visit, established patient (10 minutes)

    Procedure code(s) _____

7. Diagnosis: Tachycardia, neonatal

    Diagnostic code(s) _____

    Procedure: Hospital visit, 2 days, inpatient subsequent care (25 minutes)

    Procedure code(s) _____

8. Diagnosis: Pernicious anemia

    Diagnostic code(s) _____

    Procedure: Office visit, established patient (25 minutes); sedimentation rate, automated; CBC, automated

    Procedure code(s) _____

9. Diagnosis: Attention deficit disorder with hyperactivity; acute cystitis

   Diagnostic code(s) _____

   Procedure: Office visit, established patient (15 minutes); urinalysis

   Procedure code(s) _____

10. Diagnosis: Mastitis after delivery of a baby

    Diagnostic code(s) _____

    Procedure: Office visit, established patient (5 minutes)

    Procedure code(s) _____

CASE STUDY

Research the history of the CMS-1500 claim form. Determine when it was first used and the changes the form has undergone since its inception. Prepare a report that details these changes, including the most recent modifications to the CMS-1500 (08/05). Present the report to the class.

WORKPLACE APPLICATIONS

Collect several blank encounter forms from various medical specialties. Distribute the forms to classmates, sharing and trading the various forms. Mark several procedures on the forms and at least two diagnoses codes. Prepare a CMS-1500 claim based on information on the encounter forms. Share the information in class and explain the coding choices made on each claim.

INTERNET ACTIVITIES

1. Review the National Uniform Claim Committee Web site. Find the User Manual for the CMS-1500 claim form (08/05).

2. Find three companies that sell the CMS-1500 claim form. Compare costs and determine the least expensive place to order the form.

3. Research software applications available for completing CMS-1500 forms. Determine which of the applications would be good investments for a physician's office.

22 Professional Fees, Billing, and Collecting

VOCABULARY REVIEW

Fill in the blanks with the correct vocabulary terms from this chapter.

1. Jesse has a(n) _____ _____ of $464, which represents the total amount she owes after her insurance paid a portion of her bill.

2. Mrs. Ramone has a(n) _____ on her account for an overpayment, so the office manager sent her a check for that amount.

3. Robert's mother is the _____ of his bill, because she promised to pay the full amount for her son.

4. Julia had to _____ collections proceedings on several accounts last month, because the patients had not made payments as promised.

5. One of the tasks Pamela enjoys is _____ payments that arrive in the mail to patient accounts.

6. _____ _____ are used more and more often for payments in the physician's office.

7. An organization under contract to the government to handle insurance claims from providers is called a(n) _____ _____.

8. Mrs. Richland called the office to get the balance on her _____.

9. The office staff has been debating whether they should continue to offer _____ _____ to other healthcare providers and their staff members.

10. A business _____, which is any exchange or transfer of goods, services, or funds, must always be recorded.

11. Anna made several _____ for various bills that were due last week.

12. Dr. Taylor's fee _____ is a compilation of the fees he has charged over the past fiscal year.

13. The Peete family was considered _____ _____, because they could not afford medical care even though they were able to pay basic living expenses.

14. Deb sometimes confuses a credit with a(n) _____, which is a deduction from a revenue, net worth, or liability account.

15. Jessica totaled the _____ for the day, which came from patient and insurance payments.

16. State Farm is considered a(n) _____ _____ _____, because Bethany's injuries were sustained in a car accident and State Farm will pay her medical bills.

17. Dr. Martin reviewed his fee _____, which is a compilation of pre-established fee allowances for given services or procedures.

18. The balances due to a creditor on an account are called _____.

19. The Blackburn Clinic uses a computer to determine patient account balances, but June remembers when they used a manual _____ _____.

20. When Madelyn received the denial from Mr. Paul's insurance company, she wondered if he had paid his _____.

SKILLS AND CONCEPTS

Part I: Fee Schedules and Billing Forms

1. Examine the fee schedule on the next page and answer the following questions.

   a. What is the charge for a consultation? _____

   b. What is the charge for a 99203? _____

   c. Why is the charge different for a 99213? _____

   d. What is the most expensive procedure on the list? CPT code _____

   e. Which injection is more expensive, insulin or vitamin B_{12}? _____

Use the same fee schedule to complete the billing forms in Work Products 22-1, 22-2, and 22-3 (See pp. 203-208 of the Procedures Checklists). Circle the codes and fill in the charges for each patient. Assume that all the patients have a previous balance of zero.

2. Work Product 22-1: Marilyn Westmoreland, established patient, straightforward, penicillin injections (75 mg), diagnosis—acute tonsillitis.

3. Work Product 22-2: Jane Wells, consultation, high complexity, ECG, diagnosis—chest pain.

4. Work Product 22-3: Paula Johnson, new patient, detailed, Solu-Medrol injection IM, diagnosis—osteoarthritis.

FEE SCHEDULE

BLACKBURN PRIMARY CARE ASSOCIATES, PC
1990 Turquiose Drive
Blackburn, WI 54937
608-459-8857

Federal Tax ID Number:	00-0000000	**BCBS Group Number:**	14982
		Medicare Group Number:	14982

OFFICE VISIT, NEW PATIENT

Focused, 99201	$45.00
Expanded, 99202	$55.00
Intermediate, 99203	$60.00
Extended, 99204	$95.00
Comprehensive, 99205	$195.00
Consultation, 99245	$250.00

OFFICE VISIT, ESTABLISHED PATIENT

Minimal, 99211	$40.00
Focused, 99212	$48.00
Intermediate, 99213	$55.00
Extended, 99214	$65.00
Comprehensive, 99215	$195.00

OFFICE PROCEDURES

EKG, 12 lead, 93000	$55.00
Stress EKG, Treadmill, 93015	$295.00
Sigmoidoscopy, Flex; 45330	$145.00
Spirometry, 94010	$50.00
Cerumen Removal, 69210	$40.00
Collection & Handling	
Lab Specimen, 99000	$9.00
Venipuncture, 35415	$9.00
Urinalysis, 81000	$20.00
Urinalysis, 81002 (Dip Only)	$12.00
Influenza Injection, 90724	$20.00
Pneumococcal Injection, 90732	$20.00
Oral Polio, 90712	$15.00
DTaP, 90700	$20.00
Tetanus Toxoid, 90703	$15.00
MMR, 90707	$25.00
HIB, 90737	$20.00
Hepatitis B, newborn to age 11 years, 90744	$60.00
Hepatitis B, 11-19 years, 90745	$60.00
Hepatitis B, 20 years and above 90746	$60.00
Intramuscular Injection, 90788	
Penicillin	$30.00
Cephtriaxone	$25.00
Solu-Medrol	$23.00
Vitamin B-12	$13.00
Subcutaneous Injection, 90782	
Epinephrine	$18.00
Susphrine	$25.00
Insulin, U-100	$15.00

COMMON DIAGNOSTIC CODES

Ischemic Heart Disease	414.9
w/o myocardial infarction	411.89
w/coronary occlusion	411.81
Hypertension, Malignant	401.0
Benign	401.1
Unspecified	401.9
w/congest. heart failure	402.91
Asthma, Bronchial	493.9
w/COPD	493.2
allergic, w/S.A.	493.91
allergic, w/o S.A.	493.90
Kyphosis	737.10
w/osteoporosis	733.0
Osteoporosis	733.00
Otitis Media, Acute	382.9
Chronic	382.9

Part II: Ledgers and Computing Patient Balances

Work through the following information and record it on the ledger cards presented in the corresponding work product pages. Use one ledger for each exercise.

Ledger 1—Work Product 22-4 (see p. 209 of the Procedures Checklists)

Meagan Joy Reynolds
5534 Joe Pool Lake Road #233
Cedar Hill, Texas 75884
972-334-0423 (home)
972-331-0934 (cell)
meaganjoy@internet4.com
MR# REYM3341

Entry #	Transaction
1	Meagan comes to the Blackburn Primary Care Clinic on April 12 as a new patient. Her initial charge is $375, because she had a series of x-ray examinations, which were used to diagnose a blockage in her small intestine. Dr. Lupez recommends that she have surgery to correct the blockage as soon as possible. Meagan pays her bill in full with check #7110, although she has insurance coverage through her own policy with Prudential and her husband's policy through Southwest United Healthcare.
2	Meagan checks into Mercy Hospital and has surgery on April 21. Dr. Lupez charges $7,500 for the surgery. This charge will be filed with Meagan's insurances.
3	Meagan returns to the clinic on April 30 for a follow-up office visit. The charge is $150, which she pays in full with check #7261. Dr. Lupez says that she is doing very well since her surgery and asks her to return in mid-May for another checkup.
4	On May 2 the clinic receives an insurance payment from Prudential in the amount of $6,200. This money is applied to Meagan's account. The check number is 617761.
5	On May 3 the clinic receives check #7313 in the mail from Meagan for $300, which is applied to her account.
6	Meagan returns to the clinic on May 14 for an office visit. The charge is $75, and she pays $50 with check #7512.
7	Southwest United sends a check to the clinic for $800 on May 27, which is applied to her account. The check number is 8710.
8	Meagan sends a check for $125 to be put toward her account. The check, #7915, is posted on June 2.
9	Meagan returns to the clinic for an office visit and laboratory work on June 17. Her charges total $352, and she pays $150 with check #8116.
10	On June 20 the clinic receives Meagan's check toward her account for $100. Her check number is 8411.
11	Meagan visits the clinic for treatment of a migraine headache on June 26. Her charge is $85, and she pays $50 with check #8626. She schedules a follow-up visit with Dr. Lupez for June 30.
12	When Meagan returns for her follow-up visit on June 30, her office visit is $85, but she is unable to make a payment.
13	On July 5 the clinic receives a payment from Prudential on behalf of Meagan for $276. The Prudential check number is 721146.
14	On July 18 the clinic receives a check #9210 from Southwest United on behalf of Meagan for $124.
15	On July 31 the clinic refunds Meagan's credit balance to her using clinic check #9425.
16	The previous transaction brings Meagan's account to zero.

How much was the refund check? _____

Ledger 2—Work Product 22-5 (see p. 211 of the Procedures Checklists)

Zachary Paul Staley
2324 Hill Avenue Plaza
Grosse Pointe, MI 48230
313-445-9987 (home)
313-565-6623 (cell)
zachattack@aol.com
MR# STAZ9823

Entry #	Transaction
1	Zachary Staley visited the clinic on June 6 as a new patient and was diagnosed with diabetes. His charge was $215. He paid his $15 co-pay with check #126.
2	On June 12 a check arrived from Permian Health for $180 on Zachary's account. The check number was 21617.
3	Zachary returned to the clinic on June 15 for an office visit and laboratory work. The total charge was $128, and Zachary paid his $15 co-pay with check #214.
4	On June 16 Zachary returned to the clinic without an appointment, because he felt extremely dizzy and nauseated. He was seen by Dr. Hughes, who determined that his blood sugar had dropped substantially. After his condition was stabilized, his wife picked him up and took him home. She paid his $15 co-pay with check #217. The total charge for the visit was $70.
5	On July 7 check #36171 arrived from Permian Health on Zachary's account in the amount of $142.
6	Bethany, an insurance biller, realized that a $7 charge was not allowed for a laboratory test on Zachary's account. The office policy allows disallowed charges under $10 to be written off, so Bethany adjusts his account by $7 on July 7.
7	Zachary returns to the clinic for a routine visit on July 26 and has laboratory work done. The total charge is $156, and Zachary pays his $15 co-pay with check #310.
8	On August 1 Zachary has a brief office visit and is charged $70. Zachary forgot his checkbook, so he did not pay his co-pay.
9	On August 16 Permian sends check #41217 in the amount of $102 toward Zachary's account.
10	On August 21 Permian sends check #42168 in the amount of $55 toward Zachary's account.
11	On August 30 the clinic receives check #561 from Zachary in the amount of $40 to be placed toward his account.
12	September 6 is Zachary's next office visit, and he is charged $70. He pays his $15 co-pay with check #587.
13	Zachary sends $40 toward his account, which is received by the clinic on September 9. His check number is 620.
14	Permian Health sends check #53121 in the amount of $98 to the clinic to be applied to Zachary's account on September 15.
15	On October 3 the clinic receives check #681 from Zachary, who remembers that he did not pay his co-pay on August 1. He guesses that he owes about $40 total but is unsure, so he sends $20.
16	The clinic realizes that Zachary has overpaid on his account and sends him a refund for his credit balance using check #6116 on October 4.

How much was the refund check? _____

Ledger 3—Work Product 22-6 (see p. 213 of the Procedures Checklists)

Lynn Annette Wilson
755 South Wheeley #4A
Sacramento, CA 94203
209-552-5437 (home)
209-553-7789 (cell)
lynnannw@yahoo.com
MR# WILL8845

Entry #	Transaction
1	Lynn Annette is a single mother of four who has had a difficult year. She lost a job after contracting infectious mononucleosis and missing 3 weeks of work. She had barely recovered from that illness when she was diagnosed with ulcerative colitis. Her medical bills have become increasingly difficult to pay, although she did find a new job and recently became eligible for coverage through Aetna. She is a determined woman with the best of intentions but often must put rent, utilities, and food costs before the payment of her medical bills. She comes to the clinic for a regular office visit on July 7. Her charges are $125, and she is able to pay the entire bill, since she has been saving the money for several weeks. She pays with check #1205.
2	On July 12 Lynn Annette returns to the office and has laboratory work. Her charges are $89, and she pays her $20 co-pay with check #1314.
3	Bethany in the insurance office notices that Lynn Annette was charged $9 for a single laboratory chemistry test that is not covered by her insurance. Because Bethany knows that Lynn Annette has faced financial difficulties this year, she adjusts the bill so that Lynn Annette will not be responsible for the charge. She also makes a note for the physicians that Lynn Annette's insurance does not cover that particular laboratory test and explains that an alternate chemistry test that will produce the same results is covered. The adjustment is made on July 19.
4	Aetna sends an insurance payment (check #7611493) toward Lynn Annette's account that is received on July 23. The payment is for $85.
5	Bethany processes a refund for Lynn Annette and sends her check #5612 from the clinic account on July 24. This brings her balance to zero.
6	Lynn Annette comes to the office for a regular visit on August 1. Her charges are $284, and she pays her co-pay of $20 with check #1517.
7	On August 18 the clinic receives a check from Aetna for $200 toward Lynn Annette's account. The check number is 8267484.
8	Lynn Annette sends check #1622 in the amount of $64 to clear her account on August 31.
9	On September 12 Lynn Annette's recent check payment is returned by her bank for insufficient funds. The clinic adds a charge of $30 to her account as a returned check fee.
10	Lynn Annette comes to the clinic and apologizes for her recent returned check. She explains that she missed getting her paycheck into the bank in time to cover the payment. She brings a cashier's check to cover the check and the fee. The date is September 20.
11	Lynn Annette has minor surgery in the office on October 15. The charge is $750, and she pays a co-pay of $20 in cash.
12	On February 12 Lynn Annette sends a $20 payment on her account, using check #2612. She encloses a note that says she is still having financial difficulties and will send another payment as soon as she can.
13	On April 10 Lynn Annette sends a payment of $5 using check #2711.
14	On May 12 the clinic receives a payment from Lynn Annette in the amount of $5, using check #2781.
15	In accordance with the clinic policy of reporting accounts to a collection agency after 3 months of nonpayment, Bethany reluctantly reports Lynn Annette's account to Smith Collections. The full balance is written off.
16	On September 12 a payment of $100 is received from Lynn Annette. Bethany forwards the payment to the collection agency.

How much was written off of this account? _____

How is the payment noted on the account that was received after the write-off? _____

Chapter 22 Professional Fees, Billing, and Collecting

Completing a Day Sheet

Complete the proofs in Work Product 22-7 (see p. 215 of the Procedures Checklists) using the figures given.

Part III: Short Answers

1. Define the following terms.

   a. Usual

   b. Customary

   c. Reasonable

2. List two billing methods commonly used in the physician's office.

   a.

   b.

3. What notation should be made under the return address on statement envelopes?

4. Briefly explain cycle billing.

5. What are the pitfalls of fee adjustments?

6. What three values are considered in determining professional fees?

   a.

   b.

   c.

7. Why are estimates useful in patient treatment?

8. List five general rules for telephone collecting.

   a.

   b.

   c.

   d.

   e.

9. List four ways payment for medical services is accomplished.

   a. _____

   b. _____

   c. _____

   d. _____

10. Explain why patients sometimes fail to pay their accounts.

    _____

    _____

    _____

11. What is professional courtesy, and why is it less common now than in years past?

    _____

    _____

    _____

12. Briefly explain how "skips" can be traced.

    _____

    _____

    _____

CASE STUDY

Read back through the information about Lynn Annette Wilson in Ledger 3. How could the medical assistant help Ms. Wilson keep her account out of collections? What could be said to her during a friendly phone call to encourage her to be regular with her payments? Write two collection letters to Ms. Wilson. Make the first letter a gentle reminder. The second letter should express that the account will be placed for collection if regular payments are not forthcoming. Use the stationery provided in Work Products 22-8 and 22-9 (See pp. 217-220 of the Procedures Checklists) to write the collection letters.

WORKPLACE APPLICATIONS

Mr. Sanchez comes to the desk to check out after seeing the physician. When Sarah tells him that his bill is $95, he complains that he only saw the physician for 10 minutes. The fee is in accordance with the evaluation and management guidelines. Explain the fees to Mr. Sanchez. Write what you would say to him as an explanation of his fees.

_____

_____

_____

_____

_____

Write a dialog that could be used to ask a patient for payment as the person is checking out.

_____
_____
_____
_____
_____
_____
_____

INTERNET ACTIVITIES

1. Research medical billing companies on the Internet and compare the costs of the various services they offer. Prepare a report or presentation for the class.

2. Search for patient accounting software and explore the options available for the physician's office. Write a brief report on one software product and present it to the class.

23 Banking Services and Procedures

VOCABULARY REVIEW

Fill in the blanks with the correct vocabulary terms from this chapter.

1. Judy was unaware that checks were processed through _____ before they arrived at her bank.

2. Because Alicia was the person who wrote the check, she was considered the _____.

3. When the Blackburn Clinic purchased the ultrasound machine, they paid $10,000 toward the _____ so that they would be charged less interest.

4. Pamela wrote a check to Samantha, so Pamela is the _____ and Samantha is the _____.

5. The _____ of a check is the person who presents it for payment and may not be the person named as the payee.

6. Grace studied the _____ _____ _____, which is a series of laws that regulates sales of goods, commercial paper, secured transactions in personal property, and many aspects of banking.

7. First National Bank is considered the _____ for Dr. Lupez' business checking accounts.

8. Instruments that are legally transferable to another party are considered _____.

9. Rhonda made several _____ from the clinic checking account to pay monthly bills and order supplies.

10. As soon as the monthly bank statement arrives, Rhonda does a(n) _____ _____ to make sure the statement and checkbook balance are in agreement.

SKILLS AND CONCEPTS

Part I: Short Answers

1. List the requirements of a negotiable instrument.

   a. _____

   b. _____

   c. _____

   d. _____

2. Name several advantages to online banking.

   _____

   _____

   _____

3. Why is customer service such an important aspect of today's medical offices?

4. List four types of checks.
   a.
   b.
   c.
   d.

5. Describe each type of endorsement.
   a. Blank

   b. Restrictive

   c. Special

   d. Qualified

6. List five reasons checks should be deposited promptly.
   a.
   b.
   c.
   d.
   e.

7. Provide five guidelines for check acceptance.
   a.
   b.
   c.
   d.
   e.

8. List three reasons an individual might stop payment on a check.

    a. _____

    b. _____

    c. _____

9. Explain the ABA number and what each part of the number means.

    _____

    _____

    _____

10. List the three basic steps for preparing a deposit slip.

    a. _____

    b. _____

    c. _____

11. Where is the routing number found on a check?

    _____

Part II: Writing Checks for Disbursement of Funds

Write checks to pay the following bills. The beginning balance in the checkbook is $4,562.79. Use the checks numbered 5648 to 5651. Determine the balance after the check is written.

1. Write check #5648 to the American Medical Association for $356 for new coding books. Balance _____

2. Write check #5649 to the Blackburn Utility Company for $46.90 to pay the water bill. Balance _____

3. Write a check for the office mortgage payment to First National Bank in the amount of $1,700. Use check #5650. Balance _____

4. Write check #5651 to pay a bill to United Drug and Supply of $98.34. Balance _____

5. A deposit of $1,358 was made. Balance _____

Part III: Writing Refund Checks

Write checks for the following refunds. Use the ending balance from Part II, question 5, to determine the final balance in the checking account. Use the checks numbered 5652 to 5655.

1. Ms. Patty Bailey should receive a refund in the amount of $34.55 for an overpayment. Use check #5652. Balance _____

2. Write a check for Julie Smithy for $224.12. Her insurance company paid more than expected, so she is entitled to a refund. Use check #5653. Balance _____

3. Cindy Chan paid $10 more than she owed when she was seeing Dr. Hughes. Refund her money using check #5654. The office manager deposited $7,246.12 in checks. Balance _____

4. Carter Graves decided to postpone his knee surgery when his wife suddenly became ill. Use check #5655 to refund his $500 deposit. Balance _____

Part IV: Preparing a Bank Deposit

Prepare a bank deposit detail using the following information. Record your answers on the figure in Work Product 23-1.

1. Cash includes six (6) $20 bills; one (1) $100 bill; one (1) $50 bill; two (2) $10 bills; one (1) $5 bill; and one (1) $1 bill. Total cash ~~XXX~~ 296

2. Check payments were #2387 for $67 from Sue Patrick and #460 for $50 from Ronald Rodriguez. Total personal checks 117

3. Credit card payments were $100 and $250. Total credit cards 350

4. An insurance payment for Alejandro Sanchez arrived in the amount of $1,374.32. The payment was from Aetna and the check was #309. Total deposit 1374.32

Part V: Reconciling a Bank Statement

Reconcile the bank statement using the following facts and figures. Use the worksheet on page 171 to show your work. The checkbook balance is $4,616.96. The statement balance is $6,792.79 (this amount includes the deposit of $2,137.32—do not add that amount in again).

1. Three checks are outstanding: check #5648 for $356; check #5649 for $46.90; and check #5650 for $1,770. What is the total for outstanding checks? 2172.90

2. Does the checkbook reconcile with the statement? no

3. What is the ending balance? 4619.85

Chapter 23 Banking Services and Procedures

5652

DATE	
TO	
FOR	

BALANCE BROUGHT FORWARD		
DEPOSITS		
BALANCE		
AMT THIS CK		
BALANCE CARRIED FORWARD		

BLACKBURN PRIMARY CARE ASSOCIATES, PC
1990 Turquoise Drive
Blackburn, WI 54937
608-459-8857

5652
94-72/1224

DATE _____

PAY TO THE ORDER OF Patty Bailey $ 34.55
                                                     DOLLARS

DERBYSHIRE SAVINGS Member FDIC
P.O. BOX 8923
Blackburn, WI 54937

FOR overpymt refund

⑈055003⑈ 446782011⑈ 678800470

5653

DATE	
TO	
FOR	

BALANCE BROUGHT FORWARD		
DEPOSITS		
BALANCE		
AMT THIS CK		
BALANCE CARRIED FORWARD		

BLACKBURN PRIMARY CARE ASSOCIATES, PC
1990 Turquoise Drive
Blackburn, WI 54937
608-459-8857

5653
94-72/1224

DATE _____

PAY TO THE ORDER OF Julie Smithy $ 224.12
                                                     DOLLARS

DERBYSHIRE SAVINGS Member FDIC
P.O. BOX 8923
Blackburn, WI 54937

FOR refund

⑈055003⑈ 446782011⑈ 678800470

5654

DATE	
TO	
FOR	

BALANCE BROUGHT FORWARD		
DEPOSITS		
BALANCE		
AMT THIS CK		
BALANCE CARRIED FORWARD		

BLACKBURN PRIMARY CARE ASSOCIATES, PC
1990 Turquoise Drive
Blackburn, WI 54937
608-459-8857

5654
94-72/1224

DATE _____

PAY TO THE ORDER OF Cindy Chen $ 10.00
                                                     DOLLARS

DERBYSHIRE SAVINGS Member FDIC
P.O. BOX 8923
Blackburn, WI 54937

FOR refund

⑈055003⑈ 446782011⑈ 678800470

5655

DATE	
TO	
FOR	

BALANCE BROUGHT FORWARD		
DEPOSITS		
BALANCE		
AMT THIS CK		
BALANCE CARRIED FORWARD		

BLACKBURN PRIMARY CARE ASSOCIATES, PC
1990 Turquoise Drive
Blackburn, WI 54937
608-459-8857

5655
94-72/1224

DATE _____

PAY TO THE ORDER OF Carter Graves $ 5.00
                                                     DOLLARS

DERBYSHIRE SAVINGS Member FDIC
P.O. BOX 8923
Blackburn, WI 54937

FOR deposit refund

⑈055003⑈ 446782011⑈ 678800470

THIS WORKSHEET IS PROVIDED TO HELP YOU BALANCE YOUR ACCOUNT

1. Go through your register and mark each check, withdrawal, Express ATM transaction, payment, deposit, or other credit listed on this statement. Be sure that your register shows any interest paid into your account, and any service charges, automatic payments, or Express Transfers withdrawn from your account during this statement period.

2. Using the chart below, list any outstanding checks, Express ATM withdrawals, payments, or any other withdrawals (including any from previous months) that are listed in your register but are not shown on this statement.

3. Balance your account by filling in the spaces below.

ITEMS OUTSTANDING		
NUMBER	AMOUNT	
5648	356	00
5649	46	90
5650	1,770	00
TOTAL	$ 2172	90

ENTER

The NEW BALANCE shown on this statement ___6792.79___ $

ADD

Any deposits listed in your register or transfers into your account which are not shown on this statement.
$ ~~~~~
$ ~~~~~
+ $ ~~~~~

TOTAL

CALCULATE THE SUBTOTAL ___6792.79___ $

SUBTRACT

The total outstanding checks and withdrawals from the chart at left ___2172.90___ -$

CALCULATE THE ENDING BALANCE

This amount should be the same as the current balance shown in your check register ___4619.89___ $

CASE STUDY

The Internet has changed the way business is conducted, both in the United States and beyond U. S. borders. Some individuals are quite comfortable making purchases and paying bills online. How safe are these practices? How can the medical assistant know that online bill paying services are safe and secure? Research this information and prepare a report for the class.

WORKPLACE APPLICATIONS

The more versatile the medical assistant is, the more valuable he or she will be to the physician employer. Often new graduates hesitate to ask patients to pay their accounts. However, a medical assistant who is able to collect patient accounts increases the cash flow in the office. How might the medical assistant succinctly explain the various ways a patient can make a payment?

INTERNET ACTIVITIES

1. Explore several types of billing software. Determine which seems to be the best option for a medium-sized family practice clinic. Pay special attention to software that has banking features.

2. Investigate the history of banking and prepare a report for the class.

3. Research safety measures designed to keep confidential banking information private. How do privacy policies affect Internet banking? How can the medical assistant ensure that private information remains private? Prepare a paper or report for the class on this subject.

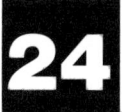

24 Financial and Practice Management

VOCABULARY REVIEW

Fill in the blanks with the correct vocabulary terms from this chapter.

1. Jenna told Andrea that a(n) _____ year is often different from a calendar year.

2. Julia works with the accounts _____ _____, which is the money that is owed to the physicians.

3. Anna works with the accounts _____ _____, which is the money the physicians owe to others.

4. Once a year Dr. Medina has his accountant total his _____ _____, which include the entire properties subject to the payment of debts.

5. Larry is the supervisor of the _____ _____ department, which records all business and accounting transactions.

6. The _____ _____ in question was sent last month, but the equipment never arrived, so Julia questions whether she should pay the entire balance due.

7. The Rosales Clinic uses the _____ _____ basis of accounting, in which income is recorded when received and expenses are recorded when paid.

8. When the total ending balance of patient ledgers equals the total of accounts receivable control, the two are said to be _____ _____.

9. The accountant prepared a(n) _____ _____ sheet for December 31, which showed the total assets, liabilities, and capital for the clinic.

10. The Tyler Clinic uses the _____ _____ basis of accounting, in which income is recorded when earned and expenses are recorded when incurred.

11. Alice keeps a(n) _____ _____ on her desk that summarizes accounts paid out.

12. Each patient receives a(n) _____ _____ every month if the balance on his or her account is more than $5.

13. Running a(n) _____ _____ is one method of checking the accuracy of accounts.

14. Joy takes minor expenses, such as those for sodas and small donations, from the _____ _____ fund.

15. Dr. Lupez asked his accountant to prepare a statement of _____ and _____ for the previous fiscal year.

16. A standard of comparison to make sure answers obtained are accurate is a(n) _____.

17. A(n) _____ _____ _____ is a summary for a specific period that shows a beginning balance, an ending balance, and all the expenditures during that particular period.

18. Angelique keeps a record of all accounts paid out in a(n) _____ _____.

19. Something that is owed, or a debt, is called a(n) _____.

20. The monetary value of a property or of an interest in a property in excess of claims or liens against it is called _____.

SKILLS AND CONCEPTS

Part I: Short Answers

1. The financial records of any business should show the following at all times:

    a. _____

    b. _____

    c. _____

    d. _____

2. When writing numbers, keep the columns straight and write _____ _____ _____.

3. The manual disbursement journal must show the following:

    a. _____

    b. _____

    c. _____

4. Name two common accounting systems used in medical offices.

    a. _____

    b. _____

5. Differentiate between accounting and bookkeeping.

    _____

    _____

    _____

6. List three cardinal rules of bookkeeping.

    a. _____

    b. _____

    c. _____

7. List two disadvantages of a single-entry system.

    a. _____

    b. _____

8. The IRS requires that complete records be kept on all employees, including the following:

    a. _____

    b. _____

    c. _____

    d. _____

9. What is Form 940 used for and when must it be filed?

10. List seven expense categories often found in a physician's office budget.

    a.
    b.
    c.
    d.
    e.
    f.
    g.

Part II: Bookkeeping Systems
Briefly explain the three types of bookkeeping systems.

1. Single-entry system

2. Double-entry system

3. Pegboard/write-it-once system

4. Which of the three systems do you think would be the easiest to work with in the medical office? Why?

Part III: Forms
Briefly explain the use of each of the following forms.

1. SS-5

2. W-2

_____

_____

3. W-3

_____

_____

4. W-4

_____

_____

CASE STUDY

Read the case study and complete the exercise following it.

Kristy Stephens works for Dr. Mitchell, who has a small office in a suburban area just outside Birmingham, Alabama. The longer that Kristy works for Dr. Mitchell, the more she learns about accounting and the business side of running a successful medical practice. Kristy is a very organized person and wants to make sure she follows the right procedures and understands why a certain task must be done a certain way. She wants to establish a calendar that shows what duties should be done at what times.

Determine when all the forms in Part III must be turned in or filed. Add tax day to the calendar. Print the calendar, showing all filing dates on it. If a template will help, use one from the Microsoft Office home page.

WORKPLACE APPLICATIONS

Complete the following math review test. Turn it in to your instructor for grading or grade it in class.

Solve the following addition problems.

1. 99 + 104 = _____
2. 78 + 57 = _____
3. 98 + 128 = _____
4. 187 + 233 = _____
5. 284 + 440 = _____
6. 306 + 291 = _____
7. 204 + 278 = _____
8. 409 + 246 = _____
9. 15 + 74 = _____
10. 181 + 369 = _____

Solve the following subtraction problems.

1. 290 − 303 = _____
2. 231 − 263 = _____
3. 453 − 156 = _____
4. 459 − 325 = _____
5. 318 − 105 = _____
6. 398 − 294 = _____

Solve the following multiplication problems.

1. 46 × 24 = _____
2. 11 × 49 = _____
3. 48 × 17 = _____
4. 26 × 24 = _____
5. 42 × 15 = _____
6. 5 × 49 = _____
7. 47 × 12 = _____
8. 26 × 34 = _____
9. 45 × 21 = _____

Solve the following division problems:

1. 1,950 ÷ 13 = _____
2. 50,350 ÷ 53 = _____
3. 12105 ÷ 15 = _____
4. 9,712 ÷ 16 = _____
5. 13,500 ÷ 20 = _____

INTERNET ACTIVITIES

1. Investigate bookkeeping software on the Internet and use any tutorials or trial software available. Determine a good program for use in the medical office and be able to defend your decision in a class presentation.

2. Look for math worksheet sites and work through some of the sheets for practice.

25 Medical Practice Management and Human Resources

VOCABULARY REVIEW

Fill in the blank with the correct vocabulary term from this chapter.

1. Dr. Hughes enjoys offering _____ to employees who perform over and above the call of duty.
2. Lucia told a _____ lie to her supervisor, which almost resulted in termination of her employment.
3. The staff enjoys _____ talks and recently traveled to North Dallas to hear Zig Ziglar speak.
4. Employee _____ can indicate the working conditions at a facility; when the staff is happy with their jobs, they tend to remain in their positions for a number of years.
5. Mrs. Gordon has always been a great promoter of employee _____, never failing to offer her smile and a kind word to others.
6. Ruth Ann was written up for _____ after she and Sue Lynn, her supervisor, had a rather loud and tense discussion last week.
7. The marketers _____ young women in their latest advertisements to promote the hospital expansion in the labor and delivery department.
8. New employees may find it helpful to be assigned a _____, who will assist them as they learn the office routines and responsibilities.
9. The office manager assigned several new duties to Ann, including development of meeting _____.
10. Sandy had 17 performance _____ to give over the course of the week.
11. People in the medical field sometimes experience _____ and feel a need to separate themselves from the profession for a time.
12. Paul was charged with _____ after he took money from the physical therapy clinic where he formerly worked.
13. The doctors and management personnel have worked hard to develop such a _____ team.
14. A _____ of _____ is necessary in any organization, even smaller ones.
15. Barbara is _____ with her paperwork and very seldom makes an error.

SKILLS AND CONCEPTS

Part I: Office Managers

1. Why is it a good idea to have one person in charge of office operations?

   _____

   _____

   _____

2. Most management problems can be prevented by carefully defining the areas of:

   a. _____

   b. _____

3. What usually happens if a manager helps employees get what they want and need from a job?

   _____

   _____

   _____

4. Managers who have a group of outstanding employees are usually looked upon as _____

   _____.

5. List the three basic types of leaders.

   a. _____

   b. _____

   c. _____

6. List and explain three types of power.

   a. _____

   b. _____

   c. _____

7. The office manager must always have enough written _____ when terminating an employee.

8. List five ways to motivate employees.

   a. _____

   b. _____

   c. _____

   d. _____

   e. _____

9. What is a "yes" person?

   _____

   _____

10. What is one of the most effective ways to improve employee morale?

    _____

    _____

Part II: Hiring and Terminating Employees

Fill in the blank with the best answer.

1. One of the most effective methods of finding new employees is through word of _____.

2. When calling a job candidate to schedule an interview, the office manager has an opportunity to judge how well the person speaks on the _____.

3. The job candidate should fill out the application at the office by hand so that the applicant's _____ can be evaluated.

4. If the job candidate feels at _____, he or she will be able to share strengths and will communicate better during the interview.

5. Relationships with those who work in the medical office should, above all else, be _____.

6. Candidates may be required to submit to a _____ check, especially if they will be handling office finances.

7. One of the most critical errors in bringing a new staff member to the team is not providing fair and adequate _____ and _____.

8. Well-written job _____ list the essential functions of the job and specify the chain of command that should be followed in the office.

9. A dismissed employee should never be left in the office _____.

10. Always check at least _____ references when hiring a new employee.

Part III: Leading During Transitions and Change

Add the appropriate word to the following sentences about change.

1. Change _____.
2. _____ with the change.
3. _____ change.
4. _____ to change quickly.
5. _____ change.
6. Anticipate _____.

Part IV: Meeting Agendas

Number these activities in the correct order for a staff meeting.

_____ Discussion of unfinished business

_____ Adjournment

_____ Discussion of problems in the administrative area

_____ Discussion of new business

_____ Reading of the minutes from the last meeting

_____ Discussion of problems in the clinical area

_____ Discussion of problems in the common areas

Part V: Word Find

Find the words on the list in the puzzle.

```
R I P B U T S S M E N T O R T Y M X H U E J I S P Z G L A M
E N C O S T Q D U V M Z P C U R M W I X H Y A E Q N A D E Y
T S K J F U I M N B N B W U O A A O Q D M Z D J I S N T Q F
E U U B C K P L N A O V V Q N L V M N C A D J G I E I M C J
N B O K G P A U I I M R T W R L D S O I E Q A A G C N J V M
T O R Z F Z M X Q M W I D I U I A M M R X R R A U Z O N C W
I R N O I T A V I T O M R I B C A I M G A P R L U U U X Q C
O D X N P B G W M V B P I P N N H Q M P P L O L X F F B H E
N I V I T J L E G R I K I E E A L Q S A W U E V O G H A E L
X N F T A Z M R E A Y W N F G R T I L A S D L I I O I N Z B
U A Y V L B O A F F A F C A X V D E H H R Z T T F N A Y G A
S T U X U X W C B U R S E R C O U H T K F N P D O I L M X R
D I E L B A F F A Y K B N V R G U F D H R T Z F J T S P D T
S O L Z N F D S O U N I T K Q J Y L Y L B B C E N R G A Z E
L N Q D F L T K T A P K I E R K F S N M C O R X U A Q D E N
X C P E X T R I N S I C V H J O B P R K M I M A M A A X Q E
P O U Q T U E J A A U C E N Q W H B Z M B H O G H Q L V Z P
K R U N I V Q Q Y C Q J S V S K Q P A R V M Y H F V N X N M
R W E X J N S T I P Y H Z Z D B W N W E W Z F F V D T S B I
L G J E G R T X N J H W P P A L D N A L S O P S C H G M Q F
Y G Z K D A H R C E K B P Y R G N A B H Y O Q L B N X K Y T
X M V F J V D N I A M G M P Q D A V Q I A G M W Q B B B H D L
L U B O S G X T K N P E V E S M Z J H G C O P T G W M T H N
H F F D Y O P E U P S C L A J O J V I O B Z Z Z N T E W G J
N O I T N E V M U C R I C Z C C B X H C M Q Z O E A N R P W
L L G K N F Y R B Y A Q C X Z K S E P X X H Z S R J T X U G
P L S G Q M I C R O M A N A G E S V N D B D V S C C J A J W
B T S Q L M U T J H B B G N Z I B P B B P K S D Q U K U L O
O S H D V K Y A T B B W U I V G L M A C X V F B F T E F V B
R K X C E F X E D X D T U E B S C Q E C E G Z D Z I P B G L
```

Affable	Disparaging	Meticulous
Agenda	Embezzlement	Micromanage
Ancillary	Extrinsic	Morale
Appraisal	Impenetrable	Motivation
Blatant	Incentives	Reprimands
Burnout	Insubordination	Retention
Chain of command	Intrinsic	Subordinate
Circumvention	Mentor	
Cohesive		

CASE STUDY

Read the case study and perform the exercise following it.

Belinda is a single mom with two children. She recently was divorced from her husband and is in the process of rebuilding her life. She enrolled in medical assisting school 8 months ago and is now preparing for graduation. Throughout her time in classes, she has researched medical facilities on the Internet and found several that are close to her apartment complex.

Belinda has several goals in life, and the most important ones involve her family. She wants to find a job that will allow her to take care of her children, provide them a good education, and save for their college education. She knows that she needs to find a job that offers health benefits. Belinda is a loyal employee and has a work history, so she is hopeful that her positions from graduation forward will be such that she is able to make steady progress toward reaching her goals.

What goals do you have for your life after graduation? Assess your own personal situation and determine five long-term (life) goals, five short-term goals (1 year or more away), and 10 immediate goals for the next 6 months. Write the goals down. For the long- and short-term goals, include a few sentences that explain why the goal is important to you. Make sure all the immediate goals are attainable in a 6-month period.

Look over your list daily. Write down all the progress you have made toward the goals and celebrate when each one is attained. It may be beneficial to keep a journal that details the progress you make toward your goals, as well as the new ones you set as the original goals are met.

WORK APPLICATIONS

1. Revise or write a new patient information booklet and assign different groups of classmates to work on different sections of the booklet. Plan a staff meeting, sending a memo to each classmate who should attend. Write an agenda for the meeting, set a time limit, and determine a general subject to discuss. Each group should discuss their part of the booklet during the meeting.

2. Compose a rough draft of your résumé. Allow three different classmates to proof the document and make suggestions. Draft a final copy and turn it in to the instructor for a grade.

INTERNET ACTIVITIES

1. Perform a job search for medical assisting positions in your area. Look for the 15 most interesting opportunities and print the job descriptions. Compare the job requirements to the skills you have learned. If appropriate, apply for the positions.

2. Research a person you consider a leader on the Internet. Read about this person's life and write a report about the individual's abilities as a leader. Share the report with the class.

3. Investigate budgeting ideas by researching the Internet. Determine what items must be included in the budget and then list all the bills and payments that must be made each month. A budget template may be available on the Microsoft Web site and can be downloaded for use. Make the estimates as close as possible to your actual income and expenses. Turn the budget in to the instructor.

26 Medical Practice Marketing and Customer Service

VOCABULARY REVIEW

Fill in the blanks with the correct vocabulary terms from this chapter.

1. Dr. Julie Todd and Dr. Robert Todd truly enjoy _____, because it provides an opportunity to reach and involve diverse audiences using key messages and effective programs.

2. Monica has identified several _____ _____ and has a strong plan for marketing efforts that she plans to implement over the next year.

3. When you are developing a marketing plan, clearly establish _____ and think about the long- and short-term goals for the practice.

4. Monica wants to develop a(n) _____ business plan that is workable and will be flexible if changes become necessary.

5. One area Monica hopes to improve is the _____ laboratory, because much of the equipment is outdated and needs to be replaced.

SKILLS AND CONCEPTS

Part I: Short Answers

1. List the three steps generally followed in preparing to implement or change medical marketing strategies.

   a. _____

   b. _____

   c. _____

2. What is meant by "reaching the target market"?

   _____

   _____

   _____

3. List five specific planning steps that are effective in developing marketing strategies.

   a. _____

   b. _____

   c. _____

   d. _____

   e. _____

4. List several phrases that should never be used with patients, especially when attempting to provide exceptional customer service.

   a. _____

   b. _____

   c. _____

   d. _____

5. Explain the concept that good customer service is a commitment.

   _____

   _____

   _____

6. What are the four Ps of marketing?

   a. _____

   b. _____

   c. _____

   d. _____

7. How does the provider determine what services to offer at the practice?

   _____

   _____

   _____

8. Provide five examples of community involvement that may help a medical practice grow.

   a. _____

   b. _____

   c. _____

   d. _____

   e. _____

9. What is the difference between advertising and public relations?

   _____

   _____

   _____

10. List the four basic steps of creating a Web site.

    a. _____

    b. _____

    c. _____

    d. _____

11. What is the goal of any business?

   _____
   _____
   _____

12. Why is it necessary for medical assistants to provide a high level of customer service to those who visit the physician's office?

   _____
   _____
   _____

Part II: Web Site Evaluation

Research various Web sites for healthcare organizations, preferably in your geographic area. Rate the Web sites from 1 to 10 (10 being the best), by putting your ranking on the line to the left of the Web site name. Then fill in the chart that follows, putting the Web sites in the order in which you ranked them.

Rank	Web Site Name	Rank	Web Site Name
_____	_____	_____	_____
_____	_____	_____	_____
_____	_____	_____	_____
_____	_____	_____	_____
_____	_____	_____	_____

Web Site	Overall Appeal	Content	Ease of Navigation	Fonts	Consistency	Comments
1						
2						
3						
4						
5						
6						
7						
8						
9						
10						

Part III: Customers in the Physician's Office

1. Who are some of the customers who visit the medical office?

2. Explain how to provide patients and other guests in the office with exceptional customer service.

Part IV: Ethics, Marketing, and Public Relations

1. Do you think that any advertising for medical services is ethical? Why or why not?

2. Why has advertising become necessary in today's health industry?

CASE STUDY

Read the case study and answer the question at the end.

Lorendia has worked for Dr. Johnson for more than 15 years. Recently she was forced to cut her hours from 40 a week to 35, because she has been diagnosed with chronic fatigue syndrome, and she struggles toward the end of the week because of the symptoms of the disease. Lorendia has become more and more impatient with the people who come to the physician's office, and she often makes a snippy remark when she is behind in her duties. Her attitude has alienated her from most of the clinic's staff. Although her job performance is not acceptable now, for most of her career her work has been above reproach.

1. How can this situation be resolved so that Lorendia can keep her job yet improve her performance?

WORKPLACE APPLICATIONS

Providing exceptional customer service can actually interfere with job duties. Some workers use customer service as an excuse to chat with patients and avoid other duties. How can the medical assistant strike a balance between providing the customer service that patients deserve and completing all the tasks required each day?

INTERNET ACTIVITIES

1. Research customer service and develop your own, original definition of the concept of customer service. Present your thoughts to the class by creating a professional presentation.

2. Research public relations and make a list of the various "free" ways publicity can be generated for the office. Choose five ideas you feel are the best. E-mail these ideas to each of your classmates. If the entire class participates, everyone will have numerous fresh ideas to use once they begin their career. Write the ideas on index cards and keep them in a box or develop a portfolio of ideas.

3. Design a fictional Web site using free software on the Internet. If appropriate, share the site with classmates and compare ideas.

27 Emergency Preparedness and Assisting with Medical Emergencies

VOCABULARY REVIEW

Define the following terms.

1. cyanosis

2. dyspnea

3. ecchymosis

4. emetic

5. fibrillation

6. hematuria

7. mediastinum

8. myocardium

9. necrosis

10. photophobia

11. polydipsia

12. polyuria

13. transient ischemic attack

Fill in the blanks with the correct terms.

14. _____ is defined as the immediate care given to a person who has been injured or has suddenly become ill.

15. AED stands for _____.

16. CPR stands for _____.

17. CVA stands for _____.

18. TIA stands for _____.

19. MI stands for _____.

20. _____ is the most dangerous form of heat-related injury and results in a shutdown of body systems.

21. _____ are the initial signs of a heat-related emergency.

22. Patients with _____ appear flushed and report headaches, nausea, vertigo, and weakness.

23. _____ are medications that may be administered to dissolve a blood clot.

24. A patient who has experienced a sudden cardiac arrest will show a(n) _____ pattern on the ECG.

25. The medical term for extensive bruising of the skin is _____.

26. If the physician diagnoses a disease that has no known cause, it is called _____.

27. _____ is a pulse rate below 60 beats per minute.

SKILLS AND CONCEPTS

1. List five classic symptoms of a heart attack.

    a. _____
    b. _____
    c. _____
    d. _____
    e. _____

2. What is the difference between classic myocardial signs and symptoms and those that may be experienced by female patients?

    _____

3. List and explain seven types of shock.

    a. _____
    b. _____
    c. _____
    d. _____
    e. _____
    f. _____
    g. _____

4. Sprains and strains are treated with:

   a. _____

   b. _____

   c. _____

   d. _____

5. Give five examples of situations in which patients with abdominal pain should be seen by a healthcare provider immediately.

   a. _____

   b. _____

   c. _____

   d. _____

   e. _____

6. Screening emergency telephone calls is an important role of the medical assistant in the ambulatory care setting. List below a minimum of two questions the medical assistant should ask for the following health problems.

   a. Syncope

   _____

   _____

   b. Head injury

   _____

   _____

   c. Insect bites or stings

   _____

   _____

   d. Burns

   _____

   _____

   e. Wounds

   _____

   _____

7. Summarize a minimum of four methods of maintaining a safe environment for both staff and patients.

   _____

   _____

   _____

   _____

8. Explain the procedure for effectively discharging a fire extinguisher.

   _____

   _____

   _____

9. List the criteria that should be included in a healthcare facility's evacuation plan.

   _____
   _____
   _____
   _____

10. Ambulatory care practitioners should be prepared to contact community emergency services as needed. Identify five resources available in your community for emergency preparedness. Include the services provided and contact information for each.

    a. _____
       _____

    b. _____
       _____

    c. _____
       _____

    d. _____
       _____

    e. _____
       _____

11. Standard Precautions are crucial for preventing the transmission of diseases associated with bioterrorism. Summarize infection control procedures that should be implemented in the event a bioterrorism incident may have occurred.

    _____
    _____
    _____

12. Summarize the CDC's recommendations to help minimize the negative psychological effects of an emergency situation on both staff members and patients.

    _____
    _____
    _____

13. OSHA recommends multiple factors that can help promote staff safety. Explain six accident prevention behaviors that should be followed in a healthcare setting.

    a. _____
    b. _____
    c. _____
    d. _____
    e. _____
    f. _____

14. You are responsible for placing and labeling biohazard waste containers in the physician's office where you work. Explain the methods for proper disposal of hazardous material in the physician's office.

15. Discuss the role of medical assistants in emergency preparedness and the ways they can help if a natural disaster or other emergency occurs in their community.

CASE STUDIES

1. Sally calls the office complaining of lumbar pain that has been present for the past 2 weeks. What type of screening questions should you ask the patient? When should the patient be seen in the office? Provide the appropriate documentation.

2. Mr. Walker, a 64-year-old patient of Dr. Bendt, calls the office complaining of shortness of breath, pressure in the chest, and sweating for the past hour. Upon checking the patient's chart, you find that Mr. Walker is a smoker and obese. What advice should you give the patient? Show your documentation.

    The physician refers Mr. Walker to the emergency department, but he refuses to go, stating, "I don't feel well enough to drive to the hospital." What should be done to meet the needs of the patient? Document your conversation.

3. A patient calls, stating that she has found a tick on her left forearm. Explain the proper technique for removal of the tick. Also, you should advise the patient to watch for what signs and symptoms? Document your conversation.

4. A 19-year-old patient sitting in the waiting room experiences a grand mal seizure. What should Cheryl, the medical assistant, do to prevent injury to the patient? After the seizure the patient needs to be placed in the recovery position to maintain her airway. Explain how to place her in this position.

WORKPLACE APPLICATIONS

1. You learned in your text about factors that are crucial for patient safety and a few of the most common mistakes that can be made by healthcare workers that result in injury to a patient. Develop a handout that summarizes patient safety factors and share it with the class.

2. At a recent office meeting, telephone screening difficulties were addressed. Dr. Bendt asks you to review the current procedures and policies that are followed when patients call the office with emergencies and offer suggestions on how possible questions might be improved. In addition, the physician would like you to make a list of "home care advice" to go along with the symptoms. The work should also include "if" and "how soon" the patient should be seen in the office or under what circumstances the patient should be referred to the emergency department. Include the following situations in your project.

Asthma	Insect bites and stings
Wounds	Head injuries
Burns	Chest pain
Diabetic coma	Hypoglycemia
Back pain	Dysuria
Burns	Syncope
Hyperglycemia	High blood pressure

3. As a medical assistant, you understand that medical emergencies have many different signs and symptoms. Dr. Bendt has asked you to create an informative brochure to educate patients about the importance of early detection and treatment. The brochure should include the following:
   a. Definition of illness
   b. Importance of early detection
   c. Signs and symptoms
   d. Risk factors
   e. Prevention recommendations
   f. What patients should do if they think they are experiencing this condition

4. Cheryl is in charge of establishing the office crash cart. What type of supplies should the cart have? What medications should be included? How should the cart and supplies be maintained? Where should the cart be kept?

5. The medical assistant can play an integral role in a community's response to natural or human-created disasters. Summarize how the medical assistant can contribute to the community response to an emergency.

INTERNET ACTIVITIES

1. You notice that your CPR certification is about to expire. Search for a list of certification sites in your area. Make a list of the contact information and share the locations with your classmates.

2. Perform a search for the Poison Control Center in your area. Search for and create a list of ideas for ways to prevent poisoning. Create an informative poster to display in your physician's office.

3. Investigate the CDC's site for emergency preparedness planning: *www.bt.cdc.gov/planning/#healthcare*

4. Search the CDC's site for coordinating emergency response: *www.bt.cdc.gov/cotper/*

MEDICAL RECORD ACTIVITIES

Documentation of an on-site emergency includes the following:

- Patient's name, address, age, and health insurance information
- Allergies, current medications, and pertinent health history
- Name and relationship of any person with the patient
- Vital signs and chief complaint
- Sequence of events, beginning with how the problem occurred, any changes in the patient's overall condition, and any observations made regarding the patient's condition
- Details of procedures or treatments performed on the patient

Document the details of the following cases.

1. Charise Mourning calls at 4 PM, just after the physician has left for the day, and reports that her husband, Sam, fell going down the steps and can't bear weight on his left leg. Mrs. Mourning is 78 years old and does not know how to drive. What questions should you ask? How should you handle the situation? Document pertinent information in Mr. Mourning's medical record.

2. Lynne Franklin, the 17-year-old mother of a 9-month-old son, calls, hysterical and crying. She states that the baby is "jerking and shaking all over the crib." She states, "I tried to hold him down, and I heard something snap! What should I do? He looks like he is turning blue!" Lynne tells you he had a fever all night. The last time she took his temperature it was 103° F axillary. She is alone with the baby. How should the situation be handled? Document the details in the baby's medical record.

3. Charles Drysden, a 42-year-old patient, calls when the rest of the office is out to lunch. He is at work and is experiencing heaviness in his chest, difficulty breathing, indigestion, sweating, and minor jaw discomfort. He reports that the discomfort in his chest started about 30 minutes ago, after he ate a large lunch. Mr. Drysden took Mylanta for the indigestion but is not feeling any better. He wants to drive himself to the office even though a co-worker has offered to take him to the emergency department (ED). His pain is getting worse, but he doesn't think he needs to go to the ED. What should you do? Document the important details in Mr. Drysden's medical record.

4. You are working in the administrative area of the office when a patient enters the waiting room screaming for attention. She insists the physician ordered her the wrong medication, and she wants to talk to the doctor immediately. The physician is not in the office today, so you attempt to handle this very angry patient. Using the skills discussed in Procedure 36-3, try to work out a solution with the patient. Document the patient interaction in the woman's health record.

28 Career Development and Life Skills

VOCABULARY REVIEW

Fill in the blanks with the correct vocabulary terms from this chapter.

1. Jerri wrote a(n) _____ of the facts that she knew related to the theft of petty cash.
2. June found Daniel's attitude to be _____ and finally made a complaint to the office manager.
3. Because Allen was continuing his studies at night and was taking 12 credit hours, he was able to place his student loan in _____.
4. Medical assisting is one of the most versatile _____ a person can enter.
5. The physician asked Merri to _____ the documents for grammar and spelling.
6. Andrea found that _____ provided her with many more job leads than simply looking in the newspaper.
7. Ms. Moore, the office manager, attempted to get the employees to bring up only the _____ facts related to the conflict.
8. Joel tried to _____ his error by placing an amendment in the medical record.
9. Dr. McDonald gave the information to Selinda to rewrite, because she could take the regulations and convert them into a(n) _____, clear document.
10. Mack called his lender to report that he had returned to school full-time so that he would not _____ on his loan.

SKILLS AND CONCEPTS

Part I: Short Answers

1. List three ways job search training helps the newly graduated medical assistant.

   a. _____

   b. _____

   c. _____

2. What are employers' three basic desires when looking for a new employee?

   a. _____

   b. _____

   c. _____

3. Define *job skills* and give two examples.

   _____

   _____

4. Define *self-management skills* and give two examples.

5. Define *transferable skills* and give two examples.

6. What is meant when it is said that a medical assistant knows his or her personal needs?

7. List and define the two best job search methods.
    a.
    b.

8. Explain at least three ways the Internet can be helpful in a job search.
    a.
    b.
    c.

9. List five items that should be included on a résumé.
    a.
    b.
    c.
    d.
    e.

10. List two things that should never be included on a résumé.
    a.
    b.

Part II: Cover Letters

Write a professional cover letter, following the suggestions in the textbook. Turn in the cover letter to the instructor, along with the assignment in Part III.

Part III: Job Applications

1. Complete the job application found on the following pages. Make sure it is legible, accurate, and complete.

DIAMONTE HOSPITAL

APPLICATION FOR EMPLOYMENT

This application is not a contract. It is intended to provide information for evaluating your suitability for employment. Please read each question carefully and give an honest and complete answer. Qualified applicants receive consideration for employment without unlawful discrimination because of sex, religion, race, color, national origin, age, disability, or other classification protected by law. Applications will remain active for three months.

PLEASE TYPE OR PRINT ALL INFORMATION

Date: _____

Position(s) applying for: _____

How did you learn about us? ☐ Walk-in ☐ Friend ☐ Relative ☐ Job hotline ☐ Employee ☐ Other
☐ Advertisement (Please state name of publication) _____ Referred by: _____

Name: _____
          Last   First   Middle initial

Mailing address: _____
          City   State   Zip code

Phone: (____) _____ (____) _____ Social Security #: _____
          Home   Message

If related to anyone in our employ, state name and department: _____

If you have been employed under another name, please list here: _____

Are you under 18 years of age? .... ☐ Yes ☐ No

Are you currently employed? .... ☐ Yes ☐ No

May we contact your present employer? .... ☐ Yes ☐ No

Do you have legal rights to work in this country?
    (Proof of legal rights to work in this country will be required upon employment) ..... ☐ Yes ☐ No

Have you ever been employed with us before? .... ☐ Yes ☐ No *If "yes," give date(s):* _____

Are you available to work: .... ☐ Full-time ☐ Part-time ☐ Shift work ☐ Temporary

Are you available to work overtime if required? .... ☐ Yes ☐ No

How flexible are you in accepting varying scheduled hours? .... ☐ Very flexible ☐ Somewhat flexible
          ☐ Need set schedule

Minimum salary desired: _____

Have you ever been discharged from a job or forced to resign? .... ☐ Yes ☐ No
    Explain: _____

Have you ever been convicted of a felony?
    If "yes," please explain: _____ ☐ Yes ☐ No
    Criminal convictions are not an absolute bar to employment but will be considered with respect to the specific requirements of the job for which you are applying.

EDUCATION

High school: _____ High school graduate/GED: ☐ Yes ☐ No
_____ Date: _____

College: _____ Graduated: ☐ Yes ☐ No
Major/field(s) of study: _____ Degree: _____
Date: _____

College: _____ Graduated: ☐ Yes ☐ No
Major/field(s) of study: _____ Degree: _____
Date: _____

Technical, business, or
correspondence school: _____ Graduated: ☐ Yes ☐ No
Major/field(s) of study: _____ Degree: _____
Date: _____

Describe any specialized training, apprenticeship, and skills such as computer, office equipment, etc. _____
_____
_____
_____
_____

LICENSES AND CERTIFICATIONS

Type of license(s)/certification(s): _____ Expiration date: _____
Type of license(s)/certification(s): _____ Expiration date: _____
Type of license(s)/certification(s): _____ Expiration date: _____
Verified by: _____
Date: _____

REFERENCES

(Give name, address, and telephone number of three references that you have known for at least one year who are not related to you.)

Name: _____ Phone: _____ Years acquainted: _____
Address: _____ Business: _____

Name: _____ Phone: _____ Years acquainted: _____
Address: _____ Business: _____

Name: _____ Phone: _____ Years acquainted: _____
Address: _____ Business: _____

EMPLOYMENT EXPERIENCE

(Please list all employment experience, with most recent employment first. If more space is needed, please use the Additional Employment form.)

Employer: _____ Duties and skills performed: _____
Address: _____ _____
Phone number(s) _____ _____
Job title: _____ _____
Supervisor's name/title: _____ _____
Reason for leaving: _____ _____
Salary received: _____ hourly / weekly / monthly _____
Employed from: _____ to _____ _____
                   month / year   *month / year*

Employer: _____ Duties and skills performed: _____
Address: _____ _____
Phone number(s) _____ _____
Job title: _____ _____
Supervisor's name/title: _____ _____
Reason for leaving: _____ _____
Salary received: _____ hourly / weekly / monthly _____
Employed from: _____ to _____ _____
                   month / year   *month / year*

Employer: _____ Duties and skills performed: _____
Address: _____ _____
Phone number(s) _____ _____
Job title: _____ _____
Supervisor's name/title: _____ _____
Reason for leaving: _____ _____
Salary received: _____ hourly / weekly / monthly _____
Employed from: _____ to _____ _____
                   month / year   *month / year*

Do you expect any of the employers listed above to give you a poor reference? ☐ Yes ☐ No
If yes, explain: _____
_____

APPLICANT'S STATEMENT

I hereby certify that the statements and information provided are true, and I understand that any false statements or omissions are cause for termination. I agree to submit to a drug test and physical following any conditional offer of employment, and I grant permission to Diamonte Hospital to investigate my criminal history, education, prior employment history, and references, and hereby release all persons or agencies from all liability or any damage for issuing this information.

I understand that this application is current for only **three months**. At the end of that time, if I do not hear from Diamonte Hospital and still wish to be considered for employment, it will be necessary to update my application.

_____   _____
Signature of Applicant   Date

_____
Print Name

DIAMONTE HOSPITAL

Part IV: Résumés

1. Write a professional résumé, following the suggestions in the textbook. Turn in the résumé and cover letter to your instructor.

Part V: Interviews

1. Set up an interview with a physician's office. Perhaps the interview can lead to an externship or a position after graduation. Use the *Record of a Job Lead* form and the *Record of an Interview* form to record pertinent information.

Part VI: Follow-up Activities

1. Write a thank you card to the person with whom you interviewed. If a job opportunity exists, continue follow-up activities with the clinic.

Part VII: Goals

1. Set some realistic goals for your career in medical assisting by answering the following questions.

    a. Where am I today?

    _____
    _____
    _____

    b. Where will I be in 5 years?

    _____
    _____
    _____

    c. Where will I be in 10 years?

    _____
    _____
    _____

    d. What additional skills do I need to get to where I want to be?

    _____
    _____
    _____
    _____

Part VIII: Budgeting

1. Plan a budget for yourself using your actual living expenses.

The Guideline Budget

MONTHLY INCOME	AMOUNT
Net Income	
Spouse Net Income	
Child Support	
Other Income	

MONTHLY EXPENSES	AMOUNT
Rent	
Gas	
Electric	
Home/Renters Insurance	
Water/Sewage	
Trash	
Home Telephone	
Cell Telephone	
Pager	
Cable TV/Satellite	
Internet/DSL	
Child Care	
Lawn Care	
Clothing	
Food-Home	
Food-Work or School	
Food-Eating Out	
Laundry/Dry Cleaning	
Medical Expenses	
Dental Expenses	
Life Insurance	
Medical Insurance	
Dental Insurance	
Eyeglasses	
Prescriptions	
Automobile Payment	
Automobile Insurance	
Repairs	
Gas/Oil	
Furniture	
Beauty/Barber Shop	
Pet Expenses	
Student Loan	
Other Loans	
Credit Cards	
Church/Charities	
Birthdays	
Anniversaries	
Christmas	
Vacation Planning	
Entertainment	

Part IX: Mail Address

1. Open an e-mail account that reflects a professional electronic address using a free service (e.g., Yahoo!, MSN, Hotmail). Make sure the mail address you choose is appropriate for professional resumes and job applications.

CASE STUDY

Monica was an exceptional student during school and graduated with a high GPA. After a successful externship and 1 month looking for employment, she has been unable to secure a job. She calls the placement officer at her school, who sends her on several interviews, which are also unsuccessful. The placement officer asks Monica to come to the school dressed for an interview and to bring her résumé. The placement officer is impressed with Monica's appearance and her communications skills during the interview. However, when she looks down at Monica's résumé, she realizes why Monica has not been hired. What problem did the placement officer probably discover? What can Monica do to be more likely to secure employment?

WORKPLACE ACTIVITIES

Make a list of 20 potential employers. Use the Internet to obtain information about the facilities. Make a list of five points about each potential employer that could be discussed in an interview. Also, find five ways you qualify for a position in the facility. If appropriate, visit the facilities and make appointments for interviews. Obtain and complete a job application from each facility. Submit the application and a résumé if you are close to the end of your training.

INTERNET ACTIVITIES

1. Research potential employers in your geographic area. Find out as much information about the employers as possible. Keep a record of the information using the job lead forms provided in the text.

2. Use the Internet to locate potential job opportunities. Have your résumé in electronic form ready to attach so that you can apply for the jobs that interest you.

3. Look for job search sites other than those in the textbook. Share the sites with your classmates.

4. Form a group on a social networking site, such as Facebook, that includes each classmate. Share e-mails and stay in touch with one another after graduation. Share leads that might result in employment.

Name _____ Date _____ Score _____

Procedure 5-1 Recognize and Respond to Verbal Communications

MAERB/CAAHEP COMPETENCIES: IV.P.IV.11, IV.A.IV.1, IV.A.IV.2, IV.A.IV.4, IV.A.IV.5, IV.A.IV.7, IV.A.IV.8, IV.A.IV.9
ABHES COMPETENCIES: 8.bb, 8.cc, 8.ii

Task: To be able to recognize verbal communication and respond to it in a professional manner.

Equipment and Supplies
- Cards with various patient scenarios

Standards: Complete the procedure and all critical steps in _____ minutes with a minimum score of 85% within three attempts.

Scoring: Divide the points earned by the total possible points. Failure to perform a critical step, indicated by an asterisk (*), results in an unsatisfactory overall score.

Time began _____ Time ended _____ Total minutes: _____

Steps	Possible Points	Attempt 1	Attempt 2	Attempt 3
1. Choose a partner and select a scenario.	5	_____	_____	_____
*2. Communicate the assigned message to the partner.	20	_____	_____	_____
3. Allow the partner to respond, using active listening skills.	10	_____	_____	_____
*4. Restate the understood message from the partner.	20	_____	_____	_____
*5. Clarify issues that required it.	10	_____	_____	_____
*6. Use professional wording without slang.	20	_____	_____	_____
*7. Continue effective communication throughout the exercise.	15	_____	_____	_____

Did the student:	Yes	No
Demonstrate sensitivity appropriate to the message being delivered?	_____	_____
Demonstrate empathy and impartiality when communicating with patients, family, and staff members?	_____	_____
Demonstrate awareness of the territorial boundaries of the person with whom he or she was communicating?	_____	_____

Did the student:	Yes	No
Recognize and protect personal boundaries in communication with others?	_____	_____
Apply active listening skills?	_____	_____
Demonstrate recognition of the patient's level of understanding in communications?	_____	_____
Communicate on the patient's level of understanding	_____	_____
Analyze communications in providing appropriate responses and feedback?	_____	_____

Comments:

Points earned _____ ÷ 100 possible points = Score _____ % Score

Instructor's signature _____

Name _____ Date _____ Score _____

Procedure 5-2 Recognize and Respond to Nonverbal Communications

MAERB/CAAHEP COMPETENCIES: IV.P.IV.11, IV.A.IV.3, IV.A.IV.10, X.A.X.3
ABHES COMPETENCIES: 8.bb, 8.cc, 8.ii

Task: To be able to recognize nonverbal communication and respond to it in a professional manner.

Equipment and Supplies
- Cards with various statements or emotions that can be communicated nonverbally.

Standards: Complete the procedure and all critical steps in _____ minutes with a minimum score of 85% within three attempts.

Scoring: Divide the points earned by the total possible points. Failure to perform a critical step, indicated by an asterisk (*), results in an unsatisfactory overall score.

Time began _____   **Time ended** _____   **Total minutes:** _____

Steps	Possible Points	Attempt 1	Attempt 2	Attempt 3
1. Choose a partner and select a card.	5			
*2. Communicate the assigned nonverbal message to the partner.	20			
3. Allow the partner to respond, using active listening skills.	10			
*4. Restate the understood message from the partner verbally.	20			
*5. Clarify issues that require it.	10			
*6. Use professional gestures and avoiding slang when interpreting the message.	20			
*7. Continue effective communication throughout the exercise.	15			

Did the student:	Yes	No
Use appropriate body language and other nonverbal skills while communicating?		
Demonstrate respect for individual diversity, incorporating awareness of personal bias in areas such as gender, race, religion, age, and economic status?		

Demonstrate awareness of diversity when providing patient care and avoiding offending patients of different cultures?

Remain impartial and show empathy when dealing with patients?

Comments:

Points earned _____ ÷ 100 possible points = Score _____ % Score

Instructor's signature _____

Name _____ Date _____ Score _____

Procedure 6-1 Respond to Issues of Confidentiality

MAERB/CAAHEP COMPETENCIES: IX.P.IX.2
ABHES COMPETENCIES: 11.b(3)

Task: To ensure that medical assistants treat all information regarding patient care as completely confidential.

Equipment and Supplies
- Copy of the Code of Ethics of the American Association of Medical Assistants
- Copy of the Medical Assistant Creed
- Copy of the Oath of Hippocrates
- Copy of the guidelines from the Health Insurance Portability and Accountability Act (HIPAA)
- Notepad and pen
- Patient's medical record

Standards: Complete the procedure and all critical steps in _____ minutes with a minimum score of 85% within three attempts.

Scoring: Divide the points earned by the total possible points. Failure to perform a critical step, indicated by an asterisk (*), results in an unsatisfactory overall score.

Time began _____ Time ended _____ Total minutes: _____

Steps	Possible Points	Attempt 1	Attempt 2	Attempt 3
1. Talk with each patient about medical care.	5			
*2. Greet patients by name and attend to their needs and questions.	20			
*3. Make sure discussions with the patient are held in a private area.	10			
*4. Use active listening and other communications skills.	20			
*5. Clarify issues that required it.	10			
*6. Reassure patients that their health information is private and confidential.	20			
*7. Explain that information cannot be kept from the physician.	10			
8. Document as required and ensure patient confidentiality.	5			

Did the student:	Yes	No
Use ethical behavior, including honesty and integrity, in performing the duties of the medical assistant's practice?	_____	_____

Comments:

Points earned _____ ÷ 100 possible points = Score _____ % Score

Instructor's signature _____

Name _____ Date _____ Score _____

Procedure 6-2 Develop a Plan for Separation of Personal and Professional Ethics

MAERB/CAAHEP COMPETENCIES: X.P.X.2
ABHES COMPETENCIES: 11.b(4)

Task: To determine one's ethical views before one is faced with the requirement to make an ethical decision.

Equipment and Supplies
- Pen and paper

Standards: Complete the procedure and all critical steps in _____ minutes with a minimum score of 85% within three attempts.

Scoring: Divide the points earned by the total possible points. Failure to perform a critical step, indicated by an asterisk (*), results in an unsatisfactory overall score.

Time began _____ **Time ended** _____ **Total minutes:** _____

Steps	Possible Points	Attempt 1	Attempt 2	Attempt 3
1. Study the ethical issues outlined in the chapter.	5			
*2. For each issue, make notes about personal beliefs, paying particular attention to whether you agree or disagree with the opinions of the Council on Ethical and Judicial Affairs.	10			
*3. Apply the ethical decision-making process to each issue.	20			
*4. Determine your personal stand on the issue.	20			
*5. Determine the appropriate professional stance on each issue.	20			
*6. Discuss one of the issues with a classmate, using the professional stance rather than the personal stance.	20			
*7. Interact with each classmate professionally, regardless of that individual's ethical views.	5			

Did the student: Yes No

Examine and consider the impact personal ethics and morals may have on the medical assistant's practice? _____ _____

Comments:

Points earned _____ ÷ 100 possible points = Score _____ % Score

Instructor's signature _____

Name _____ Date _____ Score _____

Procedure 7-1 Perform Within the Scope of Practice

MAERB/CAAHEP COMPETENCIES: IX.P.IX.2, IX.A.IX.2
ABHES COMPETENCIES: 11.b(9), 1.e

Task: To perform duties within legal boundaries and within the scope of practice in the state where one is employed as a medical assistant.

Equipment and Supplies
- Computer with Internet access
- Access to text of laws and regulations affecting the scope of practice for a medical assistant

Standards: Complete the procedure and all critical steps in _____ minutes with a minimum score of 85% within three attempts.

Scoring: Divide the points earned by the total possible points. Failure to perform a critical step, indicated by an asterisk (*), results in an unsatisfactory overall score.

Time began _____   Time ended _____   Total minutes: _____

Steps	Possible Points	Attempt 1	Attempt 2	Attempt 3
1. Read the laws and regulations that apply to medical practice as assigned by the instructor.	10	_____	_____	_____
*2. Determine whether the law or regulation is applicable in your local area.	20	_____	_____	_____
*3. Read and discuss with the class one article from the Internet on relevant laws and regulations.	20	_____	_____	_____
*4. Define for the instructor the scope of practice of a medical assistant.	20	_____	_____	_____
*5. Explain the consequences of not performing within the legal scope of practice to the instructor.	20	_____	_____	_____
*6. State for the instructor three ways to stay up-to-date on applicable laws and regulations.	10	_____	_____	_____

Did the student:

	Yes	No
Demonstrate an awareness of the consequences of not working within the legal scope of practice?	_____	_____

Comments:

Points earned _____ ÷ 100 possible points = Score _____ % Score

Instructor's signature _____

Name _____ Date _____ Score _____

Procedure 7-2 Practice Within the Standard of Care for a Medical Assistant

MAERB/CAAHEP COMPETENCIES: IX.P.IX.4
ABHES COMPETENCIES: 11.b(9)

Task: To perform duties within the standard of care in the state where one is employed as a medical assistant.

Equipment and Supplies
- Computer with Internet access
- Access to text of laws and regulations affecting the standard of care for a medical assistant.

Standards: Complete the procedure and all critical steps in _____ minutes with a minimum score of 85% within three attempts.

Scoring: Divide the points earned by the total possible points. Failure to perform a critical step, indicated by an asterisk (*), results in an unsatisfactory overall score.

Time began _____ **Time ended** _____ **Total minutes:** _____

Steps	Possible Points	Attempt 1	Attempt 2	Attempt 3
1. Research the standard of care expected of a medical assistant in your state.	5	_____	_____	_____
2. With a classmate, role-play an encounter with a patient.	10	_____	_____	_____
*3. During the introduction, identify yourself as a medical assistant.	20	_____	_____	_____
4. Use reasonable care, attention, and diligence during the encounter.	20	_____	_____	_____
*5. Treat the patient carefully and professionally.	20	_____	_____	_____
6. Make accurate judgments about actions if indicated by the role-play scenario.	10	_____	_____	_____
*7. Treat the patient with a sense of equality.	10	_____	_____	_____
*8. Document the encounter with the patient as required.	5	_____	_____	_____

Comments:

Points earned _____ ÷ 100 possible points = Score _____ % Score

Instructor's signature _____

Name _____ Date _____ Score _____

Procedure 7-3 Incorporate the Patients' Bill of Rights into Personal Practice and Medical Office Policies and Procedures

MAERB/CAAHEP COMPETENCIES: IX.P.IX.5, IX.A.IX.1

Task: To make sure that patients' rights are honored in the daily procedures performed and policies enacted in the physician's office.

Equipment and Supplies
- Copy of the Patients' Bill of Rights
- Sample office policy and procedures manual

Standards: Complete the procedure and all critical steps in _____ minutes with a minimum score of 85% within three attempts.

Scoring: Divide the points earned by the total possible points. Failure to perform a critical step, indicated by an asterisk (*), results in an unsatisfactory overall score.

Steps	Possible Points	Attempt 1	Attempt 2	Attempt 3
1. Review the Patients' Bill of Rights.	10			
*2. Select a partner to play the role of a patient.	10			
*3. Briefly explain each article of the Patients' Bill of Rights to the patient.	20			
*4. Use active listening skills to address the patient's questions.	10			
*5. Ask whether the patient understands the Patients' Bill of Rights.	20			
*6. Determine whether the patient has any questions about the Patients' Bill of Rights.	20			
*7. Interact with the patient professionally.	5			
*8. Document the encounter with the patient as required.	5			

Did the student:

Demonstrate a sensitivity to the patient's rights?

Yes   **No**
_____   _____

Comments:

Points earned _____ ÷ 100 possible points = Score _____ % Score

Instructor's signature _____

Name _____ Date _____ Score _____

Procedure 7-4 Complete an Incident Report

MAERB/CAAHEP COMPETENCIES: IX.P.IX.6
ABHES COMPETENCIES: 4.a

Task: To fill out an accurate, complete incident report that provides all legally required information.

Equipment and Supplies
- OSHA Form 301 (or other incident report form)
- Pen
- Notes taken regarding incident

Standards: Complete the procedure and all critical steps in _____ minutes with a minimum score of 85% within three attempts.

Scoring: Divide the points earned by the total possible points. Failure to perform a critical step, indicated by an asterisk (*), results in an unsatisfactory overall score.

Time began _____ **Time ended** _____ **Total minutes:** _____

Steps	Possible Points	Attempt 1	Attempt 2	Attempt 3
1. Select a partner to play the role of a patient/employee involved in an incident.	5			
*2. Interview the patient/employee about the incident.	20			
*3. Use active listening skills, asking questions to obtain a complete and accurate report.	20			
*4. Take notes as the patient/employee relates the incident.	10			
5. Read through the incident report form before entering any information.	5			
*6. Complete the incident report form without leaving any blank spaces, using professional terminology and phrasing.	20			
*7. Proofread the report for errors and omissions.	10			
*8. Review the report with the instructor.	5			
*9. Document the encounter with the patient as required.	5			

Comments:

Points earned _____ ÷ 100 possible points = Score _____ % Score

Instructor's signature _____

Name _____ Date _____ Score _____

Procedure 7-5 Apply Local, State, and Federal Healthcare Laws and Regulations That Affect the Medical Assisting Practice Setting

MAERB/CAAHEP COMPETENCIES: IX.P.IX.8, IX.A.IX.3
ABHES COMPETENCIES: 5.g

Task: To be aware of local, federal, and state laws and regulations that apply to the employer's facility and recognize the importance of compliance with such laws and regulations.

Equipment and Supplies
- Computer with Internet access
- Access to organizational websites that have established legislation and regulations that pertain to medical facilities
- Information about changes to and new federal and state legislation and regulations

Standards: Complete the procedure and all critical steps in _____ minutes with a minimum score of 85% within three attempts.

Scoring: Divide the points earned by the total possible points. Failure to perform a critical step, indicated by an asterisk (*), results in an unsatisfactory overall score.

Time began _____   Time ended _____   Total minutes: _____

Steps	Possible Points	Attempt 1	Attempt 2	Attempt 3
1. Review federal regulations that apply to healthcare workers.	20	____	____	____
2. Review state regulations that apply to healthcare workers.	20	____	____	____
*3. Prepare a report on one of the laws that affects the medical profession and practice, focusing on compliance issues.	25	____	____	____
*4. Present the report to the class.	25	____	____	____
5. Provide a copy of the report to the instructor.	10	____	____	____

Did the student: **Yes**   **No**

Recognize the importance of local, state, and federal legislation and regulations in the practice setting, as shown in the report given to the class?   _____   _____

Comments:

Points earned _____ ÷ 100 possible points = Score _____ % Score

Instructor's signature _____

Name _____ Date _____ Score _____

Procedure 7-6 Report Illegal and/or Unsafe Behaviors That Affect the Health, Safety, and Welfare of Others to Proper Authorities

MAERB/CAAHEP COMPETENCIES: X.P.X.1
ABHES COMPETENCIES: 4.f

Task: To provide a proper procedure for the medical assistant to follow when legal or ethical regulations have been breached.

Equipment and Supplies
- Contact information for regulatory and law enforcement agencies at the local, state, and federal level
- Written reports or documentation of breaches of regulations, if available

Standards: Complete the procedure and all critical steps in _____ minutes with a minimum score of 85% within three attempts.

Scoring: Divide the points earned by the total possible points. Failure to perform a critical step, indicated by an asterisk (*), results in an unsatisfactory overall score.

Time began _____ Time ended _____ Total minutes: _____

Steps	Possible Points	Attempt 1	Attempt 2	Attempt 3
1. Compile a list of all regulatory and law enforcement agencies that have jurisdiction over medical facilities in the local area.	20	____	____	____
*2. Design a document describing the agencies, to be used as a reference guide in the medical facility.	25	____	____	____
*3. Design a form to use when reporting illegal and/or unsafe behaviors that affect the health, safety, and welfare of others.	25	____	____	____
*4. Compile a list of the types of behaviors that should be reported to authorities.	25	____	____	____
*5. Provide a copy of all documents to the instructor.	5	____	____	____

Comments:

Points earned _____ ÷ 100 possible points = Score _____ % Score

Instructor's signature _____

WORK PRODUCT 7-1

Name: _____

Complete an Incident Report

Corresponds to Procedure 7-4

<u>MAERB/CAAHEP COMPETENCIES:</u> IX.P.IX.5.

<u>ABHES COMPETENCIES:</u> 5.a.

OSHA's Form 301
Injury and Illness Incident Report

U.S. Department of Labor
Occupational Safety and Health Administration

Form approved OMB no. 1218-0176

Attention: This form contains information relating to employee health and must be used in a manner that protects the confidentiality of employees to the extent possible while the information is being used for occupational safety and health purposes.

This *Injury and Illness Incident Report* is one of the first forms you must fill out when a recordable work-related injury or illness has occurred. Together with the *Log of Work-Related Injuries and Illnesses* and the accompanying *Summary*, these forms help the employer and OSHA develop a picture of the extent and severity of work-related incidents.

Within 7 calendar days after you receive information that a recordable work-related injury or illness has occurred, you must fill out this form or an equivalent. Some state workers' compensation, insurance, or other reports may be acceptable substitutes. To be considered an equivalent form, any substitute must contain all the information asked for on this form.

According to Public Law 91-596 and 29 CFR 1904, OSHA's recordkeeping rule, you must keep this form on file for 5 years following the year to which it pertains.

If you need additional copies of this form, you may photocopy and use as many as you need.

Information about the employee

1) Full name
2) Street
   City   State   ZIP
3) Date of birth ___/___/___
4) Date hired   ___/___/___
5) ☐ Male
   ☐ Female

Information about the physician or other health care professional

6) Name of physician or other health care professional

7) If treatment was given away from the worksite, where was it given?
   Facility
   Street
   City   State   ZIP

8) Was employee treated in an emergency room?
   ☐ Yes
   ☐ No

9) Was employee hospitalized overnight as an in-patient?
   ☐ Yes
   ☐ No

Information about the case

10) Case number from the Log _____ *(Transfer the case number from the Log after you record the case.)*
11) Date of injury or illness ___/___/___
12) Time employee began work _____ AM / PM
13) Time of event _____ AM / PM ☐ Check if time cannot be determined

14) **What was the employee doing just before the incident occurred?** Describe the activity, as well as the tools, equipment, or material the employee was using. Be specific. *Examples:* "climbing a ladder while carrying roofing materials"; "spraying chlorine from hand sprayer"; "daily computer key-entry."

15) **What happened?** Tell us how the injury occurred. *Examples:* "When ladder slipped on wet floor, worker fell 20 feet"; "Worker was sprayed with chlorine when gasket broke during replacement"; "Worker developed soreness in wrist over time."

16) **What was the injury or illness?** Tell us the part of the body that was affected and how it was affected; be more specific than "hurt," "pain," or sore." *Examples:* "strained back"; "chemical burn, hand"; "carpal tunnel syndrome."

17) **What object or substance directly harmed the employee?** *Examples:* "concrete floor"; "chlorine"; "radial arm saw." *If this question does not apply to the incident, leave it blank.*

18) *If the employee died, when did death occur?* Date of death ___/___/___

Completed by _____
Title _____
Phone (___) ___ - ____   Date ___/___/___

Public reporting burden for this collection of information is estimated to average 22 minutes per response, including time for reviewing instructions, searching existing data sources, gathering and maintaining the data needed, and completing and reviewing the collection of information. Persons are not required to respond to the collection of information unless it displays a current valid OMB control number. If you have any comments about this estimate or any other aspects of this data collection, including suggestions for reducing this burden, contact: US Department of Labor, OSHA Office of Statistics, Room N-3644, 200 Constitution Avenue, NW, Washington, DC 20210. Do not send the completed forms to this office.

Name _____ Date _____ Score _____

Procedure 8-1 Use Office Hardware and Software to Maintain Office Systems

MAERB/CAAHEP COMPETENCIES: V.P.V.6
ABHES COMPETENCIES: 8.II

Task: To use the office computer system at maximum capacity to run the various aspects of the physician's office.

Equipment and Supplies
- Computer system
- Computer software applications, loaded on the computer
- Software and instruction manuals, if needed
- Description of office computer systems
- Patient data
- Business data

Standards: Complete the procedure and all critical steps in _____ minutes with a minimum score of 85% within three attempts.

Scoring: Divide the points earned by the total possible points. Failure to perform a critical step, indicated by an asterisk (*), results in an unsatisfactory overall score.

Time began _____   Time ended _____   Total minutes: _____

Steps	Possible Points	Attempt 1	Attempt 2	Attempt 3
1. Compile a list of the ways a computer system is used in the medical office to make the practice more efficient.	5			
2. Choose one of these uses to research.	5			
*3. Research the ways the computer system can be used efficiently in the selected area.	10			
*4. Prepare a report about the system, detailing the ways the office uses it to maintain information about patients, employees, equipment, and/or supplies.	20			
*5. Prepare a class demonstration of the use of a computer office system in a medical practice.	20			
*6. Present the report and demonstration to the class.	20			
*7. Provide the instructor with a copy of the report.	20			

Comments:

Points earned _____ ÷ 100 possible points = Score _____ % Score

Instructor's signature _____

Name _____ Date _____ Score _____

Procedure 9-1 Demonstrate Telephone Techniques

MAERB/CAAHEP COMPETENCIES: IV.P.IV.7, IV.A.IV.2
ABHES COMPETENCIES: 8.ee

Task: To answer the phone in a physician's office in a professional manner and to respond to a request for action.

Equipment and Supplies
- Telephone
- Message pad
- Pen or pencil
- Appointment book
- Computer
- Notepad

Standards: Complete the procedure and all critical steps in _____ minutes with a minimum score of 85% within three attempts.

Scoring: Divide the points earned by the total possible points. Failure to perform a critical step, indicated by an asterisk (*), results in an unsatisfactory overall score.

Time began _____   Time ended _____   Total minutes: _____

Steps	Possible Points	Attempt 1	Attempt 2	Attempt 3
*1. Answer the phone before the third ring.	5	_____	_____	_____
*2. Speak distinctly into the mouthpiece while holding it in the correct (i.e., approximately 1 inch from the mouth).	5	_____	_____	_____
*3. Identify yourself and give the name of the office.	10	_____	_____	_____
*4. Determine the information or service the caller is requesting, taking notes, if necessary.	10	_____	_____	_____
*5. Use active listening skills.	10	_____	_____	_____
6. Screen the call, if necessary.	10	_____	_____	_____
7. Provide the caller with the requested information or service.	20	_____	_____	_____
8. If necessary, correctly transfer the call to another person.	20	_____	_____	_____
*9. Terminate the call in a pleasant manner and hang up after the caller.	10	_____	_____	_____

Comments:

Points earned _____ ÷ 100 possible points = Score _____ % Score

Instructor's signature _____

Name _____ Date _____ Score _____

Procedure 9-2 Take a Telephone Message

MAERB/CAAHEP COMPETENCIES: IV.P.IV.7, IV.A.IV.2
ABHES COMPETENCIES: 8.ee

Task: To take an accurate telephone message and follow up on the requests made by the caller.

Equipment and Supplies
- Telephone
- Computer
- Message pad
- Pen or pencil
- Notepad

Standards: Complete the procedure and all critical steps in _____ minutes with a minimum score of 85% within three attempts.

Scoring: Divide the points earned by the total possible points. Failure to perform a critical step, indicated by an asterisk (*), results in an unsatisfactory overall score.

Time began _____ Time ended _____ Total minutes: _____

Steps	Possible Points	Attempt 1	Attempt 2	Attempt 3
1. Answer the telephone correctly.	5	____	____	____
2. Using a message pad or the computer system, obtain the following information from the caller, using active listening skills:	5	____	____	____
a. The name of the person to whom the call is directed	5	____	____	____
b. The name of the caller	5	____	____	____
c. The caller's telephone number	5	____	____	____
d. The reason for the call	5	____	____	____
e. The action to be taken	5	____	____	____
f. The date and time of the call	5	____	____	____
g. The initials of the person taking the call	5	____	____	____
*3. Repeat the information back to the caller to verify its accuracy.	20	____	____	____
*4. Provide the caller with an approximate time and date the call will be returned.	10	____	____	____
*5. End the call pleasantly, allowing the caller to hang up first.	20	____	____	____
*6. Deliver the phone message to the appropriate person.	5	____	____	____

Comments:

Points earned _____ ÷ 100 possible points = Score _____ % Score

Instructor's signature _____

Name _____ Date _____ Score _____

Procedure 9-3 Call the Pharmacy with New or Refill Prescriptions

MAERB/CAAHEP COMPETENCIES: IV.P.IV.7, IV.A.IV.2
ABHES COMPETENCIES: 8.ee

Task: To call in an accurate prescription to the pharmacy for a patient in the most efficient manner.

Equipment and Supplies
- Prescription information
- Notepad
- Patient's medical record
- Telephone
- Computer and/or fax machine

Standards: Complete the procedure and all critical steps in _____ minutes with a minimum score of 85% within three attempts.

Scoring: Divide the points earned by the total possible points. Failure to perform a critical step, indicated by an asterisk (*), results in an unsatisfactory overall score.

Time began _____ Time ended _____ Total minutes: _____

Steps	Possible Points	Attempt 1	Attempt 2	Attempt 3
1. Receive the call or fax requesting a new or refill prescription from the patient or pharmacy, using appropriate telephone technique.	5	_____	_____	_____
2. Obtain the following information from the patient:	5	_____	_____	_____
*a. The patient's name	5	_____	_____	_____
*b. The telephone number where the patient can be reached	5	_____	_____	_____
*c. The patient's symptoms and current condition	5	_____	_____	_____
*d. The history of this condition, if applicable	5	_____	_____	_____
*e. Treatments the patient has tried	5	_____	_____	_____
*f. The pharmacy's name, phone number and fax number	5	_____	_____	_____
*3. Determine the action desired by the physician per office policy.	10	_____	_____	_____
*4. Document the request and action in the patient's medical record.	10	_____	_____	_____
*5. Call the pharmacy staff with the prescription information or fax the information back to the pharmacy.	20	_____	_____	_____

Steps	Possible Points	Attempt 1	Attempt 2	Attempt 3
*6. Document the time and date action on the request was completed in the patient's medical record.	10			
*7. Call the patient and relate the action taken on the request.	10			

Comments:

Points earned _____ ÷ 100 possible points = Score _____ % Score

Instructor's signature _____

Name _____ Date _____ Score _____

Procedure 10-1 Manage Appointment Scheduling Using Established Procedures

MAERB/CAAHEP COMPETENCIES: V.P.V.1, V.A.V.2
ABHES COMPETENCIES: 8.c

Task: To establish the matrix of the appointment page and enter information according to office policy.

Equipment and Supplies
- Appointment book or computer
- Office procedures manual
- Information about the physician's office hours and availability
- Clerical supplies
- Calendar

Standards: Complete the procedure and all critical steps in _____ minutes with a minimum score of 85% within three attempts.

Scoring: Divide the points earned by the total possible points. Failure to perform a critical step, indicated by an asterisk (*), results in an unsatisfactory overall score.

Time began _____ Time ended _____ Total minutes: _____

Steps	Possible Points	Attempt 1	Attempt 2	Attempt 3
*1. Mark the times the physician will not be available to see patients to establish the matrix.	20			
2. Check the list of patients who need appointments and their chief complaints.	10			
*3. Consult guidelines to determine the time each patient will need with the physician.	10			
*4. Allot appointment times according to the patient's complaint and the facilities available.	20			
*5. Enter the patient's name and contact information in the appointment book or computer program.	20			
*6. Allow for buffer time in the morning and the afternoon for sick calls and emergencies.	20			

Did the student implement time management principles to maintain efficient office function?

Comments:

Points earned _____ ÷ 100 possible points = Score _____ % Score

Instructor's signature _____

Name _____ Date _____ Score _____

Procedure 10-2 Schedule and Monitor Appointments

MAERB/CAAHEP COMPETENCIES: V.P.V.1
ABHES COMPETENCIES: 8.c

Task: To manage appointments as they are cancelled, no showed, or rescheduled throughout the business day.

Equipment and Supplies
- Appointment book or computer
- Office procedure manual
- Appointment cards
- Clerical supplies
- Telephone

Standards: Complete the procedure and all critical steps in _____ minutes with a minimum score of 85% within three attempts.

Scoring: Divide the points earned by the total possible points. Failure to perform a critical step, indicated by an asterisk (*), results in an unsatisfactory overall score.

Time began _____   Time ended _____   Total minutes: _____

Steps	Possible Points	Attempt 1	Attempt 2	Attempt 3
1. Check the appointment schedule for the next day.	10			
2. Confirm all appointments.	10			
*3. Document a patient's late arrival in the appointment book or on the computer.	10			
*4. Document a "no show" in the appointment book or on the computer.	10			
*5. Document a late arrival and a "no show" in the patient's medical record.	10			
*6. Attempt to call the patient who did not show for the appointment and document the results of the call in the medical record.	10			
*7. Set a new appointment for the "no show" patient.	10			
*8. Inform patients that the physician is running behind schedule by 15 minutes.	10			

241

Procedure **10-2** Schedule and Monitor Appointments

Steps	Possible Points	Attempt 1	Attempt 2	Attempt 3
*9. Mark the appointment book or computer when patients arrive for their appointments.	10			
*10. Have patients sign in when they arrive for their appointment.	10			

Comments:

Points earned _____ ÷ 100 possible points = Score _____ % Score

Instructor's signature _____

Name _____ Date _____ Score _____

Procedure 10-3 Schedule New Patients

MAERB/CAAHEP COMPETENCIES: V.P.V.1
ABHES COMPETENCIES: 8.c

Task: To schedule a new patient for a first office visit.

Equipment and Supplies
- Appointment book or computer
- Scheduling guidelines
- Appointment card
- Telephone

Standards: Complete the procedure and all critical steps in _____ minutes with a minimum score of 85% within three attempts.

Scoring: Divide the points earned by the total possible points. Failure to perform a critical step, indicated by an asterisk (*), results in an unsatisfactory overall score.

Time began _____ Time ended _____ Total minutes: _____

Steps	Possible Points	Attempt 1	Attempt 2	Attempt 3
*1. Obtain the patient's full name (verify the spelling), birth date, address, and telephone number.	10	_____	_____	_____
2. Determine whether the patient was referred by another physician.	10	_____	_____	_____
*3. Determine the patient's chief complaint and when the first symptoms occurred.	10	_____	_____	_____
*4. Search the appointment book for the first available time and an alternate time.	10	_____	_____	_____
*5. Offer the patient a choice of these dates and times.	20	_____	_____	_____
*6. Enter the chosen time in the appointment book, followed by the patient's telephone number, noting NP to indicate the new patient status.	10	_____	_____	_____
*7. Explain the financial arrangements expected of new patients.	10	_____	_____	_____

Steps	Possible Points	Attempt 1	Attempt 2	Attempt 3
*8. Offer travel and parking directions and e-mail or mail the paperwork the new patient must complete.	10	_____	_____	_____
*9. Repeat the day, date, and time of the appointment before saying goodbye to the patient.	10	_____	_____	_____

Comments:

Points earned _____ ÷ 100 possible points = Score _____ % Score

Instructor's signature _____

Name _____ Date _____ Score _____

Procedure 10-4 Schedule Appointments with Established Patients or Visitors

MAERB/CAAHEP COMPETENCIES: V.P.V.1
ABHES COMPETENCIES: 8.c

Task: To schedule a general appointment either by telephone or in person.

Equipment and Supplies
- Appointment book or computer
- Office procedure manual
- Clerical supplies
- Appointment cards
- Telephone

Standards: Complete the procedure and all critical steps in _____ minutes with a minimum score of 85% within three attempts.

Scoring: Divide the points earned by the total possible points. Failure to perform a critical step, indicated by an asterisk (*), results in an unsatisfactory overall score.

Time began _____   **Time ended** _____   **Total minutes:** _____

Steps	Possible Points	Attempt 1	Attempt 2	Attempt 3
*1. Answer the phone by the third ring.	10			
*2. Identify the patient on the phone and obtain his or her phone number.	10			
*3. Ask the reason for making the appointment.	10			
4. Determine whether the appointment is for the person on the phone or a family member.	5			
5. Determine which provider or employee the person wishes to see.	5			
*6. Give the caller a choice of two appointment days.	10			
*7. Give the caller a choice of morning or afternoon.	10			
*8. Give the caller a choice of times.	10			
*9. Write the chosen time in the appointment book or enter it into the computer.	10			
*10. Repeat the appointment day, date, and time back to the caller and thank the person for calling.	10			

Steps	Possible Points	Attempt 1	Attempt 2	Attempt 3
*11. Allow the caller to hang up first.	5	_____	_____	_____
*12. Prepare an appointment card for appointments made in person.	5	_____	_____	_____

Comments:

Points earned _____ ÷ 100 possible points = Score _____ % Score

Instructor's signature _____

Name _____ Date _____ Score _____

Procedure 10-5 Document Appropriately and Accurately

MAERB/CAAHEP COMPETENCIES: IX.P.IX.7
ABHES COMPETENCIES: 4.a

Task: To document appropriately and accurately on all patient medical records and other office paperwork that concerns the patient.

Equipment and Supplies
- Any medical document
- Clerical supplies
- Computer
- Office policy and procedure manual

Standards: Complete the procedure and all critical steps in _____ minutes with a minimum score of 85% within three attempts.

Scoring: Divide the points earned by the total possible points. Failure to perform a critical step, indicated by an asterisk (*), results in an unsatisfactory overall score.

Time began _____   Time ended _____   Total minutes: _____

Steps	Possible Points	Attempt 1	Attempt 2	Attempt 3
1. Determine the information that needs to be added to the medical document.	10			
2. Make sure the information is factual, timely, and accurate.	10			
*3. Document the information by writing or typing it into the record.	10			
*4. Review the entry for errors, legibility, and clarity.	10			
*5. Date and sign the entry.	10			
*6. Make sure the entry is made so that it complies with all legal regulations.	10			
*7. Make sure the entry is made in such a way that it complies with office policy.	10			
*8. If corrections are necessary, make them according to the office policy and procedures manual.	10			
*9. Make sure the correction has not obliterated any part of the medical record.	10			
*10. Initial and date the entry.	10			

Comments:

Points earned _____ ÷ 100 possible points = Score _____ % Score

Instructor's signature _____

Name _____ Date _____ Score _____

Procedure 10-6 Schedule Outpatient Admissions and Procedures

MAERB/CAAHEP COMPETENCIES: V.P.V.2
ABHES COMETENCIES: 8.f

Task: To schedule a patient for outpatient admission or procedure within the time frame needed by the physician, confirm with the patient, and issue all required instructions.

Equipment and Supplies
- Diagnostic test order from physician
- Name, address, and telephone number of diagnostic facility
- Patient's demographic information
- Patient's medical record
- Test preparation instructions
- Telephone
- Consent form

Standards: Complete the procedure and all critical steps in _____ minutes with a minimum score of 85% within three attempts.

Scoring: Divide the points earned by the total possible points. Failure to perform a critical step, indicated by an asterisk (*), results in an unsatisfactory overall score.

Time began _____   Time ended _____   Total minutes: _____

Steps	Possible Points	Attempt 1	Attempt 2	Attempt 3
1. Obtain an oral or written order from the physician for the exact procedure to be performed.	10			
*2. Determine the patient's availability.	10			
*3. Telephone the diagnostic facility to: a. Order the specific test needed b. Determine the time and date for the procedure c. Give the patient's name, age, address, and contact information d. Determine whether the patient should be given any specific instructions e. Notify the facility of the urgency of results, if applicable.	20			
*4. Notify the patient of the arrangements, including: a. Name, address, and telephone number of the facility b. Date and time to report for the test c. Instructions on preparation for the test (e.g., eating restrictions, fluids, medications, enemas) d. What to take (e.g., identification, insurance cards, orders)	20			

Steps	Possible Points	Attempt 1	Attempt 2	Attempt 3
*5. Ask the patient to repeat the instructions to verify that the person understands them.	10			
*6. Note the arrangements in the patient's medical record.	20			
*7. If necessary, put a reminder in a "tickler" file to follow up on the patient's testing to ensure that results are received.	10			

Comments:

Points earned _____ ÷ 100 possible points = Score _____ % Score

Instructor's signature _____

Name _____ Date _____ Score _____

Procedure 10-7 Schedule Inpatient Admissions

MAERB/CAAHEP COMPETENCIES: V.P.V.2
ABHES COMPETENCIES: 8.f

Task: To schedule a patient for inpatient admission within the time frame needed by the physician, confirm with the patient, and issue all required instructions.

Equipment and Supplies
- Admission orders from the physician
- Name, address, and telephone number of inpatient facility
- Patient's demographic information
- Patient's medical record
- Any preparation instructions for the patient
- Telephone
- Admission packet

Standards: Complete the procedure and all critical steps in _____ minutes with a minimum score of 85% within three attempts.

Scoring: Divide the points earned by the total possible points. Failure to perform a critical step, indicated by an asterisk (*), results in an unsatisfactory overall score.

Time began _____ **Time ended** _____ **Total minutes:** _____

Steps	Possible Points	Attempt 1	Attempt 2	Attempt 3
1. Obtain an oral or written order from the physician for the admission.	20			
*2. Precertify the admission with the patient's insurance company, if necessary.	20			
*3. Determine the physician's and the patient's availability if the admission is not an emergency.	10			
*4. Telephone the facility and schedule the admission, providing the following information: a. Testing to be done b. Admitting diagnosis c. Date and time of admission d. Patient's room preferences e. Demographic information, including insurance coverage f. Special instructions for the patient g. Urgency of test results	20			
*5. Notify the patient of the arrangements, including: a. Name, address, and phone number of the facility b. Date and time to report for admission c. Instructions on preparation for procedures, if necessary (e.g., diet restrictions, fluids, medications) d. Preadmission testing requirements	20			

Steps	Possible Points	Attempt 1	Attempt 2	Attempt 3
*6. Ask the patient to repeat the instructions to verify that the person understands them.	5			
*7. Put a reminder on the physician's calendar. If the physician keeps a list of inpatients, add the patient's name to that list.	5			

Comments:

Points earned _____ ÷ 100 possible points = Score _____ % Score

Instructor's signature _____

Name _____ Date _____ Score _____

Procedure 10-8 Schedule Inpatient Procedures

MAERB/CAAHEP COMPETENCIES: V.P.V.2
ABHES COMPETENCIES: 8.f

Task: To schedule a patient for inpatient surgery within the time frame needed by the physician, confirm with the patient, and issue all required instructions.

Equipment and Supplies
- Orders from physician
- Name, address, and telephone number of inpatient facility
- Patient's demographic information
- Patient's medical record
- Any preparation instructions for the patient
- Telephone
- Consent form

Standards: Complete the procedure and all critical steps in _____ minutes with a minimum score of 85% within three attempts.

Scoring: Divide the points earned by the total possible points. Failure to perform a critical step, indicated by an asterisk (*), results in an unsatisfactory overall score.

Time began _____   **Time ended** _____   **Total minutes:** _____

Steps	Possible Points	Attempt 1	Attempt 2	Attempt 3
1. Obtain an oral or written order from the physician for the admission.	10	_____	_____	_____
2. Precertify the admission with the patient's insurance company, if necessary.	10	_____	_____	_____
*3. Determine the physician's availability if the surgery is not an emergency. Another physician may be the surgeon, requiring coordination with his or her office.	20	_____	_____	_____
*4. Telephone the hospital surgical or diagnostic department to schedule the procedure and to: a. Order any specific tests needed b. Provide the patient's admitting diagnosis c. Establish the date and time d. Give the patient's name, age, address, and telephone number e. Provide demographic information on the patient, including insurance information f. Determine any special instructions for the patient g. Notify the facility of the urgency of the surgery or procedure, if applicable	20	_____	_____	_____

Steps	Possible Points	Attempt 1	Attempt 2	Attempt 3

*5. Notify the patient of the arrangements, if the patient has not already been admitted to the hospital, including:
  a. Name, address, and telephone number of the facility
  b. Date and time to report for admission
  c. Instructions on preparation for any procedures, if necessary (e.g., diet restrictions, fluids, medications)
  d. Preadmission testing requirements
	20	_____	_____	_____

*6. Ask the patient to repeat the instructions to verify that the person understands them.	10	_____	_____	_____
*7. Put reminder on the physician's calendar. If the physician keeps a list of inpatients, add the patient's name to that list.	10	_____	_____	_____

Comments:

Points earned _____ ÷ 100 possible points = Score _____ % Score

Instructor's signature _____

254

Procedure **10-8 Schedule Inpatient Procedures**   Copyright © 2011, 2007, 2003 by Saunders, an imprint of Elsevier Inc. All rights reserved.

WORK PRODUCT 10-1

Name: _____

Advance Preparation and Establishing a Matrix

Corresponds to Procedure 10-1

MAERB/CAAHEP COMPETENCIES: V.P.V.1.

ABHES COMPETENCIES: 8.c

Complete Appointment Page 1 using the information in Part III.

WORK PRODUCT 10-2

Name: _____

Scheduling Appointments

Corresponds to Procedure 10-1

MAERB/CAAHEP COMPETENCIES: V.P.V.1.

ABHES COMPETENCIES: 8.c

Complete Appointment Page 2 using the information in Part IV.

WORK PRODUCT 10-3

Name: _____

Scheduling Appointments

Corresponds to Procedure 10-1

MAERB/CAAHEP COMPETENCIES: V.P.V.1.

ABHES COMPETENCIES: 8.c

Complete Appointment Page 3 using the information in Part IV.

259

Work Product **10-3**

WORK PRODUCT 10-4

Name: _____

Scheduling Appointments

Corresponds to Procedure 10-1

MAERB/CAAHEP COMPETENCIES: V.P.V.1.

ABHES COMPETENCIES: 8.c

Complete Appointment Page 4 using the information in Part IV.

WORK PRODUCT 10-5

Name: _____

Scheduling Appointments

Corresponds to Procedure 10-1

MAERB/CAAHEP COMPETENCIES: V.P.V.1.

ABHES COMPETENCIES: 8.c

Complete Appointment Page 5 using the information in Part IV.

WORK PRODUCT 10-6

Name: _____

Document Appropriately and Accurately

Corresponds to Procedure 10-5

<u>MAERB/CAAHEP COMPETENCIES:</u> IX.P.IX.7.

<u>ABHES COMPETENCIES:</u> 4.a

Document the four patients listed in Part VIII using the progress note form. Use the same progress note to document all four patients' activity, although in a medical record, each would be charted in the patients' individual record.

OUTLINE FORMAT PROGRESS NOTES

Prob. No. or Letter	DATE	S Subjective	O Objective	A Assess	P Plans	Page

Patient Name _____

Start each Progress Note (Subjective, Objective, Assessment and Plans) at the appropriate shaded column to create an outline form. Write through the intervening columns to the right margin of the page.

ORDER # 26-7115 ANDRUS CLINI-REC CHART ORGANIZING SYSTEMS • 1976 BIBBERO SYSTEMS, INC. • PETALUMA, CA.
TO REORDER CALL TOLL FREE: (800) BIBBERO (800-242-2376) OR FAX (800) 242-9330 www.bibbero.com MFG IN U.S.A.

Copyright © 2011, 2007, 2003 by Saunders, an imprint of Elsevier Inc. All rights reserved.

WORK PRODUCT 10-7

Name: _____

Scheduling Inpatient and Outpatient Admissions and Procedures

Corresponds to Procedures 10-6 through 10-8

MAERB/CAAHEP COMPETENCIES: V.P.V.2

ABHES COMPETENCIES: 8.f

Complete the referral form using the information in Part VIII, question 1.

BLACKBURN PRIMARY CARE ASSOCIATES, P.C.
1990 Turquoise Drive • Blackburn, WI 54937
Phone 608-459-8857 • Fax 608-459-8860
Referral Form Effective Jan. 1, 20XX

Patient Name _____ Phone # _____
SS # _____ DOB _____
Diagnosis (ICD-9 Required) _____
Insurance Type _____
Referring Physician _____ Phone _____
Office Contact _____ Fax _____

REFERRAL FOR:
❏ Consult Only
❏ Evaluation and Treatment
❏ Inpatient Surgery
❏ Inpatient Admission
❏ Outpatient Surgery
❏ Outpatient Lab
❏ Outpatient X-ray
❏ Procedure Only
❏ Chiropractic
❏ Physical Therapy
❏ Back in Action Rehabilitation Program
❏ Psychophysiologic Evaluation
❏ Biofeedback
❏ Other _____

Comments
_____
_____
_____
_____
_____
_____

REFERRAL TIMEFRAME:
❏ First Available Appt (within 5 business days)
❏ Stat (within 24 hr)

PROVIDER:
❏ Ron Lupez, M.D.
❏ Donald Lawler, M.D.
❏ Robert Hughes, D.O.
❏ Neil Stern, D.C.
❏ Joel Lively, P.T.

PLEASE INCLUDE THE FOLLOWING:
❏ Copy of Insurance Card
❏ Demographic Information
❏ Treatment Notes
❏ Diagnostic Reports

HOSPITAL/FACILITY
❏ Mercy Hospital
❏ Presbyterian Hospital
❏ Outpatient Surgical Complex
❏ Health and Wellness Center

Scheduled By _____

Appt Date/Time _____ Physician _____

WORK PRODUCT 10-8

Name: _____

Scheduling Inpatient and Outpatient Admissions and Procedures

Corresponds to Procedures 10-6 through 10-8

<u>MAERB/CAAHEP COMPETENCIES:</u> V.P.V.2

<u>ABHES COMPETENCIES:</u> 8.f

Complete the referral form using the information in Part VIII, question 2.

BLACKBURN PRIMARY CARE ASSOCIATES, P.C.
1990 Turquoise Drive • Blackburn, WI 54937
Phone 608-459-8857 • Fax 608-459-8860
Referral Form Effective Jan. 1, 20XX

Patient Name _____ Phone # _____
SS # _____ DOB _____
Diagnosis (ICD-9 Required) _____
Insurance Type _____
Referring Physician _____ Phone _____
Office Contact _____ Fax _____

REFERRAL FOR:
- ❏ Consult Only
- ❏ Evaluation and Treatment
- ❏ Inpatient Surgery
- ❏ Inpatient Admission
- ❏ Outpatient Surgery
- ❏ Outpatient Lab
- ❏ Outpatient X-ray
- ❏ Procedure Only
- ❏ Chiropractic
- ❏ Physical Therapy
- ❏ Back in Action Rehabilitation Program
- ❏ Psychophysiologic Evaluation
- ❏ Biofeedback
- ❏ Other _____

Comments
_____
_____
_____
_____
_____

REFERRAL TIMEFRAME:
- ❏ First Available Appt (within 5 business days)
- ❏ Stat (within 24 hr)

PROVIDER:
- ❏ Ron Lupez, M.D.
- ❏ Donald Lawler, M.D.
- ❏ Robert Hughes, D.O.
- ❏ Neil Stern, D.C.
- ❏ Joel Lively, P.T.

PLEASE INCLUDE THE FOLLOWING:
- ❏ Copy of Insurance Card
- ❏ Demographic Information
- ❏ Treatment Notes
- ❏ Diagnostic Reports

HOSPITAL/FACILITY
- ❏ Mercy Hospital
- ❏ Presbyterian Hospital
- ❏ Outpatient Surgical Complex
- ❏ Health and Wellness Center

Scheduled By _____

Appt Date/Time _____ Physician _____

WORK PRODUCT 10-9

Name: _____

Scheduling Inpatient and Outpatient Admissions and Procedures

Corresponds to Procedures 10-6 through 10-8

<u>MAERB/CAAHEP COMPETENCIES:</u> V.P.V.2

<u>ABHES COMPETENCIES:</u> 8.f

Complete the referral form using the information in Part VIII, question 3.

BLACKBURN PRIMARY CARE ASSOCIATES, P.C.
1990 Turquoise Drive • Blackburn, WI 54937
Phone 608-459-8857 • Fax 608-459-8860
Referral Form Effective Jan. 1, 20XX

Patient Name _____ Phone # _____
SS # _____ DOB _____
Diagnosis (ICD-9 Required) _____
Insurance Type _____
Referring Physician _____ Phone _____
Office Contact _____ Fax _____

REFERRAL FOR:
❑ Consult Only
❑ Evaluation and Treatment
❑ Inpatient Surgery
❑ Inpatient Admission
❑ Outpatient Surgery
❑ Outpatient Lab
❑ Outpatient X-ray
❑ Procedure Only
❑ Chiropractic
❑ Physical Therapy
❑ Back in Action Rehabilitation Program
❑ Psychophysiologic Evaluation
❑ Biofeedback
❑ Other _____

Comments
_____
_____
_____
_____
_____
_____

REFERRAL TIMEFRAME:
❑ First Available Appt (within 5 business days)
❑ Stat (within 24 hr)

PROVIDER:
❑ Ron Lupez, M.D.
❑ Donald Lawler, M.D.
❑ Robert Hughes, D.O.
❑ Neil Stern, D.C.
❑ Joel Lively, P.T.

PLEASE INCLUDE THE FOLLOWING:
❑ Copy of Insurance Card
❑ Demographic Information
❑ Treatment Notes
❑ Diagnostic Reports

HOSPITAL/FACILITY
❑ Mercy Hospital
❑ Presbyterian Hospital
❑ Outpatient Surgical Complex
❑ Health and Wellness Center

Scheduled By _____

Appt Date/Time _____ Physician _____

WORK PRODUCT 10-10

Name: _____

Scheduling Inpatient and Outpatient Admissions and Procedures

Corresponds to Procedures 10-6 through 10-8

<u>MAERB/CAAHEP COMPETENCIES:</u> V.P.V.2

<u>ABHES COMPETENCIES:</u> 8.f

Complete the referral form using the information in Part VIII, Question 4.

BLACKBURN PRIMARY CARE ASSOCIATES, P.C.
1990 Turquoise Drive • Blackburn, WI 54937
Phone 608-459-8857 • Fax 608-459-8860
Referral Form Effective Jan. 1, 20XX

Patient Name _____ Phone # _____
SS # _____ DOB _____
Diagnosis (ICD-9 Required) _____
Insurance Type _____
Referring Physician _____ Phone _____
Office Contact _____ Fax _____

REFERRAL FOR:
❑ Consult Only
❑ Evaluation and Treatment
❑ Inpatient Surgery
❑ Inpatient Admission
❑ Outpatient Surgery
❑ Outpatient Lab
❑ Outpatient X-ray
❑ Procedure Only
❑ Chiropractic
❑ Physical Therapy
❑ Back in Action Rehabilitation Program
❑ Psychophysiologic Evaluation
❑ Biofeedback
❑ Other _____

Comments
_____
_____
_____
_____
_____
_____

REFERRAL TIMEFRAME:
❑ First Available Appt (within 5 business days)
❑ Stat (within 24 hr)

PROVIDER:
❑ Ron Lupez, M.D.
❑ Donald Lawler, M.D.
❑ Robert Hughes, D.O.
❑ Neil Stern, D.C.
❑ Joel Lively, P.T.

PLEASE INCLUDE THE FOLLOWING:
❑ Copy of Insurance Card
❑ Demographic Information
❑ Treatment Notes
❑ Diagnostic Reports

HOSPITAL/FACILITY
❑ Mercy Hospital
❑ Presbyterian Hospital
❑ Outpatient Surgical Complex
❑ Health and Wellness Center

Scheduled By _____
Appt Date/Time _____ Physician _____

Name _____ Date _____ Score _____

Procedure 11-1 Organize a Patient's Medical Record

MAERB/CAAHEP COMPETENCIES: V.P.V.3
ABHES COMPETENCIES: 8.b

Task: To prepare patients' medical records for the daily appointment schedule and have them ready for the physician before the patients' arrival.

Equipment and Supplies
- Appointment schedule for current date
- Patients' medical records
- Clerical supplies (e.g., pen, tape, stapler)

Standards: Complete the procedure and all critical steps in _____ minutes with a minimum score of 85% within three attempts.

Scoring: Divide the points earned by the total possible points. Failure to perform a critical step, indicated by an asterisk (*), results in an unsatisfactory overall score.

Time began _____   Time ended _____   Total minutes: _____

Steps	Possible Points	Attempt 1	Attempt 2	Attempt 3
1. Review the list of appointments for the day.	5	____	____	____
*2. Identify each patient by name and/or medical record number.	10	____	____	____
3. Pull the medical records for each established patient.	10	____	____	____
*4. Compare the records with the names on the list to make sure the correct records have been pulled.	20	____	____	____
*5. Make sure the laboratory results for all previously ordered tests are in the medical record.	10	____	____	____
*6. Replenish forms in the record so that the physician has room to write notes and/or add information.	10	____	____	____
*7. Annotate the appointment list with any special concerns.	5	____	____	____
*8. Arrange the medical records in the order the patients will be seen.	20	____	____	____
*9. Put the records in the designated place for easy retrieval once patients begin to arrive.	10	____	____	____

Comments:

Points earned _____ ÷ 100 possible points = Score _____ % Score

Instructor's signature _____

Name _____ Date _____ Score _____

Procedure 11-2 Register a New Patient

MAERB/CAAHEP COMPETENCIES: V.P.V.3
ABHES COMPETENCIES: 8.b

Task: To complete a registration form for a new patient with information for credit and insurance claims and to inform and orient the patient to the facility.

Equipment and Supplies
- Registration form
- Clerical supplies (e.g., pen, clipboard)
- Private conference area

Standards: Complete the procedure and all critical steps in _____ minutes with a minimum score of 85% within three attempts.

Scoring: Divide the points earned by the total possible points. Failure to perform a critical step, indicated by an asterisk (*), results in an unsatisfactory overall score.

Time began _____ **Time ended** _____ **Total minutes:** _____

Steps	Possible Points	Attempt 1	Attempt 2	Attempt 3
1. Determine whether the patient is new to the practice.	5			
*2. Ask the patient to complete the patient information form.	5			
3. Enter the information from the form into the computer or add the form to the patient's medical record in the prescribed place.	15			
*4. Review the entire form to make sure all information has been completed.	15			
*5. Make a copy of the insurance card, front and back.	10			
*6. Verify insurance coverage.	15			
*7. Construct the record using the materials prescribed by the medical office.	5			
*8. Add progress notes so that the physician can document information in the patient's medical record.	15			
*9. Attach an encounter form to the chart and give it to the clinical assistant for use during the patient's examination.	15			

Comments:

Points earned _____ ÷ 100 possible points = Score _____ % Score

Instructor's signature _____

Name _____ Date _____ Score _____

Procedure 12-1 Explain General Office Policies

MAERB/CAAHEP COMPETENCIES: IV.P.IV.4
ABHES COMPETENCIES: 9.p

Task: To communicate office policies and procedures effectively to patients and visitors in the office.

Equipment and Supplies
- Office policy manual
- Office procedure manual (if not included in the policy manual)
- Patient information sheets
- Office policy brochure

Standards: Complete the procedure and all critical steps in _____ minutes with a minimum score of 85% within three attempts.

Scoring: Divide the points earned by the total possible points. Failure to perform a critical step, indicated by an asterisk (*), results in an unsatisfactory overall score.

Time began _____ Time ended _____ Total minutes: _____

Steps	Possible Points	Attempt 1	Attempt 2	Attempt 3

*1. Design an office policy brochure or Web site that presents general information for patients. At a minimum, the brochure should have the following:
  a. Philosophy statement
  b. Goals
  c. Description of the medical practice
  d. Location and/or map
  e. Phone numbers
  f. Pager numbers
  g. E-mail and Web site addresses
  h. Staff names and credentials
  i. Services offered
  j. Hours of operation
  k. Appointment system
  l. Cancellation policy
  m. Prescription refill guidelines
  n. Insurances accepted
  o. Emergency procedures
  p. Alternate physician coverage
  q. Referral and records release policies
  r. Special needs accommodations
  s. Notice of privacy policies
	30			

Steps	Possible Points	Attempt 1	Attempt 2	Attempt 3
2. Offer the brochure to new patients.	5	____	____	____
*3. Sit with the patient and explain each section of the document.	20	____	____	____
*4. While explaining the brochure, look for body language and verbal statements from the patient that indicate understanding.	5	____	____	____
*5. Ask the patient whether he or she has any questions.	20	____	____	____
*6. Document that the patient received the brochure in the medical record.	20	____	____	____

Comments:

Points earned _____ ÷ 100 possible points = Score _____ % Score

Instructor's signature _____

Name _____ Date _____ Score _____

Procedure 12-2 Instruct Individuals According to Their Needs

MAERB/CAAHEP COMPETENCIES: IV.P.IV.5
ABHES COMPETENCIES: 5.b, 9.q, 8.kk

Task: To communicate office policies and procedures effectively to employees, patients, and visitors in the office so that they understand the physician's instructions.

Equipment and Supplies
- Office policy manual
- Office procedures manual (if not included in the policy manual)
- Patient information sheets (if needed)
- Physician's orders, if applicable
- Patient information brochure

Standards: Complete the procedure and all critical steps in _____ minutes with a minimum score of 85% within three attempts.

Scoring: Divide the points earned by the total possible points. Failure to perform a critical step, indicated by an asterisk (*), results in an unsatisfactory overall score.

Time began _____ **Time ended** _____ **Total minutes:** _____

Steps	Possible Points	Attempt 1	Attempt 2	Attempt 3
1. Determine the patient's communication needs.	10	_____	_____	_____
2. Arrange for an interpreter, if applicable. If no employee speaks the patient's language, make sure the patient brings an interpreter to the appointment.	10	_____	_____	_____
*3. Give the patient the physician's instructions.	10	_____	_____	_____
*4. Explain the instructions to the patient using language that the person can understand.	20	_____	_____	_____
*5. While explaining the instructions, look for verbal and nonverbal indications that the patient understands.	20	_____	_____	_____
*6. Have the patient restate the instructions to verify complete understanding.	10	_____	_____	_____
*7. Provide the patient with any written documentation available that reiterates the instructions and/or the physician's orders for tests, procedures, and/or hospital admission.	10	_____	_____	_____
*8. Document the instructions given in the patient's medical record.	10	_____	_____	_____

Comments:

Points earned _____ ÷ 100 possible points = Score _____ % Score

Instructor's signature _____

Name _____ Date _____ Score _____

Procedure 12-3 Inventory Office Supplies and Equipment

MAERB/CAAHEP COMPETENCIES: V.P.V.10
ABHES COMPETENCIES: 8.z

Task: To establish an inventory of all expendable supplies in the physician's office and to follow an efficient plan or order control using a card system.

Equipment and Supplies
- Computer
- Inventory and order control cards
- Computer spreadsheet or list of supplies on hand
- Pen or pencil

Standards: Complete the procedure and all critical steps in _____ minutes with a minimum score of 85% within three attempts.

Scoring: Divide the points earned by the total possible points. Failure to perform a critical step, indicated by an asterisk (*), results in an unsatisfactory overall score.

Time began _____   Time ended _____   Total minutes: _____

Steps	Possible Points	Attempt 1	Attempt 2	Attempt 3
1. Enter the names of each item to be inventories into a computer spreadsheet or on a note card.	5	____	____	____
*2. Write the quantity of each item on hand in the space provided.	10	____	____	____
*3. Place a notation or reorder tag at the point where the supply should be replenished.	10	____	____	____
*4. Review the spreadsheet or cards monthly to determine what supplies need to be ordered.	20	____	____	____
*5. Using supplier catalogs and the Internet, shop for the most competitive prices.	20	____	____	____
*6. When the order has been placed, note the date and quantity ordered.	20	____	____	____
*7. When the order has been received, note the date and quantity in the appropriate area on the spreadsheet, checking for backorder information.	10	____	____	____
*8. Stock the supplies, moving older items forward and placing newer items toward the back.	5	____	____	____

Comments:

Points earned _____ ÷ 100 possible points = Score _____ % Score

Instructor's signature _____

Name _____ Date _____ Score _____

Procedure 12-4 Prepare a Purchase Order

ABHES COMPETENCIES: 8.d

Task: To prepare an accurate purchase order for supplies or equipment.

Equipment and Supplies
- List or spreadsheet of current inventory
- Phone
- Purchase order
- Fax machine
- Pen

Standards: Complete the procedure and all critical steps in _____ minutes with a minimum score of 85% within three attempts.

Scoring: Divide the points earned by the total possible points. Failure to perform a critical step, indicated by an asterisk (*), results in an unsatisfactory overall score.

Time began _____   Time ended _____   Total minutes: _____

Steps	Possible Points	Attempt 1	Attempt 2	Attempt 3
*1. Review the current inventory and determine what items need to be ordered.	10	_____	_____	_____
*2. Complete the purchase order accurately, filling in all applicable spaces and blanks with the information requested.	15	_____	_____	_____
*3. List the items to be ordered, including the quantity, item numbers, size, color, price, and extended price.	15	_____	_____	_____
*4. Provide the physician's signature, DEA certificate, and medical license information when needed.	15	_____	_____	_____
*5. Call in, fax, mail, or submit the order electronically to the vendor. Keep a copy for your records. Keep any verification provided to prove that the vendor received the order.	15	_____	_____	_____
*6. Note on the inventory spreadsheet or list the items that are on order.	15	_____	_____	_____
*7. Keep a copy of the order in the appropriate place in the office filing system or in the computer business files.	15	_____	_____	_____

Comments:

Points earned _____ ÷ 100 possible points = Score _____ % Score

Instructor's signature _____

Name _____ Date _____ Score _____

Procedure 12-5 Perform and Document Routine Maintenance of Office Equipment

MAERB/CAAHEP COMPETENCIES: V.P.V.9
ABHES COMPETENCIES: 8.y

Task: To ensure that all office equipment is in good working order at all times.

Equipment and Supplies
- Spreadsheet with information on each piece of office equipment, including serial number and servicing schedule
- Pen or pencil
- Computer
- Access to all office equipment

Standards: Complete the procedure and all critical steps in _____ minutes with a minimum score of 85% within three attempts.

Scoring: Divide the points earned by the total possible points. Failure to perform a critical step, indicated by an asterisk (*), results in an unsatisfactory overall score.

Time began _____ Time ended _____ Total minutes: _____

Steps	Possible Points	Attempt 1	Attempt 2	Attempt 3

*1. Gather information about each piece of equipment, including at least the following:
  a. Name of equipment
  b. Type of equipment
  c. Manufacturer's name
  d. Manufacturer's address
  e. Contact phone numbers for technical support
  f. Contact phone numbers for manufacturer's main office
  g. Date purchased
  h. Cost of product
  i. Original receipt showing where the item was purchased
  j. Dates warranty begins and ends
  k. Addresses of where to send equipment if under warranty
	20			

Steps	Possible Points	Attempt 1	Attempt 2	Attempt 3
*2. Enter the information about each piece of equipment into a document or spreadsheet.	20			
*3. Design a document containing each month of the year.	5			
*4. Mark which equipment needs servicing in which months.	10			
*5. Check which pieces of equipment need servicing this month.	10			
*6. Schedule servicing and maintenance for the equipment on the list for the current month.	10			
*7. Make sure servicing appointments are kept.	20			
*8. Record new information and scheduling needs into the spreadsheet or list as needed.	5			

Comments:

Points earned _____ ÷ 100 possible points = Score _____ % Score

Instructor's signature _____

Name _____ Date _____ Score _____

Procedure 12-6 Use the Internet to Access Information Related to the Medical Office

MAERB/CAAHEP COMPETENCIES: V.P.V.7
ABHES COMPETENCIES: 8.II

Task: To use the Internet to research any topic related to the medical office.

Equipment and Supplies
- Computer
- Topic for research
- Printer

Standards: Complete the procedure and all critical steps in _____ minutes with a minimum score of 85% within three attempts.

Scoring: Divide the points earned by the total possible points. Failure to perform a critical step, indicated by an asterisk (*), results in an unsatisfactory overall score.

Time began _____ **Time ended** _____ **Total minutes:** _____

Steps	Possible Points	Attempt 1	Attempt 2	Attempt 3
1. Start the computer, if necessary.	10	____	____	____
2. Open a Web browser.	10	____	____	____
*3. Open a search engine (make sure you can locate at least five major search engines).	10	____	____	____
*4. Type the subject in the search box.	10	____	____	____
*5. Review the results of the search.	20	____	____	____
*6. Determine which results are from a reliable source.	10	____	____	____
*7. Decide which information is pertinent to the research project.	10	____	____	____
*8. Print the information, if desired.	10	____	____	____
*9. Create a file on the computer for storing the information.	10	____	____	____

Comments:

Points earned _____ ÷ 100 possible points = Score _____ % Score

Instructor's signature _____

Name _____ Date _____ Score _____

Procedure 12-7 Make Travel Arrangements

ABHES COMPETENCIES: 8.a, 8.d

Task: To make travel arrangements for the physician or another staff member.

Equipment and Supplies
- Travel plan or itinerary
- Telephone
- Telephone directory
- Computer with Internet access

Standards: Complete the procedure and all critical steps in _____ minutes with a minimum score of 85% within three attempts.

Scoring: Divide the points earned by the total possible points. Failure to perform a critical step, indicated by an asterisk (*), results in an unsatisfactory overall score.

Time began _____ Time ended _____ Total minutes: _____

Steps	Possible Points	Attempt 1	Attempt 2	Attempt 3
*1. Verify the dates of the planned trip.	10			
*2. Obtain the following information: a. Desired date and time of departure b. Desired date and time of return c. Preferred mode of transportation d. Number in the party e. Preferred lodging and price range f. Preferred ticketing method (electronic or paper)	10			
*3. Telephone a trusted travel agency to arrange for transportation and lodging reservations or book using the Internet.	10			
4. Arrange for travelers' checks, if needed.	10			
5. Pick up tickets, print e-tickets, or arrange for ticket delivery.	10			
*6. Check tickets to confirm conformance with the travel plan.	10			
*7. Confirm hotel and air reservations.	10			

Steps	Possible Points	Attempt 1	Attempt 2	Attempt 3

*8. Prepare an itinerary, including at least the following information:
   a. Date and time of departure
   b. Flight numbers or identifying information for other modes of transportation
   c. Mode of transportation to hotels
   d. Name, address, and telephone number of all hotels, with confirmation numbers
   e. Name, address, and emergency telephone number of travel agency
   f. Date and time of return
	10			

*9. Put one copy of the itinerary in the appropriate office file.	10			
*10. Give several copies of the itinerary to the traveler.	10			

Comments:

Points earned _____ ÷ 100 possible points = Score _____ % Score

Instructor's signature _____

Name _____ Date _____ Score _____

Procedure 12-8 Develop a Personal (Patient and Employee) Safety Plan

MAERB/CAAHEP COMPETENCIES: X.P.XI.3
ABHES COMPETENCIES: 4.e

Task: To ensure patient and employee safety during any hazard or emergency situation.

Equipment and Supplies
- Hazard assessment for facility
- Office policy manual
- Community resource information
- List of contact information for all employees
- Clerical supplies for emergency action plan

Standards: Complete the procedure and all critical steps in _____ minutes with a minimum score of 85% within three attempts.

Scoring: Divide the points earned by the total possible points. Failure to perform a critical step, indicated by an asterisk (*), results in an unsatisfactory overall score.

Time began _____ Time ended _____ Total minutes: _____

Steps	Possible Points	Attempt 1	Attempt 2	Attempt 3
*1. Complete a hazard assessment for the facility.	5	_____	_____	_____
2. Determine the roles of other area health care facilities in case of an emergency.	5	_____	_____	_____
*3. Review the information from the hazard assessment.	5	_____	_____	_____
*4. Determine the method employees will use to report their readiness for duty during a hazardous situation or an emergency.	5	_____	_____	_____
*5. Develop an emergency action plan for each type of hazard that can be reasonably anticipated.	10	_____	_____	_____
*6. Provide for patient and employee safety in the plan.	10	_____	_____	_____
*7. Determine the extent of care that can reasonably be provided in a hazardous situation or an emergency.	10	_____	_____	_____
*8. Establish a clear chain of command.	10	_____	_____	_____
*9. Provide for break and rest periods for employees.	10	_____	_____	_____
*10. Make provisions for recognizing the effects of stress on both patients and employees during an emergency.	5	_____	_____	_____

Steps	Possible Points	Attempt 1	Attempt 2	Attempt 3
*11. Determine how resources will likely be restored.	5			
*12. Consider the facility's vulnerabilities and make a plan to overcome those weaknesses.	10			
*13. Conduct regular emergency drills.	10			

Did the student:

	Yes	No
Recognize the effects of stress on all persons involved in emergency situations?		
Demonstrate self-awareness in responding to emergency situations?		

Comments:

Points earned _____ ÷ 100 possible points = Score _____ % Score

Instructor's signature _____

Procedure **12-8 Develop a Personal Safety Plan**

Name _____ Date _____ Score _____

Procedure 12-9 Maintain a Current List of Community Resources for Emergency Preparedness

MAERB/CAAHEP COMPETENCIES: X.P.XI.12
ABHES COMPETENCIES: 8.e

Task: To help patients find organizations that can assist with their needs during an emergency and to establish a list of community resources that can be used for referral purposes during any type of emergency.

Equipment and Supplies
- Phone book
- Computer with Internet access
- Library access
- Newspapers
- Local volunteer guides
- Pen or pencil
- Notepad

Standards: Complete the procedure and all critical steps in _____ minutes with a minimum score of 85% within three attempts.

Scoring: Divide the points earned by the total possible points. Failure to perform a critical step, indicated by an asterisk (*), results in an unsatisfactory overall score.

Time began _____ Time ended _____ Total minutes: _____

Steps	Possible Points	Attempt 1	Attempt 2	Attempt 3
*1. Research the resources available in the surrounding area.	25	____	____	____
*2. Prepare a document or spreadsheet containing a list of the various resources. Include the following information: a. Agency's name b. Agency's purpose or mission c. Physical address d. Mailing address, if different e. Phone numbers f. Contact name g. Hours of operation h. Services offered or performed	25	____	____	____
*3. Update the information whenever a change is necessary.	25	____	____	____
*4. Provide referrals to patients as needed.	25	____	____	____

Comments:

Points earned _____ ÷ 100 possible points = Score _____ % Score

Instructor's signature _____

Procedure **12-9 Maintain a Current List of Community Resources**

Name _____ Date _____ Score _____

Procedure 12-10 Use Proper Body Mechanics

MAERB/CAAHEP COMPETENCIES: X.P.XI.11
ABHES COMPETENCIES: 8.d

Task: To prevent workplace injuries through the use of proper body mechanics.

Equipment and Supplies
- Ergonomic brochures or instruction sheets
- Computer with Internet access
- Web sites concerned with the prevention of workplace injuries

Standards: Complete the procedure and all critical steps in _____ minutes with a minimum score of 85% within three attempts.

Scoring: Divide the points earned by the total possible points. Failure to perform a critical step, indicated by an asterisk (*), results in an unsatisfactory overall score.

Time began _____ **Time ended** _____ **Total minutes:** _____

Steps	Possible Points	Attempt 1	Attempt 2	Attempt 3
1. Evaluate the workplace and workstation for ergonomic issues.	25	_____	_____	_____
2. Test the weight of a load to be lifted and determine whether a second person should assist with the task.	25	_____	_____	_____
*3. Lift an item using ergonomic guidelines.	25	_____	_____	_____
*4. Demonstrate appropriate ergonomics while seated at a computer workstation.	25	_____	_____	_____

Comments:

Points earned _____ ÷ 100 possible points = Score _____ % Score

Instructor's signature _____

Name _____ Date _____ Score _____

Procedure 12-11 Develop and Maintain a Current List of Community Resources Related to Patients' Healthcare Needs

MAERB/CAAHEP COMPETENCIES: IV.X.P.IV.12
ABHES COMPETENCIES: 8.e

Task: To help patients find organizations that can assist with their needs beyond the physician's office and to establish a list of community resources that can be used for referral purposes.

Equipment and Supplies
- Phone book
- Computer with Internet access
- Library access
- Newspapers
- Local volunteer guides
- Pen or pencil
- Notepad

Standards: Complete the procedure and all critical steps in _____ minutes with a minimum score of 85% within three attempts.

Scoring: Divide the points earned by the total possible points. Failure to perform a critical step, indicated by an asterisk (*), results in an unsatisfactory overall score.

Time began _____ **Time ended** _____ **Total minutes:** _____

Steps	Possible Points	Attempt 1	Attempt 2	Attempt 3
*1. Research the resources available in the local community.	20	____	____	____
*2. Create a document or spreadsheet containing the following information: 　a. Agency's name 　b. Agency's purpose or mission 　c. Physical address 　d. Mailing address, if different 　e. Phone numbers 　f. Web site addresses 　g. Contact names and e-mail information 　h. Hours of operation 　i. Services offered or provided	20	____	____	____
*3. Update the information whenever necessary and at least annually.	20	____	____	____
*4. Provide referrals to agencies upon the physician's or patient's request.	20	____	____	____
*5. Document referrals in the patient's medical record.	20	____	____	____

Comments:

Points earned _____ ÷ 100 possible points = Score _____ % Score

Instructor's signature _____

WORK PRODUCT 12-1

Name: _____

Equipment Inventory

Corresponds to Procedure 12-3

<u>MAERB/CAAHEP COMPETENCIES:</u> V.P.V.10.

<u>ABHES COMPETENCIES:</u> 8.z

Complete the form below according to the instructions in Part V.

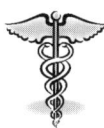

Blackburn Primary Care Associates, PC
1990 Turquoise Drive
Blackburn, WI 54937

Phone: 608-459-8857
Fax: 608-459-8860
E-mail: blackburnom@blackburnpca.com
www.blackburnpca.com

BLACKBURN PRIMARY CARE ASSOCIATES, P.C.

Equipment Inventory List

Purpose:

Date:

Description	Check/P.O. #	Purchased From	Date Purchased	Serial Number	Warranty	Value
					Total	

Copyright © 2011, 2007, 2003 by Saunders, an imprint of Elsevier Inc. All rights reserved.

WORK PRODUCT 12-2

Name: _____

Supply Inventory

Corresponds to Procedure 12-3

<u>MAERB/CAAHEP COMPETENCIES:</u> V.P.V.10.

<u>ABHES COMPETENCIES:</u> 8.z

Complete the form below page according to the instructions in Part VI.

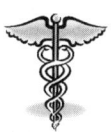

Blackburn Primary Care Associates, PC
1990 Turquoise Drive
Blackburn, WI 54937

Phone: 608-459-8857
Fax: 608-459-8860
E-mail: blackburnom@blackburnpca.com
www.blackburnpca.com

BLACKBURN PRIMARY CARE ASSOCIATES, P.C.

Supply Inventory List

Purpose:

Date:

Description and Item Number	Needed On Hand	Currently On Hand	Date Ordered	Price Per Unit	Total Price	Date Received

WORK PRODUCT 12-3

Name: _____

Equipment Maintenance Log

Corresponds to Procedure 12-5

<u>MAERB/CAAHEP COMPETENCIES:</u> V.P.V.9.

<u>ABHES COMPETENCIES:</u> 8.y

Complete the form on the next page according to the instructions in Part VIII.

EQUIPMENT INVENTORY LIST														Maintenance Schedule				
Physical Condition					Financial Information													
Asset or serial number	Item description (make and model)	Location	Condition	Vendor	Years of service left	Initial value	Down payment	Date purchased or leased	Loan term in years	Loan rate	Monthly payment	Monthly operating costs	Total monthly cost	Maintenance Date	Condition of Equipment	Out of Service?	Maintenance Performed	Date in Service
82069279P	Laptop Computer	Dr. Lopez's Office	EXC	Toshiba	5	$1,695.00	n/a	9/15/2001	n/a	n/a	$	$27.00	$27.00	9/25/2006	EXC	no	None needed	9/25/2006

WORK PRODUCT 12-4

Name: _____

Travel Expense Report

Corresponds to Procedure 12-7

<u>ABHES COMPETENCIES:</u> 8.a, 8.d

Complete the form according to the instructions in Part IX.

Date	Account	Description	Hotel	Transport	Fuel	Meals	Phone	Entertain.	Misc.	TOTAL

Subtotal
Advances
TOTAL

Expense Statement

Statement number: _____

Employee information

Name _____
Employee ID _____
Position _____

Department _____
Manager _____

Pay period

From _____
To _____

307

Work Product **12-4**

WORK PRODUCT 12-5

Name: _____

Develop a Personal (Patient and Employee) Safety Plan

Corresponds to Procedure 12-8

<u>MAERB/CAAHEP COMPETENCIES:</u> X.P.XI. 3

<u>ABHES COMPETENCIES:</u> 4.e.

MEDICAL FACILITY HAZARD ASSESSMENT FORM

This form is a general guideline for assessing hazards in the medical facility. Each facility should produce a customized form that includes any and all hazards that might be present at each facility location. Mark each item as complete (C); not complete (NC), or not applicable (NA).

Location of Facility:	
Date/Time of Inspection:	
Inspector Name:	
Inspector Signature:	

Section A: GENERAL SAFETY ISSUES

#		C	NC	NA
1	Emergency phone numbers are clearly posted in the facility.			
2	Emergency procedures are outlined in the policy/procedure manual and are located in a prominent place for reference.			
3	Emergency codes are clearly explained and posted.			
4	Emergency meeting areas are posted.			
5	Aisles, passageways, walkways, and stairwells are clear of all obstructions.			
6	No trip hazards obstruct hallways or walkways.			
7	Stairways and exits are lighted and clearly negotiable.			
8	Walkways that could be slip hazards during inclement weather are clear and mats are available when needed.			
9	Fire extinguishers are properly located and accessible.			
10	Exits and evacuation routes are clearly marked.			
11	Emergency lighting is working properly.			
12	Storage areas are neat and orderly.			
13	Trash bins are available, clean, and have disposable liners.			

Section B: Hazardous Materials

#		C	NC	NA
1	Employees have been trained on OSHA/CLIA regulations and documentation is available for review in each employee file for both intial and annual training sessions.			
2	Material Safety Data Sheets (MSDS) are available for all hazardous materials and chemicals in the facility.			
3	Spill kits are available.			
4	Hazardous materials are clearly and properly labeled.			
5	Flammable materials are stored safely.			
6	Compressed gas and oxygen cylinders are stored safely.			
7	Personal Protective Equipment (PPE) is available for all employees.			
8	Eyewash and safety showers are located in appropriate areas.			
9	Documentation is available to prove that eyewash and safety showers are tested monthly and found in good working order.			
10	Hazardous waste is located in appropriate biosafety bins.			

Section B: Hazardous Materials (continued)

		C	NC	NA
11	Documentation is available to prove proper disposal of hazardous waste.			
12	Universal waste and hazardous waste are disposed of in separate containers.			
13	Information about hazardous materials is clearly communicated to employees.			
14	The facility's Exposure Control Plan is in use.			
15	Documentation is available to prove that an annual hazard assessment has been completed.			
16	An emergency action plan is available in the facility.			
17	OSHA Form 300 is posted during the required time period.			
18	Records are available to prove that Hepatitis B immunizations were given to employees or declined by the employee.			
19	Employees are aware of procedures for reporting incidents.			
20	Needles are disposed of properly and safely.			
21	Employees are performing procedures only with proper education and training.			

Section C: Electrical Hazards

		C	NC	NA
1	Circuits are not overloaded.			
2	Equipment plugs are properly grounded and in good condition.			
3	Extension cords have a ground plug and are in good condition.			
4	Breaker box switches are clearly labeled.			
5	Surge protectors are clean, free from dust, and not overloaded.			

Section D: Emergency Preparedness

		C	NC	NA
1	An employee and patient safety plan is in place.			
2	Documentation of emergency drills is available.			
3	The role of each employee in emergency situations is delineated and communicated to the employees.			
4	Backup systems are in place for power outages.			
5	Up-to-date information is available regarding community resources.			
6	A stock of emergency supplies is available.			
7	Assessment of naturally-occuring events (e.g. weather) is determined for the geographic area and included in the employee and patient safety plan.			
8	Technological hazards are included in the safety plan.			
9	Human hazards (e.g. mass casualties, bomb threats) are included in drills and safety plans.			

Name _____ Date _____ Score _____

Procedure 13-1 Compose Professional Business Letters

MAERB/CAAHEP COMPETENCIES: IV.P.IV.10
ABHES COMPETENCIES: 7.a(1), 7.a(2), 7.b(1), 8.jj

Task: To compose a professional business letter that conveys information in an accurate and concise manner and that is easy for the reader to comprehend.

Equipment and Supplies
- Computer
- Word processing software
- Draft paper
- Letterhead
- Printer
- Pen or pencil
- Highlighter
- Envelope
- Correspondence to be answered
- Other pertinent information needed to compose a letter
- Electronic or paper dictionary and thesaurus
- Writer's handbook
- Portfolio and/or templates

Standards: Complete the procedure and all critical steps in _____ minutes with a minimum score of 85% within three attempts.

Scoring: Divide the points earned by the total possible points. Failure to perform a critical step, indicated by an asterisk (*), results in an unsatisfactory overall score.

Time began _____ Time ended _____ Total minutes: _____

Steps	Possible Points	Attempt 1	Attempt 2	Attempt 3
1. Determine the reason for sending the correspondence and the intended goals.	10	____	____	____
2. Open a document on the computer to prepare a draft of the letter and save it for future reference.	5	____	____	____
*3. Date the letter.	5	____	____	____
*4. Type the inside address.	5	____	____	____
*5. Type a subject line and list the patient's name or the subject of the correspondence.	10	____	____	____
*6. Type the body of the letter, paying strict attention to its goals.	10	____	____	____
*7. Type the closing of the letter and use the name of the person who will be considered the author.	10	____	____	____

Steps	Possible Points	Attempt 1	Attempt 2	Attempt 3
*8. Proofread the document for accuracy and spelling.	10			
*9. Make any necessary corrections to the letter.	10			
*10. Reread the letter to ensure that the goals have been met.	5			
*11. Address the envelope according to USPS OCR guidelines.	10			
*12. Affix the correct postage and mail the letter.	10			

Comments:

Points earned _____ ÷ 100 possible points = Score _____ % Score

Instructor's signature _____

Name _____ Date _____ Score _____

Procedure 13-2 Report Relevant Information to Others Succinctly and Accurately

MAERB/CAAHEP COMPETENCIES: IV.P.IV.2
ABHES COMPETENCIES: 7.b(1), 8.hh, 8.jj

Task: To compose a clearly written, grammatically correct business letter or memo that can be easily understood by the reader and to eliminate spelling and grammatical errors.

Equipment and Supplies
- Stationery
- Computer
- Correspondence to be answered or notes
- Proofreader's marks guide

Standards: Complete the procedure and all critical steps in _____ minutes with a minimum score of 85% within three attempts.

Scoring: Divide the points earned by the total possible points. Failure to perform a critical step, indicated by an asterisk (*), results in an unsatisfactory overall score.

Time began _____ **Time ended** _____ **Total minutes:** _____

Steps	Possible Points	Attempt 1	Attempt 2	Attempt 3
1. Scan the letter to be answered or the notes for the memo to be composed.	10	_____	_____	_____
*2. Compose the letter or memo, using good grammar.	10	_____	_____	_____
*3. Print a draft of the letter or memo.	10	_____	_____	_____
*4. Proofread the draft carefully, highlighting changes and noting additions to be made.	10	_____	_____	_____
*5. Revise the letter according to the notes.	20	_____	_____	_____
*6. Proofread the final draft.	10	_____	_____	_____
*7. Print the final draft.	10	_____	_____	_____
*8. Allow a co-worker to proofread the letter and make any necessary corrections.	10	_____	_____	_____
*9. Make a file copy of the letter or memo and distribute it appropriately.	10	_____	_____	_____

Comments:

Points earned _____ ÷ 100 possible points = Score _____ % Score

Instructor's signature _____

Name _____ Date _____ Score _____

Procedure 13-3 Receive, Organize, Prioritize, and Transmit Information Expediently

MAERB/CAAHEP COMPETENCIES: IV.P.IV.10, IV.P.IV.2
ABHES COMPETENCIES: 7.b(1), 8.a, 8.b, 8.hh, 8.jj

Task: To efficiently sort through the mail that arrives in the medical office on a daily basis.

Equipment and Supplies
- Computer
- Draft paper
- Letterhead stationery
- Pen or pencil
- Highlighter
- Staple remover
- Paper clips
- Letter opener
- Stapler
- Transparent tape
- Date stamp

Standards: Complete the procedure and all critical steps in _____ minutes with a minimum score of 85% within three attempts.

Scoring: Divide the points earned by the total possible points. Failure to perform a critical step, indicated by an asterisk (*), results in an unsatisfactory overall score.

Time began _____ Time ended _____ Total minutes: _____

Steps	Possible Points	Attempt 1	Attempt 2	Attempt 3
1. Clear work space on the desk.	10			
2. Sort the mail according to importance and urgency so that the most important issues can be addressed first.	10			
3. Stack the envelopes so that they all face the same direction and open them along the top edge.	10			
*4. Open the mail neatly and in an organized manner.	10			
*5. Remove the contents and paper clip the documents together, if necessary. Hold the envelope to the light or visually examine it to make sure all documents have been removed.	20			
*6. Make a note of the postmark, if necessary.	10			

Steps	Possible Points	Attempt 1	Attempt 2	Attempt 3
*7. Date stamp the letter and secure any enclosures.	20	_____	_____	_____
*8. Organize the mail for transmission to each person and distribute it at the appropriate time. Make additions to patients' medical records where indicated and/or required according to office policy and legislation.	10	_____	_____	_____

Comments:

Points earned _____ ÷ 100 possible points = Score _____ % Score

Instructor's signature _____

Name _____ Date _____ Score _____

Procedure 13-4 Address an Envelope According to Postal Service Optical Character Reader Guidelines

MAERB/CAAHEP COMPETENCIES: IV.P.IV.10, IV.P.IV.2
ABHES COMPETENCIES: 7.b(1), 8.hh, 8.jj

Task: To correctly address business correspondence so that the mail arrives at the post office and is processed by the U. S. Postal Service as efficiently as possible.

Equipment and Supplies
- Envelopes
- Computer
- Correspondence

Standards: Complete the procedure and all critical steps in _____ minutes with a minimum score of 85% within three attempts.

Scoring: Divide the points earned by the total possible points. Failure to perform a critical step, indicated by an asterisk (*), results in an unsatisfactory overall score.

Time began _____   **Time ended** _____   **Total minutes:** _____

Steps	Possible Points	Attempt 1	Attempt 2	Attempt 3
1. Place the envelope in the printer.	10	___	___	___
*2. Enter the word processing program and check the TOOLS section for envelopes. The address block should start no higher than 2¼ inches from the bottom. Leave a bottom margin of at least ⅝ inch and left and right margins of at least 1 inch.	20	___	___	___
*3. Use dark type on a light background, no script or italics, and capitalize everything in the address.	10	___	___	___
*4. Type the address in block format, using only approved abbreviations and eliminating all punctuation.	20	___	___	___
*5. Type the city, state, and ZIP code on the last line of the address.	10	___	___	___
*6. No line should have more than 27 total characters, including spaces.	10	___	___	___
*7. Leave a ⅝ × 4¾-inch blank space in the bottom right corner of the envelope.	10	___	___	___
*8. Make sure the envelope is addressed accurately, considering the requirements for overseas mailing if applicable.	10	___	___	___

Comments:

Points earned _____ ÷ 100 possible points = Score _____ % Score

Instructor's signature _____

WORK PRODUCT 13-1

Name: _____

Addressing an Envelope

Corresponds to Procedure 13-1, 13-2, and 13-4

MAERB/CAAHEP COMPETENCIES: IV.P.IV.10, IV.P.IV.2

ABHES COMPETENCIES: 7.a(1), 7.a(2), 7.b(1), 8.jj

Complete the envelopes below according to the directions in Part I, questions 1-3.

Blackburn Primary Care Associates, P.C.
1990 Turquoise Drive
Blackburn, WI 54937

Blackburn Primary Care Associates, P.C.
1990 Turquoise Drive
Blackburn, WI 54937

Blackburn Primary Care Associates, P.C.
1990 Turquoise Drive
Blackburn, WI 54937

WORK PRODUCT 13-2

Name: _____

Initiating Correspondence

Corresponds to Procedure 13-1, 13-2, and 13-4

<u>CAAHEP COMPETENCIES:</u> IV.P.IV.10, IV.P.IV.2

<u>ABHES COMPETENCIES:</u> 7.b(1), 8.a, 8.b, 8.hh, 8.jj

Using the form below, write a letter according to the directions in Part III, question A.

Blackburn Primary Care Associates
1990 Turquoise Drive
Blackburn, WI 54937
(555) 555-1234

WORK PRODUCT 13-3

Name: _____

Initiating a Memo

Corresponds to Procedure 13-1, 13-2, and 13-4

<u>CAAHEP COMPETENCIES:</u> IV.P.IV.10, IV.P.IV.2

<u>ABHES COMPETENCIES:</u> 7.b(1), 8.a, 8.b, 8.hh, 8.jj

Using the form below, write a memo according to the directions in Part III, question B.

MEMORANDUM

Date:

To:

From:

Subject:

WORK PRODUCT 13-4

Name: _____

Responding to Correspondence

Corresponds to Procedure 13-1, 13-2, and 13-3

<u>CAAHEP COMPETENCIES:</u> IV.P.IV.10, IV.P.IV.2

<u>ABHES COMPETENCIES:</u> 7.b(1), 8.a, 8.b, 8.hh, 8.jj

Using the form below, write a letter according to the directions in Part III, question C.

Blackburn Primary Care Associates
1990 Turquoise Drive
Blackburn, WI 54937
(555) 555-1234

WORK PRODUCT 13-5

Name: _____

Responding to a Memo

Corresponds to Procedure 13-1, 13-2, and 13-3

CAAHEP COMPETENCIES: IV.P.IV.10, IV.P.IV.2

ABHES COMPETENCIES: 7.b(1), 8.a, 8.b, 8.hh, 8.jj

Using the form below, write a memo according to the directions in Part III, question D.

MEMORANDUM

Date:

To:

From:

Subject:

WORK PRODUCT 13-6

Name: _____

Initiating a Fax

Corresponds to Procedure 13-1, 13-2, and 13-3

CAAHEP COMPETENCIES: IV.P.IV.10, IV.P.IV.2

ABHES COMPETENCIES: 7.b(1), 8.a, 8.b, 8.hh, 8.jj

Design a coversheet for a fax message using the form below according to the directions in Part III, question E.

Blackburn Primary Care Associates
1990 Turquoise Drive
Blackburn, WI 54937
(555) 555-1234

Name _____ Date _____ Score _____

Procedure 14-1 Organize a Patient's Medical Record

MAERB/CAAHEP COMPETENCIES: V.P.V.3
ABHES COMPETENCIES: 8.b

Task: To create a medical file for a new patient that will contain all the personal data necessary for a complete record and any other information required by the facility.

Equipment and Supplies
- Computer
- Clerical supplies (pen, clipboard)
- Registration form
- File folder
- Color-coded labels for folder
- Index label for folder tab
- Identification (ID) card, if using a numeric system
- Cross-reference card, if needed
- Financial ledger, if needed
- Routing slip
- Private conference area

Standards: Complete the procedure and all critical steps in _____ minutes with a minimum score of 85% within three attempts.

Scoring: Divide the points earned by the total possible points. Failure to perform a critical step, indicated by an asterisk (*), results in an unsatisfactory overall score.

Time began _____ Time ended _____ Total minutes: _____

Steps	Possible Points	Attempt 1	Attempt 2	Attempt 3
1. Determine that the patient is new to the office.	10	___	___	___
*2. Obtain and record the required personal data.	10	___	___	___
*3. Enter the information on the patient history form.	10	___	___	___
*4. Review the entire form.	10	___	___	___
*5. Select the label and file folder for the record.	10	___	___	___
*6. Type the caption on the label and put it on the folder.	10	___	___	___
*7. For numeric filing, prepare a cross-reference.	10	___	___	___
*8. Prepare the financial card or enter the data into a computerized ledger.	10	___	___	___

Steps	Possible Points	Attempt 1	Attempt 2	Attempt 3
*9. Put the patient history form and other required forms in the folder.	10			
*10. Clip an encounter form on the outside of the folder.	10			
11. Prepare electronic records as prescribed by the software system.	N/A			

Comments:

Points earned _____ ÷ 100 possible points = Score _____ % Score

Instructor's signature _____

Name _____ Date _____ Score _____

Procedure 14-2 Prepare an Informed Consent for Treatment Form

MAERB/CAAHEP COMPETENCIES: V.P.V.3
ABHES COMPETENCIES: 8.b

Task: To adequately and completely inform the patient about the treatment or procedure the person is to receive and to provide legal protection for the facility and the provider.

Equipment and Supplies
- Pen
- Consent form

Standards: Complete the procedure and all critical steps in _____ minutes with a minimum score of 85% within three attempts.

Scoring: Divide the points earned by the total possible points. Failure to perform a critical step, indicated by an asterisk (*), results in an unsatisfactory overall score.

Time began _____   Time ended _____   Total minutes: _____

Steps	Possible Points	Attempt 1	Attempt 2	Attempt 3
1. After the physician provides the details of the procedure to be done, prepare the consent form. Make sure the form addresses the following: a. Nature of the procedure or treatment b. Risks and/or benefits of the procedure or treatment c. Any reasonable alternatives to the procedure or treatment d. Risks and/or benefits of each alternative e. Risks and/or benefits of not performing the procedure or treatment	20	_____	_____	_____
2. Personalize the form with the patient's name and any other demographic information the form requires.	10	_____	_____	_____
*3. Give the form to the physician to use in counseling the patient about the procedure.	10	_____	_____	_____
4. Witness the patient's signature on the form, if necessary. The physician usually signs the form as well.	10	_____	_____	_____
*5. Provide the patient with a copy of the consent form.	10	_____	_____	_____

Steps	Possible Points	Attempt 1	Attempt 2	Attempt 3
6. Put the consent form in the patient's chart. The facility where the procedure is to be performed may require a copy.	10	_____	_____	_____
*7. Ask the patient if he or she has any questions about the procedure. Refer questions that you, as the medical assistant, cannot or should not answer to the physician. Make sure all the patient's questions are answered.	20	_____	_____	_____
*8. Provide the patient with the information about the date and time of the procedure.	10	_____	_____	_____

Comments:

Points earned _____ ÷ 100 possible points = Score _____ % Score

Instructor's signature _____

Name _____ Date _____ Score _____

Procedure 14-3 Add Supplementary Items to Patients' Records

MAERB/CAAHEP COMPETENCIES: V.P.V.3
ABHES COMPETENCIES: 8.a, 8.b

Task: To add supplementary documents and progress notes to patients' histories, observing standard steps in filing while creating an orderly file that facilitates ready reference to any item of information.

Equipment and Supplies
- Assorted correspondence, diagnostic reports, and progress notes
- Patients' files
- Computer
- Mending tape
- FILE stamp or pen
- Sorter
- Stapler

Standards: Complete the procedure and all critical steps in _____ minutes with a minimum score of 85% within three attempts.

Scoring: Divide the points earned by the total possible points. Failure to perform a critical step, indicated by an asterisk (*), results in an unsatisfactory overall score.

Time began _____ Time ended _____ Total minutes: _____

Steps	Possible Points	Attempt 1	Attempt 2	Attempt 3
*1. Group all papers according to the patients' names.	20			
*2. Remove any staples or paper clips.	10			
*3. Mend any damaged or torn records.	10			
*4. Attach any small items to standard-size paper.	10			
*5. Group any related papers together.	10			
*6. Put your initials or FILE stamp in the upper left corner.	10			
*7. Code the document by underlining or writing the patient's name in the upper right corner.	10			
*8. Continue steps 2 through 7 until all documents have been conditioned, released, indexed, and coded.	10			
*9. Place all documents in the sorter in filing sequence.	10			

Comments:

Points earned _____ ÷ 100 possible points = Score _____ % Score

Instructor's signature _____

Name _____ Date _____ Score _____

Procedure 14-4 Prepare a Record Release Form

MAERB/CAAHEP COMPETENCIES: IX.P. IX.3
ABHES COMPETENCIES: 4.b

Task: To provide a legal document indicating the patient's consent to the release of his or her medical records to another provider or healthcare facility following HIPAA regulations.

Equipment and Supplies
- Medical record release form
- Pen
- Envelope

Standards: Complete the procedure and all critical steps in _____ minutes with a minimum score of 85% within three attempts.

Scoring: Divide the points earned by the total possible points. Failure to perform a critical step, indicated by an asterisk (*), results in an unsatisfactory overall score.

Time began _____   **Time ended** _____   **Total minutes:** _____

Steps	Possible Points	Attempt 1	Attempt 2	Attempt 3
1. Explain to the patient that a medical record release form will be necessary to obtain records from another provider. If the patient is having records sent to another provider, a release will also be required.	20	____	____	____
*2. Review the record release form with the patient and ask if the person understands the form and if he or she has any questions about it.	20	____	____	____
*3. Have the patient sign the form in the space indicated. If other demographic information is required, (e.g., Social Security number or other names used), complete that information as well.	20	____	____	____
*4. Make a copy of the form for the file and then mail the form to the appropriate facility. Note the date the form was sent. Provide a copy to the patient if requested.	20	____	____	____
5. Follow up to make sure the requested records actually arrive.	20	____	____	____

Comments:

Points earned _____ ÷ 100 possible points = Score _____ % Score

Instructor's signature _____

Name _____ Date _____ Score _____

Procedure 14-5 File Medical Records Using an Alphabetic System

MAERB/CAAHEP COMPETENCIES: V.P.V.4
ABHES COMPETENCIES: 8.b

Task: To file records efficiently using an alphabetic system and to ensure that the records can be retrieved easily and quickly.

Equipment and Supplies
- Medical records
- Physical filing equipment
- Cart to carry records, if needed
- Alphabetic file guide
- Staple remover
- Stapler

Standards: Complete the procedure and all critical steps in _____ minutes with a minimum score of 85% within three attempts.

Scoring: Divide the points earned by the total possible points. Failure to perform a critical step, indicated by an asterisk (*), results in an unsatisfactory overall score.

Time began _____ Time ended _____ Total minutes: _____

Steps	Possible Points	Attempt 1	Attempt 2	Attempt 3
*1. Using alphabetic guidelines, put the records to be filed in alphabetic order. If a stack of documents is to be filed, place them in alphabetic order inside an alphabetic file guide or sorter. Use rules for filing documents alphabetically.	20	_____	_____	_____
*2. Go to the filing storage equipment (shelves, cabinets, or drawers) and locate the spot in the alphabet for the first file.	20	_____	_____	_____
*3. Put the file in the cabinet or drawer in correct alphabetic order.	20	_____	_____	_____
*4. If you are adding a document to a file, put it on top so that the most recent information is seen first. This puts the information in the file in reverse chronologic order.	20	_____	_____	_____
*5. Securely fasten all documents to the medical record; do not just drop the documents inside it. Refile the medical record in its proper place.	20	_____	_____	_____

Comments:

Points earned _____ ÷ 100 possible points = Score _____ % Score

Instructor's signature _____

Name _____ Date _____ Score _____

Procedure 14-6 File Medical Records Using a Numeric System

MAERB/CAAHEP COMPETENCIES: V.P.V.4
ABHES COMPETENCIES: 8.b

Task: To file records efficiently using a numeric system and ensure that the records can be easily and quickly retrieved.

Equipment and Supplies
- Medical records
- Physical filing equipment
- Cart to carry records, if needed
- Numeric file guide
- Staple remover
- Stapler
- Paper clips

Standards: Complete the procedure and all critical steps in _____ minutes with a minimum score of 85% within three attempts.

Scoring: Divide the points earned by the total possible points. Failure to perform a critical step, indicated by an asterisk (*), results in an unsatisfactory overall score.

Time began _____ Time ended _____ Total minutes: _____

Steps	Possible Points	Attempt 1	Attempt 2	Attempt 3
*1. Using numeric guidelines, put the records to be filed in numeric order. If a stack of documents is to be filed, write the chart number on the document. Use rules for filing documents alphabetically.	20			
*2. Go to the filing storage equipment (shelves, cabinets, or drawers) and locate the numeric spot for the first file.	20			
*3. Put the file in the cabinet or drawer in correct numeric order.	20			
*4. If you are adding a document to a file, put it on top so that the most recent information is seen first. This puts the information in the file in reverse chronologic order.	20			
*5. Securely fasten all documents to the medical record. Do not just drop the documents inside the medical record. Refile the medical record in its proper place.	20			

Comments:

Points earned _____ ÷ 100 possible points = Score _____ % Score

Instructor's signature _____

Name _____ Date _____ Score _____

Procedure 14-7 Maintain Organization by Filing

MAERB/CAAHEP COMPETENCIES: V.P.V.8, V.A.V.1
ABHES COMPETENCIES: 8.b

Task: To make sure various office filing systems are maintained and can be used by all staff members at the medical facility.

Equipment and Supplies
- Documents to be filed
- Various file folders
- Office filing systems (e.g., equipment maintenance, general office, and so on, if the facility's files are not kept in one general grouping)
- Clerical supplies

Standards: Complete the procedure and all critical steps in _____ minutes with a minimum score of 85% within three attempts.

Scoring: Divide the points earned by the total possible points. Failure to perform a critical step, indicated by an asterisk (*), results in an unsatisfactory overall score.

Time began _____ **Time ended** _____ **Total minutes:** _____

Steps	Possible Points	Attempt 1	Attempt 2	Attempt 3
1. Identify the correct filing system for the document.	20	_____	_____	_____
*2. Inspect the document to be added.	20	_____	_____	_____
*3. Add the document to the proper file in the correct filing system.	20	_____	_____	_____
*4. Attach the document to the file permanently or according to office policy.	20	_____	_____	_____
*5. Attach documents in the file with the most recent on top. Then place the record in the designated place in the filing system.	10	_____	_____	_____
*6. Continue the process until all documents have been filed.	10	_____	_____	_____

Did the student: **Yes**   **No**

Consider the staff's needs and limitations in establishing a filing system?   _____   _____

Comments:

Points earned _____ ÷ 100 possible points = Score _____ % Score

Instructor's signature _____

Name _____ Date _____ Score _____

Procedure 14-8 Document Patient Care Accurately

MAERB/CAAHEP COMPETENCIES: IV.P.IV.8
ABHES COMPETENCIES: 4.a

Task: To document appropriately and accurately in all medical records and other office paperwork that concerns the patient.

Equipment and Supplies
- Any medical document
- Clerical supplies
- Computer
- Office policy and procedures manual
- Progress notes

Standards: Complete the procedure and all critical steps in _____ minutes with a minimum score of 85% within three attempts.

Scoring: Divide the points earned by the total possible points. Failure to perform a critical step, indicated by an asterisk (*), results in an unsatisfactory overall score.

Time began _____ **Time ended** _____ **Total minutes:** _____

Steps	Possible Points	Attempt 1	Attempt 2	Attempt 3
*1. Determine the entry to be made into the document.	5	_____	_____	_____
*2. Make the entry in legible handwriting.	20	_____	_____	_____
*3. Check the entry for accuracy.	20	_____	_____	_____
*4. Authenticate the entry.	20	_____	_____	_____
*5. Make a correction to the same entry.	10	_____	_____	_____
*6. Authenticate the corrected entry.	10	_____	_____	_____
*7. Check the entry for accuracy.	10	_____	_____	_____
*8. Put the document in the appropriate record or file.	5	_____	_____	_____

Comments:

Points earned _____ ÷ 100 possible points = Score _____ % Score

Instructor's signature _____

WORK PRODUCT 14-1

Name: _____

Document Patient Care Accurately

Corresponds to Procedure 14-8

<u>MAERB/CAAHEP COMPETENCIES:</u> IV.P.IV.8.

<u>ABHES COMPETENCIES:</u> 4.a.

OUTLINE FORMAT PROGRESS NOTES

Patient Name _____

Prob. No. or Letter	DATE	S Subjective	O Objective	A Assess	P Plans	Page _____

Start each Progress Note (Subjective, Objective, Assessment and Plans) at the appropriate shaded column to create an outline form. Write through the Intervening columns to the right margin of the page.

ORDER # 26-7115 ANDRUS CLINI-REC CHART ORGANIZING SYSTEMS • 1976 BIBBERO SYSTEMS, INC. • PETALUMA, CA.
TO REORDER CALL TOLL FREE: (800) BIBBERO (800-242-2376) OR FAX (800) 242-9330 www.bibbero.com MFG IN U.S.A.

Name _____ Date _____ Score _____

Procedure 15-1 Document Patient Education Accurately

CAAHEP COMPETENCIES: IV.P.IV.9
ABHES COMPETENCIES: 9.r

Task: To document instructional and educational information that is offered to guide patients toward activities that will lead to good health and disease prevention.

Equipment and Supplies
- Brochures related to health information and disease prevention
- Patient information sheets (copied or computer-generated)
- Patient instruction sheets (copied or computer-generated)
- Fact sheets on various diseases and conditions
- Supplies related to the subject (e.g., needles for instruction in insulin injection)
- Patient's medical record
- Instructional DVDs, if available
- Information on websites that provide interactive educational programs

Standards: Complete the procedure and all critical steps in _____ minutes with a minimum score of 85% within three attempts.

Scoring: Divide the points earned by the total possible points. Failure to perform a critical step, indicated by an asterisk (*), results in an unsatisfactory overall score.

Time began _____ **Time ended** _____ **Total minutes:** _____

Steps	Possible Points	Attempt 1	Attempt 2	Attempt 3
1. Determine the supplies (including paperwork) needed to teach the patient according to the physician's instructions.	5			
*2. Take the patient to a quiet area where confidentiality can be reasonably expected.	10			
*3. Explain the subject of the educational session.	10			
*4. Explain that the physician wants the patient to follow certain instructions or to gain a good understanding of the condition.	10			
*5. Review each topic with the patient, one at a time.	10			
*6. Demonstrate any procedures the patient must learn and allow the patient to return the demonstration.	10			
*7. Determine whether the patient has questions about any part of the procedure. Ask the patient whether he or she feels confident in performing the procedure.	10			

Steps	Possible Points	Attempt 1	Attempt 2	Attempt 3
8. Give the handout information to the patient, if applicable.	10			
*9. Document the educational session in the patient's medical record.	10			
*10. Choose a date to follow up with the patient to address any additional questions or concerns. Document the follow-up call in the patient's medical record.	10			
*11. Encourage the patient to call the office if any questions arise.	5			

Comments:

Points earned _____ ÷ 100 possible points = Score _____ % Score

Instructor's signature _____

Name _____ Date _____ Score _____

Procedure 15-2 Execute Data Management Using Electronic Healthcare Records such as the EMR

CAAHEP COMPETENCIES: V.P.V.5
ABHES COMPETENCIES: 7.b.(2), 8.b, 8.ll

Task: To obtain and enter patient data using the electronic health record (EHR) and/or the electronic medical record (EMR).

Equipment and Supplies
- Patient's medical records
- Data to be included in medical records
- Computer

Standards: Complete the procedure and all critical steps in _____ minutes with a minimum score of 85% within three attempts.

Scoring: Divide the points earned by the total possible points. Failure to perform a critical step, indicated by an asterisk (*), results in an unsatisfactory overall score.

Time began _____ **Time ended** _____ **Total minutes:** _____

Steps	Possible Points	Attempt 1	Attempt 2	Attempt 3
*1. Welcome the patient warmly, maintaining eye contact.	10			
*2. Open the EMR.	10			
*3. Position yourself so that the computer is not between you and the patient.	10			
*4. Verify the patient's demographics.	10			
*5. Discuss the reason for the patient's visit to the physician and document the data in the EMR.	10			
*6. Keep eye contact with the patient, not the computer keyboard, especially while talking.	10			
*7. Use proper techniques for entering information into the EMR.	10			
*8. Ask the patient whether information about any other concerns should be added to the EMR.	10			
*9. Review the information entered with the patient for clarity.	10			
*10. Electronically sign all entries and save the data.	10			

Comments:

Points earned _____ ÷ 100 possible points = Score _____ % Score

Instructor's signature _____

WORK PRODUCT 15-1

Name: _____

Document Patient Education Accurately

Corresponds to Procedure 15-1

CAAHEP COMPETENCIES: IV.P.IV.9.

ABHES COMPETENCIES: 2.a., 9.r.

OUTLINE FORMAT PROGRESS NOTES

Patient Name _____

Prob. No. or Letter	DATE	S Subjective	O Objective	A Assess	P Plans	Page _____

Start each Progress Note (Subjective, Objective, Assessment and Plans) at the appropriate shaded column to create an outline form. Write through the Intervening columns to the right margin of the page.

Name _____ Date _____ Score _____

Procedure 17-1 Apply HIPAA Rules for Privacy and Release of Information

MAERB/CAAHEP COMPETENCIES: IX.P.IX.3
ABHES COMPETENCIES: 4.b

Task: To follow guidelines established by the Health Insurance Portability and Accountability Act (HIPAA) to keep patient confidentiality and to protect the patient's health information.

EQUIPMENT and SUPPLIES
- HIPAA rule
- Office policy and procedures manual
- Release of information forms
- Notice of privacy policy

Standards: Complete the procedure and all critical steps in _____ minutes with a minimum score of 85% within three attempts.

Scoring: Divide the points earned by the total possible points. Failure to perform a critical step, indicated by an asterisk (*), results in an unsatisfactory overall score.

Time began _____ **Time ended** _____ **Total minutes:** _____

Steps	Possible Points	Attempt 1	Attempt 2	Attempt 3
1. Review HIPAA rules and office policy regarding the release of patient information and confidentiality in the facility.	10	_____	_____	_____
*2. Review the notice of privacy practices for the facility.	10	_____	_____	_____
*3. Review the facility's authorization to release medical records form.	10	_____	_____	_____
*4. Thoroughly read the request for information.	10	_____	_____	_____
*5. Determine whether the document is valid.	10	_____	_____	_____
*6. Determine the exact information being requested.	10	_____	_____	_____
7. Make sure the release of information form is one designated by the facility or one that contains all the same information.	10	_____	_____	_____

Steps	Possible Points	Attempt 1	Attempt 2	Attempt 3
8. Make the requestor complete one of the facility's request forms, if necessary	10			
*9. Forward only the information requested to the person or representative of the organization who presented the authorization for release of information.	10			
*10. Release the information by mail or to the agent of the requestor.	10			

Comments:

Points earned _____ ÷ 100 possible points = Score _____ % Score

Instructor's signature _____

Name _____ Date _____ Score _____

Procedure 17-2 Perform Risk Management Procedures

ABHES COMPETENCIES: 4.e

Task: To prevent situations that may result in risks and liability in the physician's office.

Equipment and Supplies
- Copy of laws affecting the physician's practice
- Computer with Internet access
- Office policy and procedure manual

Standards: Complete the procedure and all critical steps in _____ minutes with a minimum score of 85% within three attempts.

Scoring: Divide the points earned by the total possible points. Failure to perform a critical step, indicated by an asterisk (*), results in an unsatisfactory overall score.

Time began _____ **Time ended** _____ **Total minutes:** _____

Steps	Possible Points	Attempt 1	Attempt 2	Attempt 3
*1. Become familiar with laws affecting medical practice.	20			
*2. Become familiar with office policies and procedures.	20			
*3. Choose one law to research and present risk management procedures to help the practice remain in compliance.	20			
*4. Present the report to the class.	20			
*5. Provide the instructor with a copy of the report.	20			

Comments:

Points earned _____ ÷ 100 possible points = Score _____ % Score

Instructor's signature _____

Name _____ Date _____ Score _____

Procedure 18-1 Perform ICD-9-CM Coding

MAERB/CAAHEP COMPETENCIES: IV.P.IV.3, VII.P.VII.2, VIII.P.VIII.2, VIII.A.VIII.1
ABHES COMPETENCIES: 8.r., 8.t., 8.u., 8.v.

Task: To perform accurate diagnosis coding using the ICD-9-CM manual.

Equipment and Supplies
- ICD-9-CM manual (volumes 1 and 2, current year)
- Encounter form or charge ticket
- Medical record
- Paper
- Pen or pencil

Standards: Complete the procedure and all critical steps in _____ minutes with a minimum score of 85% within three attempts.

Scoring: Divide the points earned by the total possible points. Failure to perform a critical step, indicated by an asterisk (*), results in an unsatisfactory overall score.

Time began _____ Time ended _____ Total minutes: _____

Steps	Possible Points	Attempt 1	Attempt 2	Attempt 3
Preparation				
*1. Abstract the diagnostic statement or statements from the encounter form and/or the patient's medical record.	10	___	___	___
From the Alphabetic Index				
*2. Locate the main terms taken from the diagnostic statement in the Alphabetic Index (volume 2) of the ICD-9-CM manual.	10	___	___	___
3. Locate the modifying words listed under the main term in the ICD-9-CM manual.	10	___	___	___
4. Review the conventions, punctuation, and notes in the Alphabetic Index.	10	___	___	___
5. Choose a tentative code, codes, or code range from the Alphabetic Index that matches the diagnostic statement as closely as possible.	10	___	___	___

Steps	Possible Points	Attempt 1	Attempt 2	Attempt 3

From the Tabular Index

6. Look up the codes chosen from the Alphabetic Index in the Tabular Index (volume 1).	10			
7. Review the notes, conventions, and ICD-9-CM Official Coding Guidelines associated with the code and code description in the Tabular Index.	10			
*8. Verify the tentative code's accuracy in the Tabular Index.	10			
*9. Carry the codes to the highest level of specificity.	10			
*10. Assign the code.	10			

Did the student demonstrate an ability to work with the physician to achieve the maximum reimbursement?

Comments:

Points earned _____ ÷ 100 possible points = Score _____ % Score

Instructor's signature _____

Name _____ Date _____ Score _____

Procedure 19-1 Perform Procedural Coding: CPT Coding

MAERB/CAAHEP COMPETENCIES: IV.P.IV.3, VIII.P.VIII.1, VIII.A.VIII.1
ABHES COMPETENCIES: 8.r., 8.t., 8.u., 8.v

Task: To use the steps for procedure and service coding to find the most accurate and specific CPT Category I code.

Equipment and Supplies
- CPT Coding Manual (current year)
- Encounter form (charge ticket)
- Medical record
- Paper
- Pen or pencil
- Medical dictionary or medical terminology reference book

Standards: Complete the procedure and all critical steps in _____ minutes with a minimum score of 85% within three attempts.

Scoring: Divide the points earned by the total possible points. Failure to perform a critical step, indicated by an asterisk (*), results in an unsatisfactory overall score.

Time began _____ Time ended _____ Total minutes: _____

Steps	Possible Points	Attempt 1	Attempt 2	Attempt 3
*1. Abstract the procedures and/or services performed from the medical documentation.	10			
2. Select the most appropriate main term to begin the search in the Alphabetic Index.	10			
3. Determine the main and modifying terms from the abstracted information.	10			
*4. Select a modifying term (or terms), if needed, once the main term has been located. If no modifying term produces an appropriate code or code range, repeat steps 2 and 3 using a different main term classification.	10			
5. Find the code or code ranges that include all or most of the medical record procedure or service description. Disregard any code containing descriptions or wording not included in the medical record.	5			
6. Write down the code or code ranges that best match medical documentation.	5			
*7. Turn to the main text (Tabular Index) and find the first code or code range chosen from the Alphabetic Index.	10			

Steps	Possible Points	Attempt 1	Attempt 2	Attempt 3
8. Compare the description of the code with the medical documentation. Verify that all or most of the medical record documentation matches the code description.	10	_____	_____	_____
9. Read the guidelines and notes for the section, subsection, and code to ensure that no contraindications prevent use of the code.	5	_____	_____	_____
10. Evaluate the conventions.	5	_____	_____	_____
11. Determine whether special circumstances require a modifier. Determine whether a Special Report is required.	10	_____	_____	_____
*12. Assign the code.	10	_____	_____	_____

Did the student demonstrate an ability to work with the physician to achieve the maximum reimbursement?

Comments:

Points earned _____ ÷ 100 possible points = Score _____ % Score

Instructor's signature _____

Name _____ Date _____ Score _____

Procedure 19-2 Perform Procedural Coding: Evaluation and Management (E&M) Coding

MAERB/CAAHEP COMPETENCIES: IV.P.IV.3, VIII.P.VIII.1, VIII.A.VIII.1
ABHES COMPETENCIES: 8.r., 8.t., 8.u., 8.v

Task: To use the steps for Evaluation and Management (E&M) coding to find the most accurate and specific CPT Category I E&M section code.

Equipment and Supplies
- CPT Coding Manual (current year)
- Encounter form (charge ticket)
- Medical record
- Paper
- Pen or pencil
- Medical dictionary or medical terminology reference book

Standards: Complete the procedure and all critical steps in _____ minutes with a minimum score of 85% within three attempts.

Scoring: Divide the points earned by the total possible points. Failure to perform a critical step, indicated by an asterisk (*), results in an unsatisfactory overall score.

Time began _____ **Time ended** _____ **Total minutes:** _____

Steps	Possible Points	Attempt 1	Attempt 2	Attempt 3
*1. Determine the place of service.	10			
2. Determine the patient's status.	10			
3. Review the guidelines and notes for the selected subsection, category, or subcategory.	10			
*4. Identify the subsection, category, or subcategory of service in the E&M section.	20			
*5. Review the level of E&M service descriptions for each code in the subsection, category, or subcategory chosen.	10			
6. Determine the level of service: a. Determine the extent of the history obtained. b. Determine the extent of the examination performed. c. Determine the complexity of medical decision making.	20			

Steps	Possible Points	Attempt 1	Attempt 2	Attempt 3
7. If necessary, compare the medical documentation against the examples in Appendix C (Clinical Examples) of the CPT manual.	10	_____	_____	_____
*8. Select the appropriate level of E&M service code and document it in the medical record or on the encounter form.	10	_____	_____	_____

Did the student demonstrate an ability to work with the physician to achieve the maximum reimbursement?

Comments:

Points earned _____ ÷ 100 possible points = Score _____ % Score

Instructor's signature _____

Name _____ Date _____ Score _____

Procedure 19-3 Perform Procedural Coding: Anesthesia Coding

MAERB/CAAHEP COMPETENCIES: IV.P.IV.3, VIII.P.VIII.1, VIII.A.VIII.1
ABHES COMPETENCIES: 8.r., 8.t., 8.u., 8.v

Task: To use the steps to select the most accurate and specific anesthesia code and perform the anesthesia formula calculation to determine the charge for the service.

Equipment and Supplies
- CPT coding manual (current year)
- Encounter form (charge ticket)
- Medical record
- Conversion factor list
- Paper
- Pen or pencil
- Calculator

Standards: Complete the procedure and all critical steps in _____ minutes with a minimum score of 85% within three attempts.

Scoring: Divide the points earned by the total possible points. Failure to perform a critical step, indicated by an asterisk (*), results in an unsatisfactory overall score.

Time began _____ Time ended _____ Total minutes: _____

Steps	Possible Points	Attempt 1	Attempt 2	Attempt 3
*1. Read the medical documentation to determine what procedure or service was provided.	10			
*2. Determine the anatomic site or organ system involved.	10			
3. In the Alphabetic Index, go to the heading "Anesthesia" and find the code or code range that includes all or most of the procedure or service documented in the medical record.	5			
4. Write down the code or code range found in the Alphabetic Index, under the Anesthesia heading, that best matches the medical documentation.	5			
*5. Turn to the main text (Tabular Index), Anesthesia section, and find the code or code range chosen from the Alphabetic Index.	10			
6. Read the guidelines and notes for the section, subsection, category, or subcategory.	5			
7. Evaluate the conventions, especially add-on codes (+) and exemptions from modifier –51.	5			

Steps	Possible Points	Attempt 1	Attempt 2	Attempt 3
*8. Document the code selected.	5			
9. Determine the basic unit value from the Relative Value Guide.	5			
10. Determine the patient's physical status and document the appropriate modifier.	5			
11. Determine whether a qualifying circumstance modifier should be used. If so, document the modifier.	5			
*12. Determine the total anesthesia time, divide by 15 minutes, and document the time.	10			
13. Select the appropriate geographic conversion factor.	5			
*14. Calculate the charge for the anesthesia service using the anesthesia formula.	10			
*15. Read medical documentation to determine what procedure or service was provided.	5			

Did the student demonstrate an ability to work with the physician to achieve the maximum reimbursement?

Comments:

Points earned _____ ÷ 100 possible points = Score _____ % Score

Instructor's signature _____

Name _____ Date _____ Score _____

Procedure 19-4 Perform Procedural Coding: HCPCS Coding

MAERB/CAAHEP COMPETENCIES: IV.P.IV.3, VIII.P.VIII.1, VIII.A.VIII.1
ABHES COMPETENCIES: 8.r., 8.t., 8.u., 8.v

Task: To use the steps for the procedure and service coding to find the most accurate and specific HCPCS code.

Equipment and Supplies
- HCPCS coding manual (current year)
- Medical record
- Encounter form (charge ticket)
- Paper
- Pen or pencil

Standards: Complete the procedure and all critical steps in _____ minutes with a minimum score of 85% within three attempts.

Scoring: Divide the points earned by the total possible points. Failure to perform a critical step, indicated by an asterisk (*), results in an unsatisfactory overall score.

Time began _____ Time ended _____ Total minutes: _____

Steps	Possible Points	Attempt 1	Attempt 2	Attempt 3
*1. Read the medical documentation to determine the procedures or services provided.	10			
*2. Determine the main and modifying terms from the abstracted information.	10			
3. Select modifying terms, if needed.	5			
4. Select the most appropriate main term to begin the search in the Alphabetic Index.	5			
*5. If no modifying term produces an appropriate code or code range, repeat steps 2 and 3 using a different main term classification.	10			
6. Find the code or code ranges that include all or most of the description of the procedure or service found in the medical record.	10			
7. Disregard any code or code range containing additional descriptions or modifying terms not found in the medical record.	5			

Steps	Possible Points	Attempt 1	Attempt 2	Attempt 3
*8. Write down the code that best matches the description in the medical record.	5			
9. Turn to the Main Text and find the code or code range chosen from the Alphabetic Index.	5			
*10. Compare the description of the code with the medical documentation. Verify that all or most of the medical record documentation matches the code description and that no additional element or information is present in the code description that is not found in the documentation.	10			
*11. Read the guidelines for the section, subsection, and code to make sure no contraindications prevent use of the code.	10			
12. Evaluate the HCPCS manual conventions.	5			
13. Determine whether special circumstances require a modifier.	5			
*14. Record the HCPCS code selected.	5			

Did the student demonstrate an ability to work with the physician to achieve the maximum reimbursement?

Comments:

Points earned _____ ÷ 100 possible points = Score _____ % Score

Instructor's signature _____

Name _____ Date _____ Score _____

Procedure 20-1 Apply Managed Care Policies and Procedures

MAERB/CAAHEP COMPETENCIES: IV.P.IV.3, VII.P.VII.1, IX.A.IX.2
ABHES COMPETENCIES: 1.e., 4.f., 8.r

Task: To act within the guidelines of the managed care contracts the physician and/or medical facility officials have signed.

Equipment and Supplies
- Managed care contracts (sample provided in the student workbook)
- Managed care handbooks (sample excerpt provided in the student workbook)
- Forms from managed care organizations

Standards: Complete the procedure and all critical steps in _____ minutes with a minimum score of 85% within three attempts.

Scoring: Divide the points earned by the total possible points. Failure to perform a critical step, indicated by an asterisk (*), results in an unsatisfactory overall score.

Time began _____ Time ended _____ Total minutes: _____

Steps	Possible Points	Attempt 1	Attempt 2	Attempt 3
1. Determine the managed care organization to which the patient subscribes.	10			
*2. Read and study the policies and procedures set forth by the managed care organization.	10			
3. Make sure a signature is on file for the patient.	10			
*4. Determine what procedures and services are to be billed on the claim.	20			
5. Determine whether all procedures and services to be billed are covered by the managed care plan.	20			
*6. Obtain any forms needed to process the patient's claims.	10			
7. Become familiar with the information in managed care policy manuals and handbooks.	10			
8. Determine whom to contact if questions arise about the various managed care organizations.	10			

Did the student demonstrate awareness of the consequences of not working within the legal scope of practice?

Comments:

Points earned _____ ÷ 100 possible points = Score _____ % Score

Instructor's signature _____

Name _____ Date _____ Score _____

Procedure 20-2 Apply Third-Party Guidelines

MAERB/CAAHEP COMPETENCIES: IV.P.IV.3, VII.P.VII.2
ABHES COMPETENCIES: 4.f., 8.r

Task: To ensure that claims are processed quickly and result in the highest allowable reimbursement.

Equipment and Supplies
- Insurance carrier contracts
- Insurance carrier handbooks
- Clerical supplies
- Forms from insurance carrier
- Insurance claim forms (CMS-1500)

Standards: Complete the procedure and all critical steps in _____ minutes with a minimum score of 85% within three attempts.

Scoring: Divide the points earned by the total possible points. Failure to perform a critical step, indicated by an asterisk (*), results in an unsatisfactory overall score.

Time began _____ Time ended _____ Total minutes: _____

Steps	Possible Points	Attempt 1	Attempt 2	Attempt 3
*1. Determine the patient's health insurance plan.	10	____	____	____
2. Review the rules and regulations govern that particular organization.	10	____	____	____
*3. Make sure a signature is on file for the patient.	10	____	____	____
*4. Determine the procedures and/or services to be billed on the claim.	20	____	____	____
*5. Determine whether all the procedures and/or services to be billed are covered by the health insurance plan.	20	____	____	____
*6. Inform the patient of any procedures and/or services that will not be covered.	10	____	____	____
7. Determine whether any information needs to be added to the blocks designated "for local use."	10	____	____	____
*8. Submit the claim to the correct insurance company address or clearinghouse.	10	____	____	____

Comments:

Points earned _____ ÷ 100 possible points = Score _____ % Score

Instructor's signature _____

Name _____ Date _____ Score _____

Procedure 20-3 Verify Eligibility for Managed Care Services

MAERB/CAAHEP COMPETENCIES: IV.P.IV.3; VII.P.VII.6; IX.A.IX.2
ABHES COMPETENCIES: 1.e; 4.f; 8.r

Task: To confirm that the patient's insurance is in effect and to determine what benefits are covered and what exclusions, noncovered procedures and services, and precertifications are included or required.

Equipment and Supplies
- Patient's record
- Verification of eligibility and benefits form
- Patient's insurance information
- Telephone and fax machine
- Pen

Standards: Complete the procedure and all critical steps in _____ minutes with a minimum score of 85% within three attempts.

Scoring: Divide the points earned by the total possible points. Failure to perform a critical step, indicated by an asterisk (*), results in an unsatisfactory overall score.

Time began _____ **Time ended** _____ **Total minutes:** _____

Steps	Possible Points	Attempt 1	Attempt 2	Attempt 3
*1. Determine the patient's insurance company when he or she makes the initial call for an appointment.	15			
*2. Make a copy of the front and back of the patient's insurance card (or cards).	15			
3. Complete the patient portion of the verification eligibility and benefit form, including demographic and insurance information for the patient, and the contact information for the insurance plan. Complete one form for each of the patient's insurance plans.	15			
*4. Contact the insurance carrier by phone to: • Verify that the patient is eligible for benefits and the insurance is in effect. • Determine the basic benefits, exclusions, or noncovered services of the insurance plan. • Determine whether there are deductibles, co-payments, or any other out-of-pocket expenses the patient is responsible for paying. • Determine whether preauthorization is required for referral to a specialist or for any procedures and/or services.	15			

Steps	Possible Points	Attempt 1	Attempt 2	Attempt 3
5. Obtain the name, title, and phone number of the person contacted.	20			
*6. Document all verification information in the patient's medical record.	20			

Did the student demonstrate awareness of the consequences of not working within the legal scope of practice?

Comments:

Points earned _____ ÷ 100 possible points = Score _____ % Score

Instructor's signature _____

Name _____ Date _____ Score _____

Procedure 20-4 Perform Preauthorization (Precertification) and/or Referral Procedures

MAERB/CAAHEP COMPETENCIES: IV.P.IV.3; VII.P.VII.4; VII.P.VII.5
ABHES COMPETENCIES: 8.r.; 8.s

Task: To use the information in the case study to obtain precertification from a patient's HMO for requested services or procedures.

Equipment and Supplies
- Patient's record
- Precertification/preauthorization form
- Referral form
- Patient's insurance information, including telephone and fax numbers of the insurance carrier
- Telephone and fax machine
- Pen

Standards: Complete the procedure and all critical steps in _____ minutes with a minimum score of 85% within three attempts.

Scoring: Divide the points earned by the total possible points. Failure to perform a critical step, indicated by an asterisk (*), results in an unsatisfactory overall score.

Time began _____ **Time ended** _____ **Total minutes:** _____

Steps	Possible Points	Attempt 1	Attempt 2	Attempt 3
*1. Gather the necessary documents and forms.	15			
*2. Examine the patient's record and determine the service or procedure for which preauthorization is being requested, including, if applicable, the specialist's name and phone number and the reason for the request.	15			
*3. Complete the referral form.	25			
*4. Proofread the completed form.	15			
*5. Fax the completed form to the patient's insurance carrier.	15			
*6. Place a copy of the returned approval form in the patient's medical record.	15			

Comments:

Points earned _____ ÷ 100 possible points = Score _____ % Score

Instructor's signature _____

Name _____ Date _____ Score _____

Procedure 20-5 Perform Deductible, Co-Insurance, and Allowable Amount Calculations

CAAHEP COMPETENCIES: IV.P.IV.3; VII.P.VII.2
ABHES COMPETENCIES: 8.i.; 8.m.; 8.r.; 8.v.; 8.u

Task: To calculate the patient's out-of-pocket expenses or the amount to be billed to a secondary insurance carrier and to determine what amounts, if any, are to be written off or passed on to the patient for payment.

Equipment and Supplies
- Explanation of benefits (EOB) form, explanation of Medicare benefits (EOMB) form, remittance advice (RA), or verification of eligibility and benefits form
- Patient accounts receivable ledger
- Calculator
- Pen
- Paper

Standards: Complete the procedure and all critical steps in _____ minutes with a minimum score of 85% within three attempts.

Scoring: Divide the points earned by the total possible points. Failure to perform a critical step, indicated by an asterisk (*), results in an unsatisfactory overall score.

Time began _____ Time ended _____ Total minutes: _____

Steps	Possible Points	Attempt 1	Attempt 2	Attempt 3
1. Assemble the required materials and equipment.	15			
*2. Using the EOB, EOMB, and/or RA and/or the verification of eligibility and benefits form, as well as the patient accounts receivable ledger: • Enter the total charge from the EOB and/or the patient accounts receivable ledger. • Subtract the deductible amount from the total charge.	25			
*3. If the patient has met the deductible, determine the co-insurance payment due.	15			
*4. Record the deductible and, if applicable, co-insurance amounts on separate lines in the patient balance due column of the patient ledger.	15			
5. Subtract the allowable amount of each charge from the actual billed charge.	15			
*6. Record the difference in either the adjustments or the balance due column.	15			

Comments:

Points earned _____ ÷ 100 possible points = Score _____ % Score

Instructor's signature _____

Name _____ Date _____ Score _____

Procedure 21-1 Gathering Data to Complete CMS-1500 Form

MAERB/CAAHEP COMPETENCIES: IV.P.IV.3; VII.P.VII.1; VII.P.VII.2; VII.P.VII.3; VII.P.VII.4; VII.P.VII.5; VII.P.VII.6; VIII.P.VIII.1; VIII.P.VIII.2
ABHES COMPETENCIES: 8.r.; 8.t.; 8.u.; 8.v.

Task: To gather all information and documentation required for completing an insurance claim.

Equipment and Supplies
- Patient registration form
- Photocopy of patient's insurance card or cards, driver's license or state-issued identification card, and student ID (if applicable)
- Verification of Eligibility and Benefits form
- Preauthorization and/or referral form
- Encounter form (charge ticket or superbill)
- ICD-9-CM coding manual
- CPT coding manual
- HCPCS coding manual

Standards: Complete the procedure and all critical steps in _____ minutes with a minimum score of 85% within three attempts.

Scoring: Divide the points earned by the total possible points. Failure to perform a critical step, indicated by an asterisk (*), results in an unsatisfactory overall score.

Time began _____   Time ended _____   Total minutes: _____

Steps	Possible Points	Attempt 1	Attempt 2	Attempt 3
*1. Have the patient or the patient's guardian complete the patient registration, release of information, and authorization of benefits forms in full and return them to you.	10	_____	_____	_____
*2. Ask for the patient's and the insured's driver's license and insurance card (or cards). If the patient is a student, ask for a student ID. If the patient has more than one insurance policy, get the name, address, and group and policy numbers for each company.	10	_____	_____	_____
*3. Photocopy the back and front of the patient's insurance card (or cards) and place the photocopy in the medical record and/or in the patient's insurance file.	5	_____	_____	_____
*4. Confirm the patient's and the insured's full name, address, phone number, date of birth, and gender by comparing the patient registration form with the driver's license or identification card.	5	_____	_____	_____
*5. Determine whether someone other than the patient is the guarantor.	5	_____	_____	_____

Steps	Possible Points	Attempt 1	Attempt 2	Attempt 3
*6. Call the employer and confirm the patient's employment (optional). If the patient is insured under a group health plan, workers' compensation, TRICARE, and some other types of insurance, this information can be confirmed when eligibility and benefits are verified.	5	_____	_____	_____
*7. Confirm that the patient has signed and dated the release of information form.	5	_____	_____	_____
*8. Confirm that the insured has signed the authorization of benefits form. Signatures to authorize insurance billing, supplying information to insurance companies, and acceptance of assignments of benefits (if appropriate) should be obtained from all new patients and at the beginning of each new calendar year.	10	_____	_____	_____
*9. Contact the insurance carrier and verify benefits and insurance coverage.	10	_____	_____	_____
*10. Obtain any precertification or referral authorizations required by the insurance carrier or payer.	10	_____	_____	_____
11. Code the diagnosis or diagnoses for the encounter using the ICD-9-CM coding manual.	5	_____	_____	_____
12. Select any qualifying circumstance, physical or patient status, or other modifiers as appropriate.	5	_____	_____	_____
13. Code the procedures and services provided during the encounter using the CPT and/or HCPCS coding manual.	5	_____	_____	_____
14. Select any CPT and/or HCPCS modifiers as appropriate.	5	_____	_____	_____
15. Using Table 21-1 in the textbook or a similar list of information to gather in preparation for insurance claim submission, confirm that all information needed has been obtained.	5	_____	_____	_____

Comments:

Points earned _____ ÷ 100 possible points = Score _____ % Score

Instructor's signature _____

WORK PRODUCT 21-1

Name: _____

Completing a CMS-1500 Claim Form

Corresponds to Procedure 21-2

CAAHEP COMPETENCIES: IV.P.IV.3; VII.P.VII.1; VII.P.VII.2; VII.P.VII.3; VII.P.VII.4; VII.P.VII.5; VII.P.VII.6; VIII.P.VIII.1; VIII.P.VIII.2

ABHES COMPETENCIES: 8.r.; 8.t.; 8.u.; 8.v.

Complete Claim Form 1 using the information in Part I, question 1.

WORK PRODUCT 21-2

Name: _____

Completing a CMS-1500 Claim Form

Corresponds to Procedure 21-2

<u>CAAHEP COMPETENCIES:</u> IV.P.IV.3; VII.P.VII.1; VII.P.VII.2; VII.P.VII.3; VII.P.VII.4; VII.P.VII.5; VII.P.VII.6; VIII.P.VIII.1; VIII.P.VIII.2.

<u>ABHES COMPETENCIES:</u> 8.r.; 8.t.; 8.u.; 8.v.

Complete Claim Form 2 using the information in Part I, question 2.

WORK PRODUCT 21-3

Name: _____

Completing a CMS-1500 Claim Form

Corresponds to Procedure 21-2

<u>CAAHEP COMPETENCIES:</u> IV.P.IV.3; VII.P.VII.1; VII.P.VII.2; VII.P.VII.3; VII.P.VII.4; VII.P.VII.5; VII.P.VII.6; VIII.P.VIII.1; VIII.P.VIII.2

<u>ABHES COMPETENCIES:</u> 8.r.; 8.t.; 8.u.; 8.v.

Complete Claim Form 3 using the information in Part I, question 3.

WORK PRODUCT 21-4

Name: _____

Completing a CMS-1500 Claim Form

Corresponds to Procedure 21-2

<u>CAAHEP COMPETENCIES:</u> IV.P.IV.3; VII.P.VII.1; VII.P.VII.2; VII.P.VII.3; VII.P.VII.4; VII.P.VII.5; VII.P.VII.6; VIII.P.VIII.1; VIII.P.VIII.2

<u>ABHES COMPETENCIES:</u> 8.r.; 8.t.; 8.u.; 8.v.

Complete Claim Form 4 using the information in Part I, question 4.

WORK PRODUCT 21-5

Name: _____

Completing a CMS-1500 Claim Form

Corresponds to Procedure 21-2

<u>CAAHEP COMPETENCIES:</u> IV.P.IV.3; VII.P.VII.1; VII.P.VII.2; VII.P.VII.3; VII.P.VII.4; VII.P.VII.5; VII.P.VII.6; VIII.P.VIII.1; VIII.P.VIII.2

<u>ABHES COMPETENCIES:</u> 8.r.; 8.t.; 8.u.; 8.v.

Complete Claim Form 5 using the information in Part I, question 5.

Name _____ Date _____ Score _____

Procedure 22-1 Use Computerized Office Billing Systems

CAAHEP COMPETENCIES: VI.P.VI.3
ABHES COMPETENCIES: 8.w

Task: To use the computer in such a way that office billing functions are done efficiently, accurately, and in a timely manner.

Equipment and Supplies
- Computer with billing software installed
- Physician's fee schedule
- Encounter forms
- Calculator

Standards: Complete the procedure and all critical steps in _____ minutes with a minimum score of 85% within three attempts.

Scoring: Divide the points earned by the total possible points. Failure to perform a critical step, indicated by an asterisk (*), results in an unsatisfactory overall score.

Time began _____ Time ended _____ Total minutes: _____

Steps	Possible Points	Attempt 1	Attempt 2	Attempt 3
1. Open the billing program software.	10			
*2. Generate an aging report to determine which patients need to be billed in the billing cycle.	20			
3. Review the accounts to determine whether any should be referred to a collection agency.	20			
*4. Run the software to print billing statements.	20			
*5. Determine whether any of the accounts need special handling.	10			
*6. Prepare the statements for mailing according to the billing cycle.	10			
*7. Determine the postage rate and mail the statements.	10			

Comments:

Points earned _____ ÷ 100 possible points = Score _____ % Score

Instructor's signature _____

Name _____ Date _____ Score _____

Procedure 22-2 Post Entries on a Day Sheet

CAAHEP COMPETENCIES: VI.P.VI.2.a
ABHES COMPETENCIES: 8.h

Task: To post 1 day's charges and payments and compute the daily bookkeeping cycle using a pegboard.

Equipment and Supplies
- Pegboard
- Calculator
- Pen
- Day sheet
- Receipts
- Ledger cards
- Balances from previous day

Standards: Complete the procedure and all critical steps in _____ minutes with a minimum score of 85% within three attempts.

Scoring: Divide the points earned by the total possible points. Failure to perform a critical step, indicated by an asterisk (*), results in an unsatisfactory overall score.

Time began _____   Time ended _____   Total minutes: _____

Steps	Possible Points	Attempt 1	Attempt 2	Attempt 3
1. Prepare the board: a. Place a new day sheet on the board b. Place receipts over the pegs, aligning the top receipt with the first open line on the day sheet. If you are using a computer, open the accounting program.	5	_____	_____	_____
*2. Carry forward the balances from the previous day.	5	_____	_____	_____
3. Pull the ledger cards for the patients being seen that day.	5	_____	_____	_____
*4. Insert the ledger card under the first receipt, aligning the first available writing line with the carbonized strip on the receipt.	5	_____	_____	_____
*5. Enter the patient's name, the date, the receipt number, and any existing balance from the ledger card.	5	_____	_____	_____
*6. Detach the charge slip from the receipt and clip it to the patient's medical record.	5	_____	_____	_____
*7. Accept the returned charge slip at the end of the visit.	5	_____	_____	_____
*8. Line up the receipt with the ledger card and day sheet.	5	_____	_____	_____

Steps	Possible Points	Attempt 1	Attempt 2	Attempt 3
*9. Write the service code number and fee on the receipt or, with a computer system, enter the fees in the appropriate field.	5			
*10. Accept the patient's payment and record the amount of the payment and the new balance.	5			
*11. Give the completed receipt to the patient or, with a computer system, print a receipt	5			
*12. Repeat steps 4 through 11 for each transaction of the day.	25			
*13. Total all columns of the day sheet at the end of the day.	5			
*14. Write preliminary totals in pencil where indicated at the bottom of the day sheet or, with a computer system, print an end of day summary.	5			
*15. Complete the proof of totals and enter the totals in ink.	5			
*16. Enter the figures for accounts receivable control.	5			

Comments:

Points earned _____ ÷ 100 possible points = Score _____ % Score

Instructor's signature _____

Name _____ Date _____ Score _____

Procedure 22-3 Post Adjustments

CAAHEP COMPETENCIES: VI.P.VI.2.d
ABHES COMPETENCIES: 8.m

Task: To process adjustments to patients' accounts accurately.

Equipment and Supplies
- Patient ledgers
- Office policy and procedures manual
- Explanation of benefits (EOB) or remittance advice (RA)
- Bookkeeping system
- Clerical supplies
- Payments
- Calculator

Standards: Complete the procedure and all critical steps in _____ minutes with a minimum score of 85% within three attempts.

Scoring: Divide the points earned by the total possible points. Failure to perform a critical step, indicated by an asterisk (*), results in an unsatisfactory overall score.

Time began _____   Time ended _____   Total minutes: _____

Steps	Possible Points	Attempt 1	Attempt 2	Attempt 3
1. Open the mail and set the payments aside with their corresponding EOB/RA.	10			
*2. Paper-clip the EOB/RA to the check that arrived with it as payment.	10			
*3. Post the payment to the patient's account.	10			
*4. Determine whether an adjustment is necessary on the account.	10			
*5. Review the current procedure to follow in adjusting the account.	10			
*6. If a manual system is used, make sure the ledger card is aligned properly with the day sheet.	10			
*7. Post the adjustment in the adjustment column or other specified place on the day sheet or in the computer application.	20			
*8. Check the math calculations to make sure the adjustment was figured correctly.	10			
*9. Determine the current balance on the patient's account.	10			

Comments:

Points earned _____ ÷ 100 possible points = Score _____ % Score

Instructor's signature _____

Name _____ Date _____ Score _____

Procedure 22-4 Process a Credit Balance

CAAHEP COMPETENCIES: VI.P.VI.2.e
ABHES COMPETENCIES: 8.n

Task: To return overpayments to patients in a timely manner.

Equipment and Supplies
- Patient ledgers
- Office policy and procedures manual
- Explanation of benefits (EOB) or remittance advice (RA)
- Bookkeeping system
- Clerical supplies
- Payments
- Calculator

Standards: Complete the procedure and all critical steps in _____ minutes with a minimum score of 85% within three attempts.

Scoring: Divide the points earned by the total possible points. Failure to perform a critical step, indicated by an asterisk (*), results in an unsatisfactory overall score.

Time began _____   Time ended _____   Total minutes: _____

Steps	Possible Points	Attempt 1	Attempt 2	Attempt 3
1. Review the office policy and procedures manual to determine the correct procedure for refunding a credit balance.	10			
*2. Evaluate the payment received and the EOB/RA.	20			
*3. Post the payment to the patient's account.	20			
*4. Determine whether an overpayment has been made.	10			
*5. Review the account to determine whether more insurance payments are expected on the account.	20			
*6. Adjust the credit balance off of the patient's account.	20			

Comments:

Points earned _____ ÷ 100 possible points = Score _____ % Score

Instructor's signature _____

Name _____ Date _____ Score _____

Procedure 22-5 Process Refunds

CAAHEP COMPETENCIES: VI.P.VI.2.f
ABHES COMPETENCIES: 8.o

Task: To return patient refunds in a timely manner.

Equipment and Supplies
- Patient ledgers
- Office policy and procedures manual
- Explanation of benefits (EOB) or remittance advice (RA)
- Bookkeeping system
- Clerical supplies
- Payments
- Calculator

Standards: Complete the procedure and all critical steps in _____ minutes with a minimum score of 85% within three attempts.

Scoring: Divide the points earned by the total possible points. Failure to perform a critical step, indicated by an asterisk (*), results in an unsatisfactory overall score.

Time began _____   Time ended _____   Total minutes: _____

Steps	Possible Points	Attempt 1	Attempt 2	Attempt 3
*1. Determine the amount of the refund to be processed.	20			
*2. Write a check for the amount of the refund.	20			
3. Present the check to the physician for a signature.	10			
*4. Determine the patient's correct mailing address.	20			
*5. Make a copy of the refund check and put it in the patient's medical record.	20			
*6. Mail the refund to the patient.	10			

Comments:

Points earned _____ ÷ 100 possible points = Score _____ % Score

Instructor's signature _____

Name _____ Date _____ Score _____

Procedure 22-6 Post Non-Sufficient Funds Checks

CAAHEP COMPETENCY: VI.P.VI.2.g
ABHES COMPETENCIES: 8.p

Task: To correctly note that a patient's check was returned because of insufficient funds.

Equipment and Supplies
- Patient ledgers
- Office policy and procedures manual
- Bookkeeping system
- Clerical supplies
- Calculator

Standards: Complete the procedure and all critical steps in _____ minutes with a minimum score of 85% within three attempts.

Scoring: Divide the points earned by the total possible points. Failure to perform a critical step, indicated by an asterisk (*), results in an unsatisfactory overall score.

Time began _____ Time ended _____ Total minutes: _____

Steps	Possible Points	Attempt 1	Attempt 2	Attempt 3
1. Pull the ledger card for the patient who wrote the check.	10			
*2. Determine the amount to be added back to the ledger card as a result of the returned check (usually the amount of the check plus the office returned check fee).	20			
*3. Post that amount to the patient's ledger card.	20			
*4. Send a certified letter to the patient requiring timely payment of the check and any fees assessed to the patient's account for processing.	20			
*5. Note this collection activity in the patient's financial records.	20			
*6. When the patient pays the check and fees, process it as a regular payment and return the check to the patient.	10			

Comments:

Points earned _____ ÷ 100 possible points = Score _____ % Score

Instructor's signature _____

Name _____ Date _____ Score _____

Procedure 22-7 Explain Professional Fees and Make Credit Arrangements with a Patient

CAAHEP COMPETENCIES: VI.C.VI.12
ABHES COMPETENCIES: 11.b.(3)

Task: To assist the patient in paying for services by making mutually beneficial credit arrangements according to established office policy.

Equipment and Supplies
- Patient ledger
- Calendar
- Truth in lending form
- Credit application
- Assignment of benefits form
- Private area for interview

Standards: Complete the procedure and all critical steps in _____ minutes with a minimum score of 85% within three attempts.

Scoring: Divide the points earned by the total possible points. Failure to perform a critical step, indicated by an asterisk (*), results in an unsatisfactory overall score.

Time began _____   **Time ended** _____   **Total minutes:** _____

Steps	Possible Points	Attempt 1	Attempt 2	Attempt 3
1. Answer all the patient's questions about credit thoroughly and kindly.	10			
*2. Inform the patient of the office policy regarding credit: a. Payment at the time of the first visit b. Payment by bank card c. Credit application	20			
3. Have the patient complete a credit application.	10			
*4. Check the credit application.	10			
*5. Discuss with the patient the arrangements that are possible and allow the patient to decide which arrangement is most suitable.	10			
*6. Prepare the truth in lending form and have the patient sign it if the agreement requires more than four installments.	10			

Steps	Possible Points	Attempt 1	Attempt 2	Attempt 3
*7. Have the patient execute an assignment of insurance benefits.	10			
*8. Make a copy of the patient's insurance ID and have the patient sign an assignment of benefits and release of information form, if necessary.	10			
*9. Keep the patient's credit information confidential.	10			

Comments:

Points earned _____ ÷ 100 possible points = Score _____ % Score

Instructor's signature _____

Name _____ Date _____ Score _____

Procedure 22-8 Perform Billing Procedures

CAAHEP COMPETENCIES: VI.P.VI.2.b
ABHES COMPETENCIES: 8.i

Task: To bill insurance companies for patient procedures and services and to obtain the maximum legal reimbursement.

Equipment and Supplies
- Patient ledgers
- Accounting system
- Calculator
- Claim forms
- Encounter forms
- Clerical supplies

Standards: Complete the procedure and all critical steps in _____ minutes with a minimum score of 85% within three attempts.

Scoring: Divide the points earned by the total possible points. Failure to perform a critical step, indicated by an asterisk (*), results in an unsatisfactory overall score.

Time began _____   Time ended _____   Total minutes: _____

Steps	Possible Points	Attempt 1	Attempt 2	Attempt 3
*1. Determine the procedures and/or services to be billed by reading the patient's medical record.	20			
*2. Determine the diagnosis code or codes applicable to the claim.	10			
*3. Determine the procedure code or codes applicable to the claim.	10			
*4. Complete the CMS 1500 claim form, following the directions provided for each block.	20			
5. Insert the correct amount of money to bill in the appropriate block on the claim form.	10			
6. Address the claim to the carrier's correct address for claim submissions.	10			
7. Mail the claim form.	10			
8. Follow up on the claim to ensure timely payment.	10			

Comments:

Points earned _____ ÷ 100 possible points = Score _____ % Score

Instructor's signature _____

Procedure **22-8 Perform Billing Procedures**

Name _____ Date _____ Score _____

Procedure 22-9 Perform Collection Procedures

CAAHEP COMPETENCIES: VI.P.VI.2.c
ABHES COMPETENCIES: 8.i

Task: To collect the maximum amount of funds on each account.

Equipment and Supplies
- Patient ledger
- Office policy and procedures manual
- Clerical supplies
- Scripts for telephone collections
- Letters for collection efforts
- Telephone
- Letterhead and envelopes
- Copies of claim forms previously filed

Standards: Complete the procedure and all critical steps in _____ minutes with a minimum score of 85% within three attempts.

Scoring: Divide the points earned by the total possible points. Failure to perform a critical step, indicated by an asterisk (*), results in an unsatisfactory overall score.

Time began _____ **Time ended** _____ **Total minutes:** _____

Steps	Possible Points	Attempt 1	Attempt 2	Attempt 3
1. Review the office policy for collection procedures.	10			
*2. Evaluate the patient's ledger to determine whether it needs collection activity.	10			
*3. Determine the appropriate collection activity for the account.	10			
*4. Telephone the patient or guarantor to initiate payment on the account.	10			
*5. If the patient or guarantor cannot be reached by phone, send a postcard or collection letter.	10			
*6. Send a more demanding collection letter if past efforts by phone or letter have not produced results.	10			
*7. Once all collection efforts have failed, present the account to the physician for a decision on further disposition.	10			

Steps	Possible Points	Attempt 1	Attempt 2	Attempt 3
*8. With the physician's approval, send the account to a collection agency.	10	_____	_____	_____
*9. If further payments arrive on the account, send them directly to the collection agency.	10	_____	_____	_____
*10. Document the final collection activity in the patient's medical record.	10	_____	_____	_____

Comments:

Points earned _____ ÷ 100 possible points = Score _____ % Score

Instructor's signature _____

Name _____ Date _____ Score _____

Procedure 22-10 Post Collection Agency Payments

CAAHEP COMPETENCIES: VI.P.VI.2.h
ABHES COMPETENCIES: 8.q

Task: To post payments received on an account after it has been turned over to a collection agency.

Equipment and Supplies
- Patient ledger
- Office policy and procedures manual
- Bookkeeping system
- Clerical supplies
- Calculator

Standards: Complete the procedure and all critical steps in _____ minutes with a minimum score of 85% within three attempts.

Scoring: Divide the points earned by the total possible points. Failure to perform a critical step, indicated by an asterisk (*), results in an unsatisfactory overall score.

Time began _____ **Time ended** _____ **Total minutes:** _____

Steps	Possible Points	Attempt 1	Attempt 2	Attempt 3
*1. Determine that a payment received is for an account that is currently being serviced by a collection agency.	25	___	___	___
*2. Notify the collection agency that a payment has been made on the account. Mail the payment to the collection agency.	25	___	___	___
3. Notify the patient that the payment has been forwarded to the collection agency.	25	___	___	___
*4. Instruct the patient to send any future payments to the collection agency.	25	___	___	___

Comments:

Points earned _____ ÷ 100 possible points = Score _____ % Score

Instructor's signature _____

WORK PRODUCT 22-1

Name: _____

Perform Billing Procedures

Complete the billing form below page using the information in Part I, question 2.

Corresponds to Procedure 22-8

CAAHEP COMPETENCIES: VI.P.VI.2.b.

ABHES COMPETENCIES: 8.i.

Blackburn Primary Care Associates, PC
1990 Turquoise Drive
Blackburn, WI 54937
(608) 459-8857

Howard M. Lawler, MD 11
Joanne R. Hughes, MD 21
Ralph Garcia Lopez, MD 31
TAX ID NO. 00-00000000

GUARANTOR NAME AND ADDRESS	PATIENT NO.	PATIENT NAME	DOCTOR NO.	DATE
	DATE OF BIRTH	TELEPHONE NO.	INSURANCE: CODE / DESCRIPTION	CERTIFICATE NO.

OFFICE - NEW
X	CPT	SERVICE	FEE
X	99201	Prob Foc/Straight	
	99202	Exp Prob/Straight	
X	99203	Detailed/Low	60
	99204	Compre/Moderate	
	99205	Compre/High	

OFFICE - ESTABLISHED
X	CPT	SERVICE	FEE
	99211	Nurse/Minimal	
	99212	Prob Foc/Straight	
	99213	Exp Prob/Low	
	99214	Detailed/Moderate	
	99215	Compre/High	

OFFICE - CONSULT
X	CPT	SERVICE	FEE
	99241	Prob Foc/Straight	
	99242	Exp Prob/Straight	
	99243	Detailed/Low	
	99244	Compre/Moderate	
X	99245	Compre/High	250

PREVENTIVE CARE - ADULT
X	CPT	SERVICE	FEE
	99385	18-39 Initial	
	99386	40-64 Initial	
	99387	65+ Initial	
	99395	18-39 Periodic	
	99396	40-64 Periodic	
	99397	65+ Periodic	

GASTROENEROLOGY
X	CPT	SERVICE	FEE
	45300	Sigmoidoscopy Rig	
	45305	Sigmoid Rig w/bx	
	45330	Sigmoidoscopy Flex	
	45331	Sigmoid Flex w/bx	
	45378	Colonoscopy Diag	
	45380	Colonoscopy w/bx	
	46600	Anoscopy	

CARDIOLOGY & HEARING
X	CPT	SERVICE	FEE
X	93000	EKG (Global)	55
	93015	Stress Test (Global)	
	93224	Holter (Global)	
	93225	Holter Hook Up	
	93227	Holter Interpretation	
	94010	Pulm Function Test	
	92551	Audiometry Screen	

INJECTIONS & IMMUNIZATION
X	CPT	SERVICE	FEE
	86585	TB Skin Test	
	90716	Varicella Vaccine	
	90724	Flu Vaccine	
	90732	Pneumovax	
	90718	TD Immunization	
X	J23	Solu-Medrol	
X	90782	Injection IM*	
X	90788	Injection IM Antibiot*	25
		Injection joint*	

REPAIR & DERMATOLOGY
X	CPT	SERVICE	FEE
	17110	Warts: #	
		Tags: #	
		Lesion Excis	
		Lesion Destruct	
		SIZE CM: SITE:	
		MALIG: PREMAL/BEN:	
		(Check One Above)	
		Simple Closure	
		Intermed Closure	
		SIZE CM: SITE:	
	10060	I&D Abscess	
	10080	I&D Cyst	

OTHER / SUPPLIES/DRUGS*
DRUG NAME: Penicillin
UNIT/MEASURE:
QUANTITY:
FOR ALL INJECTIONS, SUPPLY DRUG INFORMATION: Penicillin

SM MED MAJOR (circle one)

DIAGNOSTIC CODES: ICD-9-CM

- ☐ 789.0 Abdominal Pain
- ☐ 795.0 Abnormal Pap Smear
- ☐ 706.1 Acne Vulgaris
- ☐ 477.0 Allergic Rhinitis
- ☐ 285.9 Anemia, NOS
- ☐ 281.0 Pernicious
- ☐ 411.1 Angina, Unstable
- ☐ 427.9 Arythmia, NOS
- ☐ 440.9 Arteriosclerosis
- ☐ 714.0 Arthritis, Rheumatoid
- ☐ 414.0 ASHD
- ☐ 493.90 Asthma, Bronchial W/O Status Ast.
- ☐ 493.91 Asthma, Bronchial W/Status Ast.
- ☐ 466.1 Bronchiolitis, Acute
- ☐ 466.0 Bronchitis, Acute
- ☐ 727.3 Bursitis
- ☒ 786.50 Chest Pain
- ☐ 574.20 Cholelithiasis
- ☐ 372.30 Conjunctivitis, Unspecified
- ☐ 564.0 Constipation
- ☐ 496 COPD
- ☐ 692.9 Dermatitis, Allergic
- ☐ 250.01 Diabetes Mellitus, ID
- ☐ 250.00 Diabetes Mellitus, NID
- ☐ 558.9 Diarrhea
- ☐ 562.11 Diverticulitis
- ☐ 562.10 Diverticulosis

- ☐ 782.3 Edema
- ☐ 492.8 Emphysema
- ☐ V16.0 Family History Of Diabetes
- ☐ 780.6 Fever of Undetermined Origin
- ☐ 578.9 G.I. Bleeding, Unspecified
- ☐ 727.41 Ganglion of Joint
- ☐ 535.0 Gastritis, Acute
- ☐ V72.3 Arythmia, NOS
- ☐ 748.0 Headache
- ☐ 550.90 Hernia, Inguinal, NOS
- ☐ 054.9 Herpes Simplex
- ☐ 053.9 Herpes Zoster
- ☐ 708.9 Hives/Urticaria
- ☐ 401.1 Hypertension, Benign
- ☐ 401.0 Hypertension, Malignant
- ☐ 402.90 Hypertension, W/O CHF
- ☐ 244.9 Hypothyroidism, Primary
- ☐ 380.4 Impacted Cerumen
- ☐ 487.1 Influenza
- ☐ 564.1 Irritable Bowel Syndrome
- ☐ 464.0 Laryngitis, Acute
- ☐ 454.9 Leg Varicose Veins
- ☐ 424.0 Mitral Valve Prolapse
- ☐ 412 Myocardial Infarction, Old
- ☒ 715.90 Osteoarthritis, Unspec. Site
- ☐ 620.2 Ovarian Cyst

- ☐ 614.9 Pelvic Inflammatory Disease
- ☐ 685.1 Pilonidal Cyst
- ☐ 462 Pharyngitis, Acute
- ☐ 627.1 Postmenopausal Bleeding
- ☐ 625.4 Premenstrual Tension
- ☐ 782.1 Rash
- ☐ 569.3 Rectal Bleeding
- ☐ 398.90 Rheumatic Heart Disease, NOS
- ☐ 431.9 Sinusitis, Acute, NOS
- ☐ 782.1 Skin Eruption, Rash
- ☐ 845.00 Sprain, Ankle
- ☐ 848.9 Sprain, Muscle, Unspec. Site
- ☐ 785.6 Swollen Glands
- ☐ 246.9 Thyroid Disease, Unspecified
- ☒ 463 Tonsillitis, Acute

- ☐ 474.0 Tonsillitis, Chronic
- ☐ 465.9 Upper Respiratory Infection, Acute
- ☐ 599.0 Urinary Tract Infection
- ☐ V03.9 Vaccination/Bacterial Dis.
- ☐ V06.8 Vaccination/Combination
- ☐ V04.8 Vaccination, Influenza
- ☐ 616.10 Vaginitis, Vulvitis, NOS
- ☐ 780.4 Vertigo
- ☐ 787.0 Vomiting, Nausea

RETURN APPOINTMENT
_____ Days
_____ Weeks
_____ Months

Authorization Number: ▶ _____

BALANCE DUE

DATE OF SERVICE	CPT CODE	DIAGNOSIS CODE(S)	CHARGE
		423	

Place of Service:
( ) Office
( ) Emergency Room
( ) Inpatient Hospital
( ) Outpatient Hospital
( ) Nursing Home

TOTAL CHARGE	$
AMOUNT PAID	$
PREVIOUS BAL	$ 0
BALANCE DUE	$ 78

Check #: _____
(Circle Method of Payment)
CASH CHECK MC VISA

Physician's Signature
▶ _____

WORK PRODUCT 22-2

Name: _____

Perform Billing Procedures

Corresponds to Procedure 22-8

<u>CAAHEP COMPETENCIES:</u> VI.P.VI.2.b.

<u>ABHES COMPETENCIES:</u> 8.i.

Complete the billing form below using the information in Part I, question 3.

Blackburn Primary Care Associates, PC
1990 Turquoise Drive
Blackburn, WI 54937
(608) 459-8857

Howard M. Lawler, MD 11
Joanne R. Hughes, MD 21
Ralph Garcia Lopez, MD 31
TAX ID NO. 00-00000000

GUARANTOR NAME AND ADDRESS	PATIENT NO.	PATIENT NAME	DOCTOR NO.	DATE
	DATE OF BIRTH / TELEPHONE NO.	INSURANCE: CODE / DESCRIPTION	CERTIFICATE NO.	

OFFICE - NEW
X	CPT	SERVICE	FEE
	99201	Prob Foc/Straight	
	99202	Exp Prob/Straight	
	99203	Detailed/Low	
	99204	Compre/Moderate	
	99205	Compre/High	

OFFICE - ESTABLISHED
X	CPT	SERVICE	FEE
	99211	Nurse/Minimal	
	99212	Prob Foc/Straight	
	99213	Exp Prob/Low	
	99214	Detailed/Moderate	
	99215	Compre/High	

OFFICE - CONSULT
X	CPT	SERVICE	FEE
	99241	Prob/Foc/Straight	
	99242	Exp Prob/Straight	
	99243	Detailed/Low	
	99244	Compre/Moderate	
	99245	Compre/High	

PREVENTIVE CARE - ADULT
X	CPT	SERVICE	FEE
	99385	18-39 Initial	
	99386	40-64 Initial	
	99387	65+ Initial	
	99395	18-39 Periodic	
	99396	40-64 Periodic	
	99397	65+ Periodic	

GASTROENEROLOGY
X	CPT	SERVICE	FEE
	45300	Sigmoidoscopy Rig	
	45305	Sigmoid Rig w/bx	
	45330	Sigmoidoscopy Flex	
	45331	Sigmoid Flex w/bx	
	45378	Colonoscopy Diag	
	45380	Colonoscopy w/bx	
	46600	Anoscopy	

CARDIOLOGY & HEARING
X	CPT	SERVICE	FEE
	93000	EKG (Global)	
	93015	Stress Test (Global)	
	93224	Holter (Global)	
	93225	Holter Hook Up	
	93227	Holter Interpretation	
	94010	Pulm Function Test	
	92551	Audiometry Screen	

INJECTIONS & IMMUNIZATION
X	CPT	SERVICE	FEE
	86585	TB Skin Test	
	90716	Varicella Vaccine	
	90724	Flu Vaccine	
	90732	Pneumovax	
	90718	TD Immunization	
	90782	Injection IM*	
	90788	Injection IM Antibiot*	
		Injection joint*	
SM	MED	MAJOR (circle one)	
FOR ALL INJECTIONS, SUPPLY DRUG INFORMATION			

REPAIR & DERMATOLOGY
X	CPT	SERVICE	FEE
	17110	Warts: #	
		Tags: #	
		Lesion Excis	
		Lesion Destruct	
SIZE CM:		SITE:	
MALIG:		PREMAL/BEN:	
(Check One Above)			
		Simple Closure	
		Intermed Closure	
SIZE CM:		SITE:	
	10060	I&D Abscess	
	10080	I&D Cyst	

OTHER

SUPPLIES/DRUGS*
DRUG NAME:
UNIT/MEASURE:
QUANTITY

DIAGNOSTIC CODES: ICD-9-CM

- ☐ 789.0 Abdominal Pain
- ☐ 795.0 Abnormal Pap Smear
- ☐ 706.1 Acne Vulgaris
- ☐ 477.0 Allergic Rhinitis
- ☐ 285.9 Anemia, NOS
- ☐ 281.0 Pernicious
- ☐ 411.1 Angina, Unstable
- ☐ 427.9 Arythmia, NOS
- ☐ 440.9 Arteriosclerosis
- ☐ 714.0 Arthritis, Rheumatoid
- ☐ 414.0 ASHD
- ☐ 493.90 Asthma, Bronchial W/O Status Ast.
- ☐ 493.91 Asthma, Bronchial W/Status Ast.
- ☐ 466.1 Bronchiolitis, Acute
- ☐ 466.0 Bronchitis, Acute
- ☐ 727.3 Bursitis
- ☐ 786.50 Chest Pain
- ☐ 574.20 Cholelithiasis
- ☐ 372.30 Conjunctivitis, Unspecified
- ☐ 564.0 Constipation
- ☐ 496 COPD
- ☐ 692.9 Dermatitis, Allergic
- ☐ 250.01 Diabetes Mellitus, ID
- ☐ 250.00 Diabetes Mellitus, NID
- ☐ 558.9 Diarrhea
- ☐ 562.11 Diverticulitis
- ☐ 562.10 Diverticulosis

- ☐ 782.3 Edema
- ☐ 492.8 Emphysema
- ☐ V16.0 Family History Of Diabetes
- ☐ 780.6 Fever of Undetermined Origin
- ☐ 578.9 G.I. Bleeding, Unspecified
- ☐ 727.41 Ganglion of Joint
- ☐ 535.0 Gastritis, Acute
- ☐ V72.3 Arythmia, NOS
- ☐ 748.9 Headache
- ☐ 550.90 Hernia, Inguinal, NOS
- ☐ 054.9 Herpes Simplex
- ☐ 053.9 Herpes Zoster
- ☐ 708.9 Hives/Urticaria
- ☐ 401.1 Hypertension, Benign
- ☐ 401.0 Hypertension, Malignant
- ☐ 402.90 Hypertension, W/O CHF
- ☐ 244.9 Hypothyroidism, Primary
- ☐ 380.4 Impacted Cerumen
- ☐ 487.1 Influenza
- ☐ 564.1 Irritable Bowel Syndrome
- ☐ 464.0 Laryngitis, Acute
- ☐ 454.9 Leg Varicose Veins
- ☐ 424.0 Mitral Valve Prolapse
- ☐ 412 Myocardial Infarction, Old
- ☐ 715.90 Osteoarthritis, Unspec. Site
- ☐ 620.2 Ovarian Cyst

- ☐ 614.9 Pelvic Inflammatory Disease
- ☐ 685.1 Pilonidal Cyst
- ☐ 462 Pharyngitis, Acute
- ☐ 627.1 Postmenopausal Bleeding
- ☐ 625.4 Premenstrual Tension
- ☐ 782.1 Rash
- ☐ 569.3 Rectal Bleeding
- ☐ 398.90 Rheumatic Heart Disease, NOS
- ☐ 431.9 Sinusitis, Acute, NOS
- ☐ 782.1 Skin Eruption, Rash
- ☐ 845.00 Sprain, Ankle
- ☐ 848.9 Sprain, Muscle, Unspec. Site
- ☐ 785.6 Swollen Glands
- ☐ 246.9 Thyroid Disease, Unspecified
- ☐ 463 Tonsillitis, Acute

- ☐ 474.0 Tonsillitis, Chronic
- ☐ 465.9 Upper Respiratory Infection, Acute
- ☐ 599.0 Urinary Tract Infection
- ☐ V03.9 Vaccination/Bacterial Dis.
- ☐ V06.8 Vaccination/Combination
- ☐ V04.8 Vaccination, Influenza
- ☐ 616.10 Vaginitis, Vulvitis, NOS
- ☐ 780.4 Vertigo
- ☐ 787.0 Vomiting, Nausea
- ☐ _____
- ☐ _____
- ☐ _____

RETURN APPOINTMENT
_____ Days
_____ Weeks
_____ Months

Authorization Number:
▶ _____

BALANCE DUE

DATE OF SERVICE	CPT CODE	DIAGNOSIS CODE(S)	CHARGE

Place of Service:
( ) Office
( ) Emergency Room
( ) Inpatient Hospital
( ) Outpatient Hospital
( ) Nursing Home

TOTAL CHARGE	$
AMOUNT PAID	$
PREVIOUS BAL	$
BALANCE DUE	$

Check #: _____
(Circle Method of Payment)
CASH CHECK MC VISA

Physician's Signature
▶ _____

WORK PRODUCT 22-3

Name: _____

Perform Billing Procedures

Corresponds to Procedure 22-8

<u>CAAHEP COMPETENCIES:</u> VI.P.VI.2.b.

<u>ABHES COMPETENCIES:</u> 8.i.

Complete the billing form below using the information in Part I, question 4.

Blackburn Primary Care Associates, PC
1990 Turquoise Drive
Blackburn, WI 54937
(608) 459-8857

Howard M. Lawler, MD 11
Joanne R. Hughes, MD 21
Ralph Garcia Lopez, MD 31
TAX ID NO. 00-00000000

GUARANTOR NAME AND ADDRESS	PATIENT NO.	PATIENT NAME	DOCTOR NO.	DATE

	DATE OF BIRTH	TELEPHONE NO.	INSURANCE CODE	DESCRIPTION	CERTIFICATE NO.

OFFICE - NEW
X	CPT	SERVICE	FEE
	99201	Prob Foc/Straight	
	99202	Exp Prob/Straight	
	99203	Detailed/Low	
	99204	Compre/Moderate	
	99205	Compre/High	

OFFICE - ESTABLISHED
X	CPT	SERVICE	FEE
	99211	Nurse/Minimal	
	99212	Prob Foc/Straight	
	99213	Exp Prob/Low	
	99214	Detailed/Moderate	
	99215	Compre/High	

OFFICE - CONSULT
X	CPT	SERVICE	FEE
	99241	Prob/Foc/Straight	
	99242	Exp Prob/Straight	
	99243	Detailed/Low	
	99244	Compre/Moderate	
	99245	Compre/High	

PREVENTIVE CARE - ADULT
X	CPT	SERVICE	FEE
	99385	18-39 Initial	
	99386	40-64 Initial	
	99387	65+ Initial	
	99395	18-39 Periodic	
	99396	40-64 Periodic	
	99397	65+ Periodic	

GASTROENEROLOGY
X	CPT	SERVICE	FEE
	45300	Sigmoidoscopy Rig	
	45305	Sigmoid Rig w/bx	
	45330	Sigmoidoscopy Flex	
	45331	Sigmoid Flex w/bx	
	45378	Colonoscopy Diag	
	45380	Colonoscopy w/bx	
	46600	Anoscopy	

CARDIOLOGY & HEARING
X	CPT	SERVICE	FEE
	93000	EKG (Global)	
	93015	Stress Test (Global)	
	93224	Holter (Global)	
	93225	Holter Hook Up	
	93227	Holter Interpretation	
	94010	Pulm Function Test	
	92551	Audiometry Screen	

INJECTIONS & IMMUNIZATION
X	CPT	SERVICE	FEE
	86585	TB Skin Test	
	90716	Varicella Vaccine	
	90724	Flu Vaccine	
	90732	Pneumovax	
	90718	TD Immunization	
	90782	Injection IM*	
	90788	Injection IM Antibiot*	
		Injection joint*	
	SM	MED	MAJOR (circle one)
FOR ALL INJECTIONS, SUPPLY DRUG INFORMATION			

REPAIR & DERMATOLOGY
X	CPT	SERVICE	FEE
	17110	Warts: #	
		Tags: #	
		Lesion Excis	
		Lesion Destruct	
SIZE CM:		SITE:	
MALIG:		PREMAL/BEN:	
		(Check One Above)	
		Simple Closure	
		Intermed Closure	
SIZE CM:		SITE:	
	10060	I&D Abscess	
	10080	I&D Cyst	

OTHER

SUPPLIES/DRUGS*
DRUG NAME:
UNIT/MEASURE:
QUANTITY

DIAGNOSTIC CODES: ICD-9-CM

- ☐ 789.0 Abdominal Pain
- ☐ 795.0 Abnormal Pap Smear
- ☐ 706.1 Acne Vulgaris
- ☐ 477.0 Allergic Rhinitis
- ☐ 285.9 Anemia, NOS
- ☐ 281.0 Pernicious
- ☐ 411.1 Angina, Unstable
- ☐ 427.9 Arythmia, NOS
- ☐ 440.9 Arteriosclerosis
- ☐ 714.0 Arthritis, Rheumatoid
- ☐ 414.0 ASHD
- ☐ 493.90 Asthma, Bronchial W/O Status Ast.
- ☐ 493.91 Asthma, Bronchial W/Status Ast.
- ☐ 466.1 Bronchiolitis, Acute
- ☐ 466.0 Bronchitis, Acute
- ☐ 727.3 Bursitis
- ☐ 786.50 Chest Pain
- ☐ 574.20 Cholelithiasis
- ☐ 372.30 Conjunctivitis, Unspecified
- ☐ 564.0 Constipation
- ☐ 496 COPD
- ☐ 692.9 Dermatitis, Allergic
- ☐ 250.01 Diabetes Mellitus, ID
- ☐ 250.00 Diabetes Mellitus, NID
- ☐ 558.9 Diarrhea
- ☐ 562.11 Diverticulitis
- ☐ 562.10 Diverticulosis

- ☐ 782.3 Edema
- ☐ 492.8 Emphysema
- ☐ V16.0 Family History Of Diabetes
- ☐ 780.6 Fever of Undetermined Origin
- ☐ 578.9 G.I. Bleeding, Unspecified
- ☐ 727.41 Ganglion of Joint
- ☐ 535.0 Gastritis, Acute
- ☐ V72.3 Arythmia, NOS
- ☐ 748.0 Headache
- ☐ 550.90 Hernia, Inguinal, NOS
- ☐ 054.9 Herpes Simplex
- ☐ 053.9 Herpes Zoster
- ☐ 708.9 Hives/Urticaria
- ☐ 401.1 Hypertension, Benign
- ☐ 401.0 Hypertension, Malignant
- ☐ 402.90 Hypertension, W/O CHF
- ☐ 244.9 Hypothyroidism, Primary
- ☐ 380.4 Impacted Cerumen
- ☐ 487.1 Influenza
- ☐ 564.1 Irritable Bowel Syndrome
- ☐ 464.0 Laryngitis, Acute
- ☐ 454.9 Leg Varicose Veins
- ☐ 424.0 Mitral Valve Prolapse
- ☐ 412 Myocardial Infarction, Old
- ☐ 715.90 Osteoarthritis, Unspec. Site
- ☐ 620.2 Ovarian Cyst

- ☐ 614.9 Pelvic Inflammatory Disease
- ☐ 685.1 Pilonidal Cyst
- ☐ 462 Pharyngitis, Acute
- ☐ 627.1 Postmenopausal Bleeding
- ☐ 625.4 Premenstrual Tension
- ☐ 782.1 Rash
- ☐ 569.3 Rectal Bleeding
- ☐ 398.90 Rheumatic Heart Disease, NOS
- ☐ 431.9 Sinusitis, Acute, NOS
- ☐ 782.1 Skin Eruption, Rash
- ☐ 845.00 Sprain, Ankle
- ☐ 848.9 Sprain, Muscle, Unspec. Site
- ☐ 785.6 Swollen Glands
- ☐ 246.9 Thyroid Disease, Unspecified
- ☐ 463 Tonsillitis, Acute

- ☐ 474.0 Tonsillitis, Chronic
- ☐ 465.9 Upper Respiratory Infection, Acute
- ☐ 599.0 Urinary Tract Infection
- ☐ V03.9 Vaccination/Bacterial Dis.
- ☐ V06.8 Vaccination/Combination
- ☐ V04.8 Vaccination, Influenza
- ☐ 616.10 Vaginitis, Vulvitis, NOS
- ☐ 780.4 Vertigo
- ☐ 787.0 Vomiting, Nausea
- ☐ _____ _____
- ☐ _____ _____
- ☐ _____ _____

RETURN APPOINTMENT
_____ Days
_____ Weeks
_____ Months

Authorization Number:
▶ _____

BALANCE DUE

DATE OF SERVICE	CPT CODE	DIAGNOSIS CODE(S)	CHARGE

Place of Service:
( ) Office
( ) Emergency Room
( ) Inpatient Hospital
( ) Outpatient Hospital
( ) Nursing Home

TOTAL CHARGE	$
AMOUNT PAID	$
PREVIOUS BAL	$
BALANCE DUE	$

Check #: _____
(Circle Method of Payment)
CASH   CHECK   MC   VISA

Physician's Signature
▶ _____

WORK PRODUCT 22-4

Name: _____

Posting to Patient Accounts

Corresponds to Procedures 22-3 through 22-6, 22-10

<u>CAAHEP COMPETENCIES:</u> VI.P.VI.2.d., VI.P.VI.2.e., VI.P.VI.2.f., VI.P.VI.2.g., VI.P.VI.2.h.

<u>ABHES COMPETENCIES:</u> 8.m., 8.n., 8.o., 8.p., 8.q.

Fill out the ledger using the information in Part II, ledger 1.

Blackburn Primary Care Associates, PC
1990 Turquoise Drive
Blackburn, WI 54937
Phone: 608-459-8857
Fax: 608-459-8860
E-mail: blackburnom@blackburnpca.com
www.blackburnpca.com

Patient Name _____

Address _____

City _____ State _____ Zip _____

Home Phone _____ Cell Phone _____

Email _____ MR# _____

Account Ledger

Entry #	Date	Reference	Service	Charge	Payment	Adj	Current Balance
1							
2							
3							
4							
5							
6							
7							
8							
9							
10							
11							
12							
13							
14							
15							
16							

WORK PRODUCT 22-5

Name: _____

Posting to Patient Accounts

Corresponds to Procedures 22-3 through 22-6, 22-10

CAAHEP COMPETENCIES: VI.P.VI.2.d., VI.P.VI.2.e., VI.P.VI.2.f., VI.P.VI.2.g., VI.P.VI.2.h.

ABHES COMPETENCIES: 8.m., 8.n., 8.o., 8.p., 8.q.

Fill out the ledger using the information in Part II, ledger 2.

Blackburn Primary Care Associates, PC
1990 Turquoise Drive
Blackburn, WI 54937
Phone: 608-459-8857
Fax: 608-459-8860
E-mail: blackburnom@blackburnpca.com
www.blackburnpca.com

Patient Name _____
Address _____
City _____ State _____ Zip _____
Home Phone _____ Cell Phone _____
Email _____ MR# _____

Account Ledger

Entry #	Date	Reference	Service	Charge	Payment	Adj	Current Balance
1							
2							
3							
4							
5							
6							
7							
8							
9							
10							
11							
12							
13							
14							
15							
16							

WORK PRODUCT 22-6

Name: _____

Posting to Patient Accounts

Corresponds to Procedures 22-3 through 22-6, 22-10

CAAHEP COMPETENCIES: VI.P.VI.2.d., VI.P.VI.2.e., VI.P.VI.2.f., VI.P.VI.2.g., VI.P.VI.2.h.

ABHES COMPETENCIES: 8.m., 8.n., 8.o., 8.p., 8.q.

Fill out the ledger using the information in Part II, ledger 3.

Blackburn Primary Care Associates, PC
1990 Turquoise Drive
Blackburn, WI 54937
Phone: 608-459-8857
Fax: 608-459-8860
E-mail: blackburnom@blackburnpca.com
www.blackburnpca.com

Patient Name _____
Address _____
City _____ State _____ Zip _____
Home Phone _____ Cell Phone _____
Email _____ MR# _____

Account Ledger

Entry #	Date	Reference	Service	Charge	Payment	Adj	Current Balance
1							
2							
3							
4							
5							
6							
7							
8							
9							
10							
11							
12							
13							
14							
15							
16							

WORK PRODUCT 22-7

Name: _____

Proof of Posting

Corresponds to Procedures 22-3 through 22-6, 22-10

<u>CAAHEP COMPETENCIES:</u> VI.P.VI.2.d., VI.P.VI.2.e., VI.P.VI.2.f., VI.P.VI.2.g., VI.P.VI.2.h.

<u>ABHES COMPETENCIES:</u> 8.m., 8.n., 8.o., 8.p., 8.q.

Today's Totals

Column A	Fees/Charges	$896.00
Column B	Payments	$1643.00
Column C	Adjustments	$36.00
Column D	New Balance	$3526.00
Column E	Old Balance	$4309.00

Daily Proof - Box One
Arithmetic Posting Proof

Column E	
Plus Column A	
Subtotal	
Minus Column B	
Subtotal	
Minus Column C	
Equals Column D	

Accounts Receivable
Previous Day 7923.00
Month to Date – Box Two
Accounts Receivable Proof

Accounts Receivable Previous Day	
Plus Column A	
Subtotal	
Minus Column B	
Subtotal	
Minus Column C	
Accounts Receivable End of Day	

Accounts Receivable
Beginning of Month $9071.00
Column A MTD $6589.00
Column B MTD $8226.00
Column C MTD $294.00
Year to Date – Box Three
Accounts Receivable Proof

Accounts Receivable Beginning of Month	
Plus Column A Month to Date	
Subtotal	
Minus Column B Month to Date	
Subtotal	
Minus Column C Month to Date	
Accounts Receivable Month to Date	

↑————TOTALS MUST EQUAL————↑

WORK PRODUCT 22-8

Name: _____

Perform Collection Procedures

PePCorresponds to Procedure 22-9

<u>CAAHEP COMPETENCIES:</u> VI.P.VI.2.c.

Blackburn Primary Care Associates
1990 Turquoise Drive
Blackburn, WI 54937
(555) 555-1234

WORK PRODUCT 22-9

Name: _____

Perform Collection Procedures

Corresponds to Procedure 22-9

CAAHEP COMPETENCIES: VI.P.VI.2.c.

Blackburn Primary Care Associates
1990 Turquoise Drive
Blackburn, WI 54937
(555) 555-1234

Name _____ Date _____ Score _____

Procedure 23-1 Write Checks in Payment of Bills

CAAHEP COMPETENCIES: VI.P.VI.2
ABHES COMPETENCIES: 8.j

Task: To write checks correctly for the payment of bills.

Equipment and Supplies
- Checkbook
- Bills to be paid

Standards: Complete the Procedure and all critical steps in _____ minutes with a minimum score of 85% within three attempts.

Scoring: Divide the points earned by the total possible points. Failure to perform a critical step, indicated by an asterisk (*), results in an unsatisfactory overall score.

Time began _____   Time ended _____   Total minutes: _____

Steps	Possible Points	Attempt 1	Attempt 2	Attempt 3
*1. Locate the bill to be paid. Then fill out the check stub first.	10			
*2. Complete the check stub and the check with a pen or use computer software.	10			
*3. Date the check.	10			
*4. Write the payee's name on the appropriate line.	10			
*5. Leave no space before the name and follow with dashes or a line so that information cannot be added to the check.	10			
6. Enter the amount correctly and in a way that prevents alteration.	20			
*7. Verify the amount with the check stub.	20			
8. On the bill being paid, note the date it was paid and the check number. Then file the bill.	10			

Comments:

Points earned _____ ÷ 100 possible points = Score _____ % Score

Instructor's signature _____

Name _____ Date _____ Score _____

Procedure 23-2 Prepare a Bank Deposit

CAAHEP COMPETENCIES: VI.P.VI.1
ABHES COMPETENCIES: 8.g

Task: To prepare a bank deposit for the day's receipts and to complete appropriate office records related to the deposit.

Equipment and Supplies
- Currency
- Checks for deposit
- Deposit slip
- Endorsement stamp
- Envelope
- Pen

Standards: Complete the Procedure and all critical steps in _____ minutes with a minimum score of 85% within three attempts.

Scoring: Divide the points earned by the total possible points. Failure to perform a critical step, indicated by an asterisk (*), results in an unsatisfactory overall score.

Time began _____ **Time ended** _____ **Total minutes:** _____

Steps	Possible Points	Attempt 1	Attempt 2	Attempt 3
1. Organize the currency.	10	_____	_____	_____
*2. Total the currency and record the amount on the deposit slip.	10	_____	_____	_____
*3. Put a restrictive endorsement on the back of each check.	20	_____	_____	_____
*4. List each check separately on the deposit slip by ABA number or the patient's last name.	20	_____	_____	_____
*5. Total the amount of currency and checks and enter the total on the deposit slip.	10	_____	_____	_____
*6. Enter the amount of the deposit in the checkbook.	10	_____	_____	_____
*7. Keep a copy of the deposit slip for office records.	10	_____	_____	_____
*8. Put the currency, checks, and deposit slip in an envelope or deposit bag for transport to the bank.	10	_____	_____	_____

Comments:

Points earned _____ ÷ 100 possible points = Score _____ % Score

Instructor's signature _____

Name _____ Date _____ Score _____

Procedure 23-3 Reconcile a Bank Statement

ABHES COMPETENCIES: 8.g

Task: To reconcile a bank statement with the checking account.

Equipment and Supplies
- Ending balance of previous statement
- Current bank statement
- Cancelled checks for current month
- Checkbook stubs
- Calculator
- Pen

Standards: Complete the Procedure and all critical steps in _____ minutes with a minimum score of 85% within three attempts.

Scoring: Divide the points earned by the total possible points. Failure to perform a critical step, indicated by an asterisk (*), results in an unsatisfactory overall score.

Time began _____ **Time ended** _____ **Total minutes:** _____

Steps	Possible Points	Attempt 1	Attempt 2	Attempt 3
*1. Compare the opening balance of the new statement with the closing balance of the previous statement.	10			
*2. Compare debits and/or cancelled checks with the items on the statement.	10			
*3. Arrange the checks in numeric order and compare them with the stubs.	10			
*4. Put a checkmark on the matching stub.	10			
*5. List and total the outstanding checks.	10			
*6. Verify that all previous outstanding checks have cleared.	10			
*7. Subtract the total of the outstanding checks from the statement balance.	10			
*8. To the total in step 7, add any deposits made but not included on the statement balance.	10			
*9. Total any bank charges that appear on the bank statement and subtract them from the checkbook balance.	10			
*10. If the checkbook and statement do not agree, match the bank statement entries with the checkbook entries to find the errors. Redo all math to check for errors.	10			

Comments:

Points earned _____ ÷ 100 possible points = Score _____ % Score

Instructor's signature _____

WORK PRODUCT 23-1

Name: _____

Prepare a Bank Deposit

Corresponds to Procedure 23-2

<u>CAAHEP COMPETENCIES:</u> VI.P.VI.2.

<u>ABHES COMPETENCIES:</u> 8.j.

Fill in the bank deposit figure using the information in Part IV, questions 1-4.

BANK DEPOSIT DETAIL

BANK NUMBER	PAYMENTS			CREDIT CARD
	BY CHECK OR PMO	BY COIN OR CURRENCY		
2387	67 00	20 00		100 00
460	50 00	20 00		250 00
309	1374 32	20 00		
		20 00		
		20 00		
		20 00		
		100 00		
		50 00		
		10 00		
		10 00		
		5 00		
		1 00		
TOTALS	1491 32	296 00		350 00
CURRENCY		296~		
COIN		~		
CHECKS		1491.32		
CREDIT CARDS		350~		
TOTAL RECEIPTS				
LESS CREDIT CARD $		350~		
TOTAL DEPOSITS		1787.32		

DEPOSIT DATE: _____ FIRM: _____

Name _____ Date _____ Score _____

Procedure 24-1 Perform Accounts Receivable Procedures

CAAHEP COMPETENCIES: VI.P.VI.2
ABHES COMPETENCIES: 8.k

Task: To collect amounts due to the physician or medical facility.

Equipment and Supplies
- Patient ledgers
- Office policy and Procedures manual
- Telephone
- Letterhead and envelopes
- Clerical supplies

Standards: Complete the Procedure and all critical steps in _____ minutes with a minimum score of 85% within three attempts.

Scoring: Divide the points earned by the total possible points. Failure to perform a critical step, indicated by an asterisk (*), results in an unsatisfactory overall score.

Time began _____ **Time ended** _____ **Total minutes:** _____

Steps	Possible Points	Attempt 1	Attempt 2	Attempt 3
*1. Prompt the computer to compile a report on the age of accounts receivables.	10			
*2. Divide the accounts into the following categories: a. 0–30 days b. 30–60 days c. 60–90 days d. 90–120 days e. over 120 days	20			
*3. If the computer program does not perform this function, manually pull all ledger cards with a balance due and divide them into the categories in step 2.	10			
*4. Examine the accounts to see which are awaiting an insurance payment or other activity. If insurance is pending and the account is not long overdue, do not take action. File these ledger cards back in the tray.	10			
*5. Follow office Procedure in taking collection activity on the account. Put collection stickers or messages on the inside of the mailing envelope.	10			
6. Attempt to call the patient and make payment arrangements.	10			
7. Bill the patient once monthly according to the individual's billing cycle.	10			

Steps	Possible Points	Attempt 1	Attempt 2	Attempt 3
8. Post payments on the day they arrive at the office.	10			
9. Demonstrate sensitivity and professionalism when handling accounts.	10			

Comments:

Points earned _____ ÷ 100 possible points = Score _____ % Score

Instructor's signature _____

Name _____ Date _____ Score _____

Procedure 24-2 Perform Accounts Payable Procedures

CAAHEP COMPETENCIES: VI.P.VI.2
ABHES COMPETENCIES: 8.j

Task: To determine the age of accounts and decide what collection activity is needed.

Equipment and Supplies
- Patient ledger cards with a balance due
- Pen
- Computer
- Calculator

Standards: Complete the Procedure and all critical steps in _____ minutes with a minimum score of 85% within three attempts.

Scoring: Divide the points earned by the total possible points. Failure to perform a critical step, indicated by an asterisk (*), results in an unsatisfactory overall score.

Time began _____ **Time ended** _____ **Total minutes:** _____

Steps	Possible Points	Attempt 1	Attempt 2	Attempt 3
1. Pull all ledger cards with a balance due and divide them into the following categories: a. 0–30 days b. 30–60 days c. 60–90 days d. 90–120 days e. over 120 days	10	_____	_____	_____
*2. Determine which accounts are awaiting an insurance payment. Return those ledgers to the ledger tray.	20	_____	_____	_____
*3. For the accounts that remain, follow the office Procedure for collections. Put collection reminder stickers on the statements sent to the patient or send a collection letter. Make sure the stickers are inside the envelope, not on the outside.	10	_____	_____	_____
*4. Call patients whose accounts are more than 90 days old. Attempt to make payment arrangements.	20	_____	_____	_____
*5. Send a collection letter to patients whose accounts are more than 120 days old.	20	_____	_____	_____
*6. Add the total accounts receivable for each category and arrive at a figure outstanding for each.	10	_____	_____	_____
7. Note in the chart and/or on the ledger any arrangements made with patients regarding payment of the accounts. Send a follow-up letter to remind the patients of their payment agreements.	10	_____	_____	_____

Comments:

Points earned _____ ÷ 100 possible points = Score _____ % Score

Instructor's signature _____

Name _____ Date _____ Score _____

Procedure 24-3 Account for Petty Cash

ABHES COMPETENCIES: 8.1

Task: To establish a petty cash fund, maintain an accurate record of expenditures for 1 month, and replenish the fund as necessary.

Equipment and Supplies
- Form for petty cash fund
- Pad of vouchers
- Disbursement journal
- Two checks
- List of petty cash expenditures

Standards: Complete the Procedure and all critical steps in _____ minutes with a minimum score of 85% within three attempts.

Scoring: Divide the points earned by the total possible points. Failure to perform a critical step, indicated by an asterisk (*), results in an unsatisfactory overall score.

Time began _____ Time ended _____ Total minutes: _____

Steps	Possible Points	Attempt 1	Attempt 2	Attempt 3
1. Determine the amount needed in the petty cash fund.	10			
*2. Write a check in the determined amount.	10			
*3. Record the beginning balance in the petty cash fund.	10			
*4. Post the amount to miscellaneous on the disbursement record.	10			
*5. Prepare a petty cash voucher for each amount withdrawn from the fund.	10			
*6. Record each voucher in the petty cash record and enter the new balance.	10			
*7. Write a check to replenish the fund as necessary, keeping in mind that the total of the vouchers plus the fund balance must equal the beginning amount in petty cash.	10			
*8. Total the expense columns and post to the appropriate accounts in the disbursement journal.	10			
*9. Record the amount added to the fund.	10			
*10. Record the new balance in the petty cash fund.	10			

Comments:

Points earned _____ ÷ 100 possible points = Score _____ % Score

Instructor's signature _____

Name _____ Date _____ Score _____

Procedure 24-4 Process an Employee Payroll

ABHES COMPETENCIES: 8.d

Task: To process payroll and compensate employees, making deductions accurately.

Equipment and Supplies
- Checkbook
- Computer and payroll software, if applicable
- Pen
- Tax withholding tables
- Federal Employers Tax Guide

Standards: Complete the Procedure and all critical steps in _____ minutes with a minimum score of 85% within three attempts.

Scoring: Divide the points earned by the total possible points. Failure to perform a critical step, indicated by an asterisk (*), results in an unsatisfactory overall score.

Time began _____ Time ended _____ Total minutes: _____

Steps	Possible Points	Attempt 1	Attempt 2	Attempt 3
*1. Make sure all information has been collected on the employees, including a copy of the Social Security card, a W-4 form, and an I-9 form.	20	_____	_____	_____
*2. Review the time cards for all employees. Determine whether any employees need counseling because of late arrivals or habitual absences.	20	_____	_____	_____
*3. Figure the salary or hourly wages due the employee for the period worked.	20	_____	_____	_____
*4. Figure the deductions that must be taken from the paycheck. These usually include but are not limited to: a. Federal, state, and local taxes b. Social Security withholdings c. Medicare withholdings d. Other deductions (e.g., insurance, savings) e. Donations to organizations (e.g., the United Way)	20	_____	_____	_____
*5. Write the check for the balance due the employee. Most software can print the checks and explanations of deductions. Put a copy in the employee's file.	20	_____	_____	_____

Comments:

Points earned _____ ÷ 100 possible points = Score _____ % Score

Instructor's signature _____

Name _____ Date _____ Score _____

Procedure 25-1 Interview Effectively

ABHES COMPETENCIES: 8.ff

Task: To evaluate job candidates fairly and choose the best person to fill an available position in the medical facility.

Equipment and Supplies
- Candidate's completed job application
- Candidate's resume
- Private area in the medical office
- Clerical supplies

Standards: Complete the Procedure and all critical steps in _____ minutes with a minimum score of 85% within three attempts.

Scoring: Divide the points earned by the total possible points. Failure to perform a critical step, indicated by an asterisk (*), results in an unsatisfactory overall score.

Time began _____ **Time ended** _____ **Total minutes:** _____

Steps	Possible Points	Attempt 1	Attempt 2	Attempt 3
*1. Review the duties the candidate will be required to perform.	5			
*2. Match each job application with the corresponding résumé.	5			
*3. Separate strong candidates from the moderate and the weak candidates.	5			
*4. Call each strong candidate and schedule an appointment for an interview.	5			
*5. Evaluate the applicant's speaking voice while making the appointment for the interview.	2			
6. Select several interview questions in advance to ask all the applicants.	5			
*7. Note whether the applicant arrives on time for the interview.	2			
*8. Introduce yourself to the applicant and proceed to a private area for the interview.	5			
*9. Make the applicant feel as much at ease as possible.	5			
*10. Ask the applicant the chosen questions.	5			

Steps	Possible Points	Attempt 1	Attempt 2	Attempt 3
*11. Evaluate the answers and make notations about the candidate that are not demeaning or unprofessional.	10			
*12. Ask the candidate whether he or she has any questions.	2			
*13. Offer the candidate a brief tour of the facility.	2			
*14. Provide a date by which a hiring decision will be made and suggest that the candidate call the facility that day, if desired.	2			
*15. Evaluate all applicants fairly according to their experience and training.	5			
*16. Select the best three candidates and call them for a second interview, if desired.	5			
*17. Discuss the final hiring decision with the physician or others who might be involved in the hiring process.	5			
*18. Make the final hiring decision.	5			
*19. Call the candidate to ask him or her to come to the office to discuss the position.	5			
*20. Negotiate salary and benefits.	5			
*21. Offer the position.	5			
*22. If the offer is declined, call the next candidate to the office to discuss the position; repeat until a satisfactory candidate accepts and agrees to a start date.	5			

Comments:

Points earned _____ ÷ 100 possible points = Score _____ % Score

Instructor's signature _____

Name _____ Date _____ Score _____

Procedure 25-2 Conduct a Performance Review

ABHES COMPETENCIES: 4.a

Task: To evaluate job performance fairly and determine the strengths and weaknesses of employees using accurate documentation.

Equipment and Supplies
- Employee's file
- Past evaluations of employee
- Notes and/or reports on employee's behavior
- Private area in the medical office
- Clerical supplies

Standards: Complete the Procedure and all critical steps in _____ minutes with a minimum score of 85% within three attempts.

Scoring: Divide the points earned by the total possible points. Failure to perform a critical step, indicated by an asterisk (*), results in an unsatisfactory overall score.

Time began _____   Time ended _____   Total minutes: _____

Steps	Possible Points	Attempt 1	Attempt 2	Attempt 3
1. Set an appointment for the review with the employee.	10	___	___	___
*2. Allow the employee to complete a self-evaluation of his or her own work.	10	___	___	___
*3. Review the self-evaluation, then document additional information about the employee and his or her performance.	15	___	___	___
4. Share the information with any other supervisor or the physician, if dictated by office policy or if needed for additional input.	10	___	___	___
*5. Complete the final written review and proofread it for accuracy and completeness.	10	___	___	___
*6. Discuss the review with the employee during the evaluation appointment.	10	___	___	___
*7. Progress through the interview and explain the results of the evaluation to the employee.	10	___	___	___
*8. Allow the employee to respond to any of the points raised during the evaluation, but do not allow an argumentative attitude.	5	___	___	___

Steps	Possible Points	Attempt 1	Attempt 2	Attempt 3
*9. Allow the employee to respond to the evaluation in writing within a limited period (e.g., 5 days).	5			
*10. Ask the employee to sign the evaluation to document that it was reviewed with the individual (the employee does not have to agree with the evaluation to sign it).	5			
*11. Give a copy of the evaluation to the employee.	5			
*12. Put a copy of the evaluation in the employee's file.	5			

Comments:

Points earned _____ ÷ 100 possible points = Score _____ % Score

Instructor's signature _____

Name _____ Date _____ Score _____

Procedure 25-3 Arrange a Group Meeting

ABHES COMPETENCIES: 4.d

Task: To plan and conduct a productive meeting that will result in achieved goals and apply concepts for office Procedures.

Equipment and Supplies
- Meeting room
- Agenda
- Visual aids and equipment
- Handouts
- Stopwatch or clock
- Computer
- Paper
- List of items for the agenda

Standards: Complete the Procedure and all critical steps in _____ minutes with a minimum score of 85% within three attempts.

Scoring: Divide the points earned by the total possible points. Failure to perform a critical step, indicated by an asterisk (*), results in an unsatisfactory overall score.

Time began _____ Time ended _____ Total minutes: _____

Steps	Possible Points	Attempt 1	Attempt 2	Attempt 3
1. Determine the purpose of the meeting and draft a list of the items to be discussed; include the desired results of the meeting.	10	_____	_____	_____
*2. Determine where the meeting will be held, the time and date of the meeting, and the individuals who should attend.	10	_____	_____	_____
*3. Send a memo, e-mail, or letter to the individuals who should attend the meeting at least 10 days in advance, if possible. Send a copy to any supervisors who should be kept informed about the issues to be raised at the meeting.	10	_____	_____	_____
*4. Make sure the notice includes the following information: a. Date b. Time c. Place d. Directions (if not a common meeting room or if held away from the office) e. Speakers and/or meeting topics f. Cost and registration information, if applicable g. List of items individuals should bring to the meeting	10	_____	_____	_____
*5. Finalize the list of items to discuss and place them in priority order.	10	_____	_____	_____

Steps	Possible Points	Attempt 1	Attempt 2	Attempt 3
*6. Delegate any tasks that others can accomplish and follow up to be sure they fulfill their duties before the meeting.	10			
*7. Assign a staff member the task of taking notes and keeping time during the meeting.	10			
*8. Make a list of all items to take to the meeting (e.g., microphones, projectors, screens, computers, disks containing presentations).	10			
*9. Compile the final agenda for the meeting.	10			
*10. On the meeting day, transport all items needed to the meeting room. Begin and end the meeting on time. Stay on track and follow the agenda.	10			

Comments:

Points earned _____ ÷ 100 possible points = Score _____ % Score

Instructor's signature _____

Name _____ Date _____ Score _____

Procedure 26-1 Design a Presentation

ABHES COMPETENCIES: 7.b.(2.)

Task: To gain skill in designing presentations that can be used for a variety of projects in the medical facility.

Equipment and Supplies
- Information about presentation subject
- Software (e.g., PowerPoint), if needed
- Computer access
- Peripheral computer equipment, if needed

Standards: Complete the Procedure and all critical steps in _____ minutes with a minimum score of 85% within three attempts.

Scoring: Divide the points earned by the total possible points. Failure to perform a critical step, indicated by an asterisk (*), results in an unsatisfactory overall score.

Time began _____ **Time ended** _____ **Total minutes:** _____

Steps	Possible Points	Attempt 1	Attempt 2	Attempt 3
*1. Determine the goals of the presentation.	10			
2. Write an outline of the entire presentation.	10			
3. Build the presentation using software (e.g., PowerPoint), highlighting the major points of the presentation.	5			
*4. Evaluate the audience and adjust the presentation to appeal to that audience.	10			
5. Rehearse the presentation several times in front of a mirror.	5			
6. Make a list of all equipment and materials to take to the presentation.	10			
*7. Arrive for the presentation 15 to 30 minutes early, depending on the preparation and setup required.	10			
8. Deliver the presentation within the prescribed period.	10			
9. Ask the audience whether they have any questions about the information in the presentation.	10			
10. Thank the audience and remove all equipment and supplies when appropriate.	10			
11. Send a thank you note to the organization for allowing the presentation, if appropriate.	10			

Comments:

Points earned _____ ÷ 100 possible points = Score _____ % Score

Instructor's signature _____

Name _____ Date _____ Score _____

Procedure 26-2 Prepare a Presentation Using PowerPoint

ABHES COMPETENCIES: 7.b.(2.)

Task: To enhance presentations using PowerPoint as a visual aid.

Equipment and Supplies
- Information about presentation subject
- Software (for this exercise, PowerPoint)
- Computer access
- Peripheral computer equipment, if needed

Standards: Complete the Procedure and all critical steps in _____ minutes with a minimum score of 85% within three attempts.

Scoring: Divide the points earned by the total possible points. Failure to perform a critical step, indicated by an asterisk (*), results in an unsatisfactory overall score.

Time began _____   Time ended _____   Total minutes: _____

Steps	Possible Points	Attempt 1	Attempt 2	Attempt 3
1. Open the PowerPoint program.	5	____	____	____
2. Have the outline of the presentation available.	5	____	____	____
3. Click on the NEW SLIDE icon on the program menu.	5	____	____	____
4. Create the title slide using the slide layout section on the right side of the screen.	5	____	____	____
5. Create additional slides using the slide layout section or design the slides manually.	5	____	____	____
*6. Limit the number of words on the slides so that a concise message results	5	____	____	____
7. Make sure the font is as large as possible on the slide, beginning with a size 18 font and increasing from there.	5	____	____	____
*8. Do not use more than three fonts per slide.	5	____	____	____
*9. Do not use more than three text-only slides in a row.	5	____	____	____
10. Insert photographs or clip art into the presentation: click on INSERT and then on PICTURE; then choose CLIP ART or FROM FILE.	5	____	____	____

Steps	Possible Points	Attempt 1	Attempt 2	Attempt 3
11. Format the background of each slide or of all slides: click on FORMAT, and then BACKGROUND; then choose a color or fill effect.	5	_____	_____	_____
12. Click on SLIDE SHOW and adjust the slide transitions so that the slides appear and disappear as desired and are timed correctly.	5	_____	_____	_____
13. Click on CUSTOM ANIMATION to change the entrance and exit of the slides to achieve the desired effect.	5	_____	_____	_____
*14. Save the presentation frequently while working on it.	5	_____	_____	_____
15. Click on VIEW in the task bar and then on SLIDE SORTER to be able to move the slides around in the presentation.	5	_____	_____	_____
16. To run the show continuously, click on SLIDE SHOW and then on SET UP SHOW; in the Show Options box, click in the box labeled Loop Continuously Until Escape.	5	_____	_____	_____
17. Make sure the presentation has been saved.	5	_____	_____	_____
*18. Practice the presentation several times to smooth all transitions and to become thoroughly familiar with the content.	5	_____	_____	_____
*19. Anticipate questions the audience may ask and have answers prepared.	5	_____	_____	_____
20. Offer other visual aids (e.g., handouts), if appropriate, when giving the presentation.	5	_____	_____	_____

Documentation in the Medical Record:

Comments:

Points earned _____ ÷ 100 possible points = Score _____ % Score

Instructor's signature _____

Name _____ Date _____ Score _____

Procedure 27-1 Develop a Patient Safety Plan: Order the Correct Medication from the Pharmacy

CAAHEP COMPETENCIES: X.PXI.3
ABHES COMPETENCIES: 6.b, 6.c, 6.d, 6.e, 9.g

Task: To telephone the correct medication prescription order into the pharmacy.

Scenario: The physician writes an order to be phoned into the pharmacy for a new patient diagnosed with depression. You think the order reads "Avinza, 30 mg PO bid." The pharmacist asks you for the physician's DEA number, because Avinza is a narcotic analgesic. You ask the physician for clarification and are told the order was for Avanza, an antidepressant. Look up both medications in a drug reference. What could have happened if a powerful narcotic had been ordered rather than the antidepressant the physician intended?

Equipment and Supplies
- Notepad with pen
- PDR or other drug reference
- Patient's record

Standards: Complete the procedure and all critical steps in _____ minutes with a minimum score of 85% in three attempts.

Scoring: Divide the points earned by the total possible points. Failure to perform a critical step, indicated by an asterisk (*), results in an unsatisfactory overall score.

Time began _____   Time ended _____   Total minutes: _____

Steps	Possible Points	Attempt 1	Attempt 2	Attempt 3
1. Review the physician's written order for a prescription or repeat the order back to the physician if it is a verbal order. For a verbal order, write down the order and have the physician review it to make sure you have the correct medication before calling the pharmacy.	20			
2. If you are unfamiliar with the medication, look up the drug in a reference book.	20			
3. Once you are familiar with a medication, if the order does not match the patient's diagnosis, ask the physician for clarification.	20			
4. Refer to the office's policy and procedures manual to review the procedure for calling in a prescription order to the pharmacy.	20			
5. Clarify any questions with the office manager to prevent any future errors.	20			

Comments:

Points earned _____ ÷ 100 possible points = Score _____ % Score

Instructor's signature _____

Name _____ Date _____ Score _____

Procedure 27-2 Evaluate the Work Environment to Identify Safe and Unsafe Working Conditions: Develop an Environmental Safety Plan

CAAHEP COMPETENCIES: X.PXI.2, X.PXI.4
ABHES COMPETENCIES: 9.e

Task: To assess the healthcare facility for possible safety issues and develop a safety plan.

Scenario: Work with a partner to evaluate environmental safety in the laboratory at your school. Record your results and discuss with the class. After the group shares their observations, develop a safety plan for your lab.

Equipment and Supplies
- Pen and paper
- Policy and procedure for environmental safety issues in the facility

Standards: Complete the procedure and all critical steps in _____ minutes with a minimum score of 85% in three attempts.

Scoring: Divide the points earned by the total possible points. Failure to perform a critical step, indicated by an asterisk (*), results in an unsatisfactory overall score.

Time began _____ Time ended _____ Total minutes: _____

Steps	Possible Points	Attempt 1	Attempt 2	Attempt 3
1. Check the floors and hallways for obstructions and possible tripping hazards, including torn carpets, possible spills, protruding electrical cords, and so on.	10			
2. Check storage areas to make sure the tops of cabinets are clear and heavier items are stored closer to the floor.	10			
3. Assess the location and security of handrails placed around the facility. They should be placed with all stairs, in bathrooms, and in any other areas staff members or patients may need assistance.	10			
4. Examine all electrical plugs and outlets to prevent electrical overload.	10			
5. Check all equipment to make sure it is in safe working condition.	10			
6. Make sure all lights are working (both inside and outside the facility). Also make sure there is adequate lighting and that light fixtures are in good condition.	10			

Steps	Possible Points	Attempt 1	Attempt 2	Attempt 3
7. Check the working condition of smoke alarms and examine all fire extinguishers.	10			
8. Make sure evacuation routes are posted throughout the facility, with clearly marked exit routes and floor plans with exits marked.	10			
9. Record your observations and share them with the class.	10			
10. Based on group discussion, develop a plan of action for improving the safety of the laboratory.	10			

Comments:

Points earned _____ ÷ 100 possible points = Score _____ % Score

Instructor's signature _____

Name _____ Date _____ Score _____

Procedure 27-3 Develop an Employee Safety Plan: Manage a Difficult Patient

CAAHEP COMPETENCIES: X.PXI.3
ABHES COMPETENCIES: 5.a, 9.e

Task: To communicate with an angry patient in a safe, therapeutic manner. The following procedure is part of an overall employee safety plan.

Scenario: You are working at the admissions desk when an extremely angry patient comes storming into the office, yelling about a mistake on his bill. Although the facility uses an outside billing center, you recognize that you should try to help the patient and attempt to diffuse the situation. Remember: Call 911 immediately and alert any available security if you or one of your co-workers is threatened with violence.

Equipment and Supplies
- Telephone
- Policy and procedures manual
- Patient's record

Standards: Complete the procedure and all critical steps in _____ minutes with a minimum score of 85% in three attempts.

Scoring: Divide the points earned by the total possible points. Failure to perform a critical step, indicated by an asterisk (*), results in an unsatisfactory overall score.

Time began _____ Time ended _____ Total minutes: _____

Steps	Possible Points	Attempt 1	Attempt 2	Attempt 3
1. Although it is important to safeguard a patient's privacy, do not ask an angry patient into an isolated room; do not close the door.	10			
2. Alert other staff members about the situation if possible.	10			
3. If you do not feel physically threatened, allow the patient to blow off steam.	10			
4. When the patient begins to slow down, offer supportive statements, such as, "I understand it is frustrating to receive a bill you think is unfair." Continue to make supportive statements until the patient is calmer (think of it as the patient screaming his way up a mountain; sooner or later he is going to run out of steam; when he begins to slow down, you can then start offering supportive statements).	10			
5. Once you can discuss the situation, ask the patient for the details of the problem. Gather as much information as possible so you can work together on a possible solution.	20			

Steps	Possible Points	Attempt 1	Attempt 2	Attempt 3
6. After determining the problem, suggest a possible solution. For example, you will contact the billing office with the information and make sure they get back to the patient as soon as possible.	10			
7. Report the incident to your supervisor. In the following Documentation in the Medical Record section, document the problem and the agreed-upon action as you would in the patient's record, being careful not to use judgmental statements.	20			
8. Discuss your approach to managing the difficult patient at the next staff meeting. With your supervisor's permission, summarize your approach and include it as part of the facility's employee safety plan.	10			

Documentation in the Medical Record:

Comments:

Points earned _____ ÷ 100 possible points = Score _____ % Score

Instructor's signature _____

Name _____ Date _____ Score _____

Procedure 27-4 Demonstrate the Proper Use of a Fire Extinguisher

CAAHEP COMPETENCIES: X.PXI.5
ABHES COMPETENCIES: 9.a

Task: To role-play the safe and proper use of a fire extinguisher.

Equipment and Supplies
- Portable, office-size ABC fire extinguisher that has been discharged

Standards: Complete the procedure and all critical steps in _____ minutes with a minimum score of 85% in three attempts.

Scoring: Divide the points earned by the total possible points. Failure to perform a critical step, indicated by an asterisk (*), results in an unsatisfactory overall score.

Time began _____ **Time ended** _____ **Total minutes:** _____

Steps	Possible Points	Attempt 1	Attempt 2	Attempt 3
1. Pull the pin from the handle of the extinguisher.	20			
2. Aim the discharge from the extinguisher toward the bottom of the flames.	20			
3. Squeeze the handle of the extinguisher so that it begins to discharge.	20			
4. Sweep the extinguisher from side to side toward the base of the fire until it is out or until fire officials arrive.	20			
5. Check on the safety of all patients and other personnel.	20			

Comments:

Points earned _____ ÷ 100 possible points = Score _____ % Score

Instructor's signature _____

Name _____ Date _____ Score _____

Procedure 27-5 Participate in a Mock Environmental Exposure Event: Evacuate a Physician's Office

CAAHEP COMPETENCIES: XI.PXI.6, XI.PXI.7
ABHES COMPETENCIES: 9.e

Task: To role-play an environmental disaster and implement an evacuation plan.

Scenario: Role-play this scenario with your lab group: The building next door to the physician's office where you work is on fire. One member of the group is the designated emergency action coordinator, two individuals are responsible for helping patients with special needs out of the facility, and one person is designated to be the last to leave after the building has been cleared. In a community emergency situation, certain staff members may be designated to provide immediate assistance to survivors. Two medical assistants are sent to help with fire victims. How could medical assistants help in this situation? After the evacuation is complete, meet in a designated spot to discuss the process and determine whether the evacuation plan could be improved in any areas. Document the steps taken throughout the mock environmental event.

Equipment and Supplies
- Pen and paper
- Policy and procedure for evacuation of the facility and response to an environmental disaster

Standards: Complete the procedure and all critical steps in _____ minutes with a minimum score of 85% in three attempts.

Scoring: Divide the points earned by the total possible points. Failure to perform a critical step, indicated by an asterisk (*), results in an unsatisfactory overall score.

Time began _____ Time ended _____ Total minutes: _____

Steps	Possible Points	Attempt 1	Attempt 2	Attempt 3
1. An emergency action coordinator is put in charge.	5	_____	_____	_____
2. The coordinator takes action to manage the emergency at the facility and notifies and works with community emergency services.	5	_____	_____	_____
3. Victims of the fire are being cared for across the street, where a triage and treatment center has been set up by the city's police, fire, and emergency responder units. Two medical assistant staff members are sent to help. They do the following: • Use therapeutic communication techniques to calm and care for victims • Implement appropriate Standard Precautions • Monitor and record vital signs • Gather pertinent health histories • Observe victims for possible complications (e.g., breathing problems, shock, angina) • Immediately report any life-threatening changes in a patient's status to emergency responders • Use first aid skills as needed.	10	_____	_____	_____

Steps	Possible Points	Attempt 1	Attempt 2	Attempt 3
4. The coordinator designates an employee to immediately shut down any combustibles (e.g., oxygen tanks).	10			
5. Using the posted evacuation routes, staff members follow floor plan diagrams to the closest safe exit. They also identify any hazardous areas in the facility to avoid during the emergency evacuation.	10			
6. Staff members provide assistance for employees and patients with special needs who may require extra help during the evacuation.	10			
7. One staff member checks to make sure everyone has left the facility and that fire doors have been closed before leaving the building.	10			
8. All evacuated personnel and patients meet in a designated area to count heads and make sure everyone exited the facility safely.	10			
9. After everyone has been accounted for and the office's patients are safe, staff members who are not needed report to the triage area to provide assistance to rescue workers and victims.	10			
10. Discuss the evacuation exercise and response to a community disaster with the class.	10			
11. Document your role in the exercise. What were the strengths and weaknesses of the group's response to an environmental emergency?	10			

Comments:

Points earned _____ ÷ 100 possible points = Score _____ % Score

Instructor's signature _____

Name _____ Date _____ Score _____

Procedure 27-6 Maintain an Up-to-Date List of Community Resources for Emergency Preparedness

CAAHEP COMPETENCIES: X.PXI.12
ABHES COMPETENCIES: 9.e

Task: To develop and maintain a list of community agencies that would respond to a natural disaster or other emergency.

Scenario: You are asked by your employer to develop a list of groups in your community who are part of the community-wide emergency preparedness plan that has been mandated by the state and federal government. Using multiple resources, develop a comprehensive list of emergency services for your area.

Equipment and Supplies
- Telephone
- Internet access
- Pen and paper
- Electronic record

Standards: Complete the procedure and all critical steps in _____ minutes with a minimum score of 85% in three attempts.

Scoring: Divide the points earned by the total possible points. Failure to perform a critical step, indicated by an asterisk (*), results in an unsatisfactory overall score.

Time began _____ **Time ended** _____ **Total minutes:** _____

Steps	Possible Points	Attempt 1	Attempt 2	Attempt 3
1. Start with an online search for the area LEMA office sponsored by the Department of Homeland Security. If the office has a Web site, check it for information about the emergency preparedness plan in your community. You can begin the search at *www.ready.gov/america*.	25			
2. Gather contact information for local police, fire, and EMS services that can be posted next to all telephones in the facility.	25			
3. Investigate services provided by your local Public Health office and the American Red Cross.	25			
4. Organize the information you gathered about community resources for emergency preparedness. With your supervisor's approval, post a copy of this information in all appropriate locations in the facility. Prepare a data base in the computer that can be updated as the information changes.	25			

Comments:

Points earned _____ ÷ 100 possible points = Score _____ % Score

Instructor's signature _____

Name _____ Date _____ Score _____

Procedure 27-7 Maintain Provider/Professional-Level CPR Certification: Use an Automated External Defibrillator

CAAHEP COMPETENCIES: X.PXI.9
ABHES COMPETENCIES: 9.e, 9.o

Task: To defibrillate adult victims with cardiac arrest. Most adult victims in sudden cardiac arrest are in ventricular fibrillation. The survival rate for victims with ventricular fibrillation is as high as 90% when defibrillation occurs within the first minute of collapse; however, the survival rate for these patients declines 7% to 10% with every minute defibrillation does not occur.

Equipment and Supplies
- Practice automated external defibrillator (AED)
- Approved mannequin

Standards: Complete the procedure and all critical steps in _____ minutes with a minimum score of 85% in three attempts.

Scoring: Divide the points earned by the total possible points. Failure to perform a critical step, indicated by an asterisk (*), results in an unsatisfactory overall score.

Time began _____ **Time ended** _____ **Total minutes:** _____

Steps	Possible Points	Attempt 1	Attempt 2	Attempt 3
1. Place the AED near the victim's left ear and then turn on the machine.	10			
2. Attach the electrode pads as pictured on the AED. Place the electrodes at the sternum and the apex of the heart. Make sure the pads are in complete contact with the victim's chest and do not overlap.	20			
3. All rescuers must clear away from the victim. Press the ANALYZE button; the AED analyzes the victim's coronary status, announces whether the victim is going to be shocked, and automatically charges the electrodes.	20			
*4. All rescuers must clear away from the victim. If the machine is not automated, press the SHOCK button. Three analyze-shock cycles may be performed.	20			
5. Deliver one shock; leave the AED attached and immediately resume CPR, starting with chest compressions.	10			

Steps	Possible Points	Attempt 1	Attempt 2	Attempt 3
6. After five cycles of CPR (about 2 minutes), repeat the AED analysis and deliver another shock if indicated. If a nonshockable rhythm is detected, the AED should instruct the rescuer to resume CPR immediately, beginning with chest compressions.	10			
7. If the machine gives the "no shock indicated" signal, assess the victim. Check the carotid pulse and the person's breathing status and keep the AED attached until emergency medical services arrive.	10			

Comments:

Points earned _____ ÷ 100 possible points = Score _____ % Score

Instructor's signature _____

Name _____ Date _____ Score _____

Procedure 27-8 Perform Patient Screening Using Established Protocols: Telephone Screening and Appropriate Documentation

CAAHEP COMPETENCIES: I.PI.6
ABHES COMPETENCIES: 9.e

Task: To assess the direction of emergency care and document information appropriately in the patient's record.

Scenario: Cheryl is working with the telephone screening staff when they receive a call from the mother of a 5-year-old patient. The mother reports that her son fell and cut his arm. What type of information should Cheryl gather about the injury? What action should be taken? How should the incident be documented?

Equipment and Supplies
- Notepad with pen or pencil
- Facility's emergency procedures manual
- Appointment book or computer program
- Area emergency numbers
- Patient's medical record

Standards: Complete the procedure and all critical steps in _____ minutes with a minimum score of 85% in three attempts.

Scoring: Divide the points earned by the total possible points. Failure to perform a critical step, indicated by an asterisk (*), results in an unsatisfactory overall score.

Time began _____ Time ended _____ Total minutes: _____

Steps	Possible Points	Attempt 1	Attempt 2	Attempt 3
1. Stay calm and reassure the caller.	10			
2. Verify the identity of the caller and the injured patient.	10			
3. Immediately record the names of the caller and the patient, their location, and the phone number.	10			
4. Determine whether the patient's condition is life-threatening. Quantify the amount of blood loss and determine whether the patient is alert and responsive and breathing is normal. Notify EMS if necessary.	10			
5. If EMS is notified, stay on the line with the caller until EMS personnel arrive at the scene.	10			

Steps	Possible Points	Attempt 1	Attempt 2	Attempt 3
6. If emergency services are not needed, gather details about the injury to determine whether the patient can be seen in the office or should be referred to an emergency department (ED). Consider the following questions: • Is there a suspected head or neck injury? • Has the patient been moved? • Is there a possible fracture? If so, where? • Are there any other symptoms? • Is there anything pertinent in the patient's health history that would complicate the situation? • Has the caller administered any first aid? If so, what type?	10			
7. Based on the information gathered, determine when the patient should be seen in the office if the person is not referred to an ED.	10			
8. At any point in this process, do not hesitate to consult the physician or experienced staff members or refer to the facility's emergency procedures manual to determine how to manage the patient's problem.	10			
9. Always allow the caller to hang up first, just in case more information or assistance is needed.	10			
10. In the following Documentation in the Medical Record section, document as you would in the patient's record the information gathered, the actions taken or recommended, any home care recommendations, and whether the physician was notified.	10			

Documentation in the Medical Record:

Comments:

Points earned _____ ÷ 100 possible points = Score _____ % Score

Instructor's signature _____

Name _____ Date _____ Score _____

Procedure 27-9 Maintain Provider/Professional-Level CPR Certification: Perform Adult Rescue Breathing and One-Rescuer CPR; Perform Pediatric and Infant CPR

CAAHEP COMPETENCIES: X.PXI.9
ABHES COMPETENCIES: 9.e, 9.o

Task: To restore a victim's breathing and circulation when respiration or pulse or both stop.

Equipment and Supplies
- Disposable gloves
- CPR ventilator mask for the adult, child, and infant
- Approved mannequins

Standards: Complete the procedure and all critical steps in _____ minutes with a minimum score of 85% within three attempts.

Scoring: Divide the points earned by the total possible points. Failure to perform a critical step, indicated by an asterisk (*), results in an unsatisfactory overall score.

Time began _____ **Time ended** _____ **Total minutes:** _____

Steps	Possible Points	Attempt 1	Attempt 2	Attempt 3
1. Establish unresponsiveness. Tap the victim and ask, "Are you OK?" Wait a moment for a response.	10	____	____	____
2. Activate the emergency response system. Put on gloves and get the ventilator mask.	5	____	____	____
3. Tilt the victim's head by placing one hand on the forehead and applying enough pressure to push the head back; with the fingers of the other hand under the chin, lift up and pull the jaw forward. Look, listen, and feel for signs of breathing. Place your ear over the mouth and listen for breathing. Watch the rising and falling of the chest for evidence of breathing. If breathing is absent or inadequate, open the airway and place the ventilator mask over the victim's mouth and nose.	10	____	____	____
4. Give 2 slow breaths (1½ to 2 seconds per breath for an adult; 1 to 2 seconds per breath for an infant or child), holding the ventilator mask tightly against the face while tilting the victim's chin up to keep the airway open. Remove your mouth from the mouthpiece between breaths to allow time for the patient to exhale between breaths.	10	____	____	____

Steps	Possible Points	Attempt 1	Attempt 2	Attempt 3

*5. Check the patient's pulse (at the carotid artery for an adult or older child; at the brachial artery for an infant). If a pulse is present, continue rescue breathing (1 breath every 4 to 5 seconds—about 10 to 12 breaths per minute for an adult; 1 breath every 3 seconds— about 12 to 20 breaths per minute for an infant or child). If no signs of circulation are present, begin cycles of 30 chest compressions (at a rate of about 100 compressions per minute for an adult) followed by 2 slow breaths. 10 _____ _____ _____

6. To deliver chest compressions, kneel at the victim's side a couple of inches from the chest. Move your fingers up the ribs to the point where the sternum and the ribs join in the center of the lower part of the sternum but above the xiphoid process. 10 _____ _____ _____

*7. Place the heel of your hand on the chest over the lower part of the sternum. 5 _____ _____ _____

*8. Place your other hand on top of the first and either interlace or lift your fingers upward off of the chest. 5 _____ _____ _____

9. 5 _____ _____ _____

10. Depress the sternum 1½ to 2 inches in an adult victim. Relax the pressure on the sternum after each compression but do not remove your hands from the sternum. 10 _____ _____ _____

11. After performing 30 compressions (at a rate of about 100 compressions per minute), perform the head tilt–chin lift maneuver to open the airway and give 2 slow rescue breaths. 5 _____ _____ _____

12. After 5 cycles of compressions and breaths (30:2 ratio, about 2 minute) recheck the breathing and carotid pulse. If a pulse is present but breathing is not, continue rescue breathing (1 breath every 5 seconds, about 10 to 12 breaths per minute) and re-evaluate the victim's breathing and pulse every few minutes. If no signs of circulation are present, continue 30:2 cycles of compressions and ventilations, starting with chest compressions. Continue giving CPR until an AED is available or EMS relieves you. 5 _____ _____ _____

Performing CPR on a child: The procedure for performing CPR on a child ages 1 through 8 years is essentially the same as that for an adult. The differences are as follows:
- Perform 5 cycles of compressions and breaths on the child (30:2 ratio, about 2 minutes) before calling 911 or the local emergency number or using an AED. If another person is available, have that person activate EMS while you care for the child.

Steps	Possible Points	Attempt 1	Attempt 2	Attempt 3

- Use only one hand to perform chest compressions.
- Breathe more gently.
- Use the same compression-to-breath ratio as used for adults, 30 compressions followed by 2 breaths per cycle; after 2 breaths, immediately begin the next cycle of compressions and breaths.
- After 5 cycles (about 2 minutes) of CPR without response, use a pediatric AED if available.
- Continue until the child responds or help arrives.

Performing CPR on an infant: Infant cardiac arrest typically is caused by a lack of oxygen from drowning or choking. If you know the infant has an airway obstruction, clear the obstruction; if you do not know why the infant is unresponsive, perform CPR for 2 minutes (about 5 cycles) before calling 911 or the local emergency number. If another person is available, have that person call for help immediately while you attend to the baby.
- Draw an imaginary line between the infant's nipples. Place two fingers on the sternum just below this intermammary line.
- Gently compress the chest.
- Compression rate should be 100 to 120 per minute.
- Administer 2 slow breaths after every 30 compressions.
- After about five 30:2 cycles, activate EMS.
- Continue CPR until the infant responds or help arrives.

Rescue breathing for an infant: Use an infant ventilator mask or cover the baby's mouth and nose with your mouth.
- Give 2 rescue breaths by gently puffing out the cheeks and slowly breathing into the infant's mouth, taking about 1 second for each breath.

13. Remove your gloves and the ventilator mask valve and discard them in the biohazard container. Disinfect the ventilator mask per the manufacturer's recommendations. Sanitize your hands.   5   ____   ____   ____

14. In the following Documentation in the Medical Record section, document the procedure and the patient's condition as you would in the patient's medical record.   5   ____   ____   ____

Documentation in the Medical Record:

Comments:

Points earned _____ ÷ 100 possible points = Score _____ % Score

Instructor's signature _____

Name _____ Date _____ Score _____

Procedure 27-10 Perform First Aid Procedures: Administer Oxygen

CAAHEP COMPETENCIES: X.PXI.10
ABHES COMPETENCIES: 9.e

Task: To provide oxygen for a patient in respiratory distress.

Equipment and Supplies
- Physician's order
- Portable oxygen tank
- Pressure regulator
- Flow meter
- Nasal cannula with connecting tubing
- Patient's chart

Standards: Complete the procedure and all critical steps in _____ minutes with a minimum score of 85% in three attempts.

Scoring: Divide the points earned by the total possible points. Failure to perform a critical step, indicated by an asterisk (*), results in an unsatisfactory overall score.

Time began _____ Time ended _____ Total minutes: _____

Steps	Possible Points	Attempt 1	Attempt 2	Attempt 3
1. Gather the necessary equipment and sanitize your hands.	10	____	____	____
2. Identify the patient and explain the procedure.	10	____	____	____
3. Check the pressure gauge on the tank to determine the amount of oxygen in the tank.	10	____	____	____
4. If necessary, open the cylinder on the tank one full counterclockwise turn; then attach the cannula tubing to the flow meter.	10	____	____	____
*5. Adjust the flow of oxygen according to the physician's order. Usually the flow meter is set at 12 to 15 liters per minute (LPM). Check to make sure oxygen is flowing through the cannula.	20	____	____	____
6. Insert the cannula tips into the patient's nostrils and adjust the tubing around the back of the ears.	10	____	____	____
7. Make sure the patient is comfortable and answer any questions the patient may have. Continue to monitor the patient throughout the procedure and document any changes in the person's condition.	10	____	____	____

Steps	Possible Points	Attempt 1	Attempt 2	Attempt 3
8. Sanitize your hands.	10	_____	_____	_____
9. In the following Documentation in the Medical Record section, document the procedure as you would in the patient's record. Include the number of liters of oxygen being administered and the patient's condition.	10	_____	_____	_____

Documentation in the Medical Record:

Comments:

Points earned _____ ÷ 100 possible points = Score _____ % Score

Instructor's signature _____

Procedure **27-10** Perform First Aid Procedures: Administer Oxygen

Name _____ Date _____ Score _____

Procedure 27-11 Perform First Aid Procedures: Respond to an Airway Obstruction in an Adult

CAAHEP COMPETENCIES: X.PXI.10
ABHES COMPETENCIES: 9.e

Task: To remove an airway obstruction and restore ventilation.

Equipment and Supplies
- Disposable gloves
- Ventilation mask (for unconscious victim)
- Approved mannequin for practicing removal of a foreign body airway obstruction (FBAO)

Standards: Complete the procedure and all critical steps in _____ minutes with a minimum score of 85% in three attempts.

Scoring: Divide the points earned by the total possible points. Failure to perform a critical step, indicated by an asterisk (*), results in an unsatisfactory overall score.

Time began _____   Time ended _____   Total minutes: _____

Steps	Possible Points	Attempt 1	Attempt 2	Attempt 3
1. Ask the victim, "Are you choking?" If the victim indicates yes, ask, "Can you speak?" If the victim is unable to speak, tell the person you are going to help.	10			
2. Stand behind the victim with your feet slightly apart.	5			
3. Reach around the victim's abdomen and place an index finger into the victim's navel or at the level of the belt buckle. Make a fist of the opposite hand (do not tuck the thumb into the fist) and place the thumb side of the fist against the victim's abdomen above the navel. If the victim is pregnant, place the fist above the enlarged uterus. If the victim is obese, you may need to place the fist higher in the abdomen. (Chest thrusts may need to be performed on a pregnant or obese victim.)	10			
*4. Place the opposite hand over the fist and give abdominal thrusts in a quick inward and upward movement.	10			
5. Repeat the abdominal thrusts until the object is expelled or the victim becomes unresponsive.	5			
Unresponsive Victim				
6. Carefully lower the patient to the ground, activate the emergency response system, and put on disposable gloves.	10			

Steps	Possible Points	Attempt 1	Attempt 2	Attempt 3
7. Immediately begin CPR with 30 compressions and 2 breath cycles using the ventilator mask.	10			
8. Each time the airway is opened to deliver a rescue breath during CPR, look for an object in the victim's mouth and remove it if visible. If no object is found, immediately return to the cycle of 30 chest compressions.	10			
9. A finger sweep should be used only if the obstruction is visible.	5			
10. Continue cycles of 30 compressions to 2 rescue breaths until either the obstruction is removed or EMS arrives.	5			
11. If the obstruction is removed, assess the victim for breathing and circulation. If a pulse is present but the patient is not breathing, begin rescue breathing.	10			
12. Once either the patient's condition has stabilized or EMS has taken over, remove your gloves and the ventilator mask valve and discard them in the biohazardous waste container. Disinfect the ventilator mask according to the manufacturer's recommendations. Sanitize your hands.	5			
13. In the following Documentation in the Medical Record section, document the procedure and the patient's condition as you would in the patient's record.	5			

Documentation in the Medical Record:

Comments:

Points earned _____ ÷ 100 possible points = Score _____ % Score

Instructor's signature _____

Name _____ Date _____ Score _____

Procedure 27-12 Perform First Aid Procedures: Care for a Patient Who Has Fainted

CAAHEP COMPETENCIES: X.PXI.10
ABHES COMPETENCIES: 9.e

Task: To provide emergency care for and assessment of a patient who has fainted.

Equipment and Supplies
- Sphygmomanometer
- Stethoscope
- Watch with second hand
- Blanket
- Foot stool or box
- Pillows
- Oxygen equipment, if ordered by the physician:
  - Portable oxygen tank
  - Pressure regulator
  - Flow meter
  - Nasal cannula with connecting tubing
- Patient's record

Standards: Complete the procedure and all critical steps in _____ minutes with a minimum score of 85% in three attempts.

Scoring: Divide the points earned by the total possible points. Failure to perform a critical step, indicated by an asterisk (*), results in an unsatisfactory overall score.

Time began _____ Time ended _____ Total minutes: _____

Steps	Possible Points	Attempt 1	Attempt 2	Attempt 3
*1. If a warning is given that the patient feels faint, have the patient lower the head to the knees to increase the blood supply to the brain. If this does not stop the episode, either have the patient lie down on the examination table or lower the patient to the floor. If the patient collapses to the floor when fainting, treat with caution because of possible head or neck injuries.	10	_____	_____	_____
2. Immediately notify the physician of the patient's condition and assess the patient for life-threatening emergencies, such as respiratory or cardiac arrest. If the patient is breathing and has a pulse, monitor the vital signs.	10	_____	_____	_____
3. Loosen any tight clothing and keep the patient warm. Cover the person with a blanket if needed.	10	_____	_____	_____
*4. If a head or neck injury is not a concern, elevate the patient's legs above the level of the heart, using a footstool with pillow if available.	20	_____	_____	_____

Steps	Possible Points	Attempt 1	Attempt 2	Attempt 3
5. Continue to monitor the vital signs. Provide oxygen via nasal cannula if ordered by the physician.	10			
6. If the vital signs are unstable or the patient does not respond quickly, activate emergency medical services.	10			
7. If the patient vomits, roll the person onto his or her side to prevent aspiration of vomitus into the lungs.	10			
8. Once the patient has recovered completely, help the person into a sitting position. Do not leave the patient unattended on the examination table.	10			
9. In the following Documentation in the Medical Record section, document the incident as you would in the patient's record: Include a description of the episode, the patient's symptoms and vital signs, the duration of the faint, and any complaints. If oxygen was administered, document the number of liters and how long it was administered.	10			

Documentation in the Medical Record:

Comments:

Points earned _____ ÷ 100 possible points = Score _____ % Score

Instructor's signature _____

Name _____ Date _____ Score _____

Procedure 27-13 Perform First Aid Procedures: Control Bleeding

CAAHEP COMPETENCIES: III.PIII.2, III.PIII.3, X.PXI.10
ABHES COMPETENCIES: 9.e

Task: To stop hemorrhaging from an open wound.

Equipment and Supplies
- Gloves (sterile if available)
- Appropriate personal protective equipment (PPE) according to OSHA guidelines, including:
  ○ Impermeable gown
  ○ Goggles or face shield
  ○ Impermeable mask
  ○ Impermeable foot covers if indicated
- Sterile dressings
- Bandaging material
- Biohazardous waste container
- Patient's record

Standards: Complete the procedure and all critical steps in _____ minutes with a minimum score of 85% in three attempts.

Scoring: Divide the points earned by the total possible points. Failure to perform a critical step, indicated by an asterisk (*), results in an unsatisfactory overall score.

Time began _____ Time ended _____ Total minutes: _____

Steps	Possible Points	Attempt 1	Attempt 2	Attempt 3
1. Sanitize your hands and put on the appropriate PPE.	10	_____	_____	_____
2. Assemble the necessary equipment and supplies.	10	_____	_____	_____
3. Apply several layers of sterile dressing material directly to the wound and exert pressure.	10	_____	_____	_____
4. Wrap the wound with bandage material. Add more dressing and bandaging material if the bleeding continues.	10	_____	_____	_____
5. If the bleeding persists and the wound is on an extremity, elevate the extremity above the level of the heart. Notify the physician immediately if the bleeding cannot be controlled.	10	_____	_____	_____

Steps	Possible Points	Attempt 1	Attempt 2	Attempt 3
6. If the bleeding still continues, maintain direct pressure and elevation; also apply pressure to the appropriate artery. If the wound is in the arm, apply pressure to the brachial artery by squeezing the inner aspect of the upper middle arm. If the wound is in the leg, apply pressure to the femoral artery on the affected side by pushing with the heel of the hand into the femoral crease at the groin. If the bleeding cannot be controlled, activate emergency medical services.	10	_____	_____	_____
7. Once the bleeding has been controlled and the patient's condition has been stabilized, dispose of contaminated materials in the biohazardous waste container.	10	_____	_____	_____
8. Disinfect the area, remove your gloves, and discard them in the biohazardous waste container.	10	_____	_____	_____
9. Sanitize your hands.	10	_____	_____	_____
10. In the following Documentation in the Medical Record section, document the incident as you would in the patient's record. Include the details of the wound, when and how it occurred, the patient's symptoms and vital signs, the treatment provided by the physician, and the patient's current condition.	10	_____	_____	_____

Documentation in the Medical Record:

Comments:

Points earned _____ ÷ 100 possible points = Score _____ % Score

Instructor's signature _____

Name _____ Date _____ Score _____

Procedure 28-1 Organize a Job Search

ABHES COMPETENCIES: 11.a

Task: To devote adequate time to the job search and organize it in an efficient way to facilitate proper follow-up.

Equipment and Supplies
- Record of a job lead form
- Record of an interview form
- Copies of your résumé
- List of interview questions
- Contact information for former employers and references
- Map of geographic area (e.g., printed from an Internet mapping program)
- Internet access
- Computer
- Job search Web links
- Local newspapers
- Contact information for friends and family

Standards: Complete the procedure and all critical steps in _____ minutes with a minimum score of 85% within three attempts.

Scoring: Divide the points earned by the total possible points. Failure to perform a critical step, indicated by an asterisk (*), results in an unsatisfactory overall score.

Time began _____   Time ended _____   Total minutes: _____

Steps	Possible Points	Attempt 1	Attempt 2	Attempt 3
*1. Format the résumé as an accurate, up-to-date document.	5	_____	_____	_____
2. Make copies of the record of job lead form and the record of interview form.	5	_____	_____	_____
*3. Research job search Web sites and newspapers for job leads.	10	_____	_____	_____
*4. Network and contact employers directly to obtain job leads.	10	_____	_____	_____
*5. Gather information on job leads and complete a record of job lead form for each one.	10	_____	_____	_____
6. Prepare a targeted copy of your résumé for each job lead.	10	_____	_____	_____
7. Take the résumé to the facility, and ask to complete an application, *or* …	5	_____	_____	_____

Steps	Possible Points	Attempt 1	Attempt 2	Attempt 3
*8. E-mail the résumé to the facility according to the directions listed in the job advertisement.	5			
*9. Document all activity pertaining to each job lead.	10			
10. Schedule interviews for as many facilities as possible.	10			
*11. Keep a record of job details on the record of interview form for later reference.	5			
*12. Send thank you notes to all professionals who grant an interview when the appointment is over.	10			
13. Compare opportunities when making a choice between offered positions.	5			

Did the student exhibit initiative in organizing the job search?

Comments:

Points earned _____ ÷ 100 possible points = Score _____ % Score

Instructor's signature _____

Name _____ Date _____ Score _____

Procedure 28-2 Prepare a Résumé

ABHES COMPETENCIES: 11.a

Task: To write an effective résumé for use as a tool in gaining employment

Equipment and Supplies
- Scratch paper
- Pen or pencil
- Former job descriptions, if available
- List of addresses of former employers, schools, and names of supervisors
- Computer or word processor
- Quality stationery and envelopes

Standards: Complete the procedure and all critical steps in _____ minutes with a minimum score of 85% within three attempts.

Scoring: Divide the points earned by the total possible points. Failure to perform a critical step, indicated by an asterisk (*), results in an unsatisfactory overall score.

Time began _____ **Time ended** _____ **Total minutes:** _____

Steps	Possible Points	Attempt 1	Attempt 2	Attempt 3
1. Perform a self-evaluation by making notes about your strengths as a medical assistant. Consider job skills, self-management skills, and transferable skills.	10			
2. Explore formatting and decide on a professional résumé appearance that best highlights your skills and experience. Use the templates available in word processing software or design your own.	10			
3. Put your name, address, and two telephone numbers where you can be contacted at the top of the résumé.	10			
4. Write a job objective that specifies your employment goals.	10			
5. Provide details about your educational experience. List degrees and/or certifications you have obtained.	10			
6. Provide details about your work experience. Include the names and contact information for all previous supervisors. Do not include salary expectations or reasons for leaving former jobs.	10			
7. Prepare a cover letter and a list of references. Send the references with the résumé only when requested.	10			
8. Type the résumé carefully and make sure it has no errors.	5			

Steps	Possible Points	Attempt 1	Attempt 2	Attempt 3
9. Proofread the résumé. Allow another person to read it and check it for missed errors.	5			
10. Print the résumé on high-quality paper. Review it again for errors and to make sure it looks attractive on the printed page.	5			
11. Target each résumé to a specific person or position. Do not send generic résumés to each prospective employer.	5			
12. For all résumés distributed, follow up with a phone call to arrange an interview.	10			

Did the student exhibit dependability, punctuality, and a positive work ethic through his or her wording of the resume?

Did the student express a responsible attitude in his or her wording of the resume?

Comments:

Points earned _____ ÷ 100 possible points = Score _____ % Score

Instructor's signature _____

Name _____ Date _____ Score _____

Procedure 28-3 Complete a Job Application

ABHES COMPETENCIES: 11.a

Task: To complete an accurate, detailed, written job application legibly so as to secure a job offer.

Equipment and Supplies
- Record of job lead form
- Record of interview form
- Copies of your résumé
- Contact information for former employers and references
- Contact information for friends and family

Standards: Complete the procedure and all critical steps in _____ minutes with a minimum score of 85% within three attempts.

Scoring: Divide the points earned by the total possible points. Failure to perform a critical step, indicated by an asterisk (*), results in an unsatisfactory overall score.

Time began _____ **Time ended** _____ **Total minutes:** _____

Steps	Possible Points	Attempt 1	Attempt 2	Attempt 3
*1. Read the entire job application before completing any part of it.	10	_____	_____	_____
2. Gather any information that may be necessary to answer all questions on the application.	10	_____	_____	_____
*3. Begin to complete the application legibly.	10	_____	_____	_____
4. Answer each question on the document or write "not applicable."	10	_____	_____	_____
5. Do not leave any space blank.	10	_____	_____	_____
6. Do not write "See résumé" anywhere on the document.	10	_____	_____	_____
*7. Be completely honest about every fact written on the document.	10	_____	_____	_____
8. Sign the document and date it.	10	_____	_____	_____
*9. Proofread the document and make sure none of the information conflicts with your résumé.	10	_____	_____	_____
10. Submit the application.	10	_____	_____	_____

Comments:

Points earned _____ ÷ 100 possible points = **Score** _____ **% Score**

Instructor's signature _____

Name _____ Date _____ Score _____

Procedure 28-4 Interview for a Job

MAERB/CAAHEP COMPETENCIES: IV.A.IV.6
ABHES COMPETENCIES: 11.a, 8.aa

Task: To project a professional appearance during a job interview and to be able to express the reasons you, the medical assistant, are the best candidate for the position.

Equipment and Supplies
- Record of job lead form
- Record of interview form
- Job application
- Copies of your résumé
- Contact information for former employers and references
- Contact information for friends and family
- Sample interview questions

Standards: Complete the procedure and all critical steps in _____ minutes with a minimum score of 85% within three attempts.

Scoring: Divide the points earned by the total possible points. Failure to perform a critical step, indicated by an asterisk (*), results in an unsatisfactory overall score.

Time began _____   **Time ended** _____   **Total minutes:** _____

Steps	Possible Points	Attempt 1	Attempt 2	Attempt 3
*1. Prepare for the interview by studying sample interview questions and learning basic information about the facility.	10	_____	_____	_____
*2. Know all the information on your résumé so that you can discuss it confidently during the interview.	10	_____	_____	_____
*3. Prepare clothing that reflects a professional image for the facility where you hope to be employed.	10	_____	_____	_____
4. Gather all materials that might be needed during the interview, such as copies of résumés, contact information, and copies of earned certificates.	5	_____	_____	_____
*5. Arrive for the interview at least 15 minutes early.	10	_____	_____	_____
6. Stand and shake hands with the interviewer when he or she enters the room.	5	_____	_____	_____
7. Listen intently as the interviewer describes the position and be ready to explain how you fit the requirements for the position.	5	_____	_____	_____
*8. Answer all of the interviewer's questions confidently, smiling when appropriate and displaying a positive attitude.	10	_____	_____	_____

Steps	Possible Points	Attempt 1	Attempt 2	Attempt 3
*9. When the interviewer has finished, ask intelligent questions.	10	____	____	____
10. Determine a day and time when the next contact will be made.	5	____	____	____
11. Express interest in the position.	5	____	____	____
*12. Send a thank you note or letter to the interviewer within 24 hours of the interview.	10	____	____	____
*13. Follow up on the interview as appropriate.	5	____	____	____

Did the student demonstrate awareness of how an individual's personal appearance affects anticipated responses?
Did the student pay attention, listen, and learn during the interview?
Did the student exhibit a positive attitude and a sense of responsibility during the interview?
Did the student express an ability to adapt to change during the interview?

Comments:

Points earned _____ ÷ 100 possible points = Score _____ % Score

Instructor's signature _____

Name _____ Date _____ Score _____

Procedure 28-5 Negotiate a Salary

ABHES COMPETENCIES: 11.a

Task: To develop negotiation skills that will help you, as a medical assistant, obtain the salary and benefits that will sustain your family.

Equipment and Supplies
- Record of job lead form
- Record of interview form
- Information about job offers received
- Contact name at medical facility

Standards: Complete the procedure and all critical steps in _____ minutes with a minimum score of 85% within three attempts.

Scoring: Divide the points earned by the total possible points. Failure to perform a critical step, indicated by an asterisk (*), results in an unsatisfactory overall score.

Time began _____ **Time ended** _____ **Total minutes:** _____

Steps	Possible Points	Attempt 1	Attempt 2	Attempt 3
1. Study the job offer made.	5			
2. Determine whether the offer is sufficient as it stands.	5			
*3. Make a list of what additional salary and/or benefits you need, at a minimum.	10			
4. Arrive at the second or subsequent interview appointment to discuss the job with the hiring supervisor.	5			
*5. Thank the supervisor for the offer presented and express interest in the position.	5			
6. State the additional salary and/or benefits desired.	10			
7. Discuss the possibilities as to whether the facility would be willing to increase the offer to match your request.	10			
*8. Give reasons the additional benefits should be offered, based on your past performance, experience, or other valid factors.	10			
9. Discuss reasonable compromises regarding the additional salary and/or benefits.	10			

Steps	Possible Points	Attempt 1	Attempt 2	Attempt 3
10. Ask what level of performance is expected for an increase in salary and/or benefits	5	_____	_____	_____
11. Express interest in the position and tell the supervisor you will be giving it serious consideration.	10	_____	_____	_____
12. Determine the next contact time with the supervisor.	5	_____	_____	_____
13. Weigh the offer and compromises to make a good decision about the job offer.	10	_____	_____	_____

Was the student courteous and diplomatic during salary negotiations?

Comments:

Points earned _____ ÷ 100 possible points = Score _____ % Score

Instructor's signature _____

English-Spanish Terms for the Medical Assistant

abscess A localized collection of pus that causes tissue destruction and may be either under the skin or deep within the body.
absceso Cantidad de pus localizada en un lugar que puede estar bajo la piel o a más profundidad en el interior del cuerpo y causa la destrucción de los tejidos.

academic degree A title conferred by a college, university, or professional school after completion of a program of study.
grado académico Título concedido por una, universidad o escuela profesional, tras completar un programa de estudios.

accommodation Adjustment of the eye for seeing various sizes of objects at different distances.
acomodación Ajuste del ojo para ver distintos tamaños de objetos a distancias diferentes.

account A statement of transactions during a fiscal period and the resulting balance.
cuenta Estado de transacciones durante un periodo fiscal y el saldo resultante.

account balance The amount owed or on hand in an account.
saldo de la cuenta Suma que se debe o que está en una cuenta.

accounts receivable ledger A record of the income and payments due from creditors on an account.
libro mayor de cuentas por cobrar Registro de cargos y pagos asentados en una cuenta.

accreditation The process by which an organization is recognized for adhering to a group of standards that meet or exceed the expectations of the accrediting agency.
acreditación Proceso por el cual se reconoce a una organización por su cumplimiento de ciertos estándares en un grado que cumple o sobrepasa las expectativas de la agencia que la acredita.

act The formal product of a legislative body; a decision or determination by a sovereign, a legislative council, or a court of justice.
ley Producto formal de un cuerpo legislativo; decisión o determinación por un soberano, un consejo legislativo o un tribunal de justicia.

acute Having a rapid onset and severe symptoms.
agudo Que tiene un comienzo rápido y síntomas serios.

adage A saying, often in metaphoric form, that embodies a common observation.
refrán Dicho, con frecuencia metafórico, que refleja una observación común.

adhesions Bands of scar tissue that bind together two anatomic surfaces that normally are separate.
adhesiones Bandas de tejido de una cicatriz que unen dos superficies anatómicas que están normalmente separadas.

adrenocorticotropic hormone (ACTH) A hormone released by the anterior pituitary gland that stimulates the production and secretion of glucocorticoids.
hormona adrenocorticotropina (ACTH) Hormona, liberada por la glándula pituitaria anterior, que estimula la producción y secreción de glucocorticoides.

advent A coming into being or use.
advenimiento Próximo a ser o a usarse.

advocate One who pleads the cause of another; one who defends or maintains a cause or proposal.
abogado Persona que defiende la causa de otro; aqel que defiende o apoya una causa o propuesta.

affable Being pleasant and at ease in talking to others; characterized by ease and friendliness.
afable Que es agradable y tiene un trato fácil con los demás; caracterizado por su trato fácil y amistoso.

agenda A list or outline of things to be considered or done.
agenda Lista o resumen de cosas a considerar o a hacer.

aggression A forceful action or procedure intended to dominate; hostile, injurious, or destructive behavior, especially when caused by frustration.
agresión Acción o procedimiento forzado, con la intención de dominar; comportamiento hostil, injurioso o destructivo, en especial cuando es causado por frustración.

albuminuria Abnormal presence of albumin in the urine.
albuminuria Presencia anómala de albúmina en la orina.

aliquot   A portion of a well-mixed sample removed for testing.
alícuota   Porción de una muestra bien mezclada, separada para ser analizada.

allegation   A statement of what a party to a legal action undertakes to prove.
alegación   Declaración por una de las partes implicadas en un proceso legal para apoyar lo que dicha parte intenta probar.

allied health fields   Areas of healthcare delivery or related services in which professionals assist physicians with the diagnosis, treatment, and care of patients in many different specialty areas.
campos relacionados con la salud   Áreas del cuidado de la salud y servicios relacionados en los cuales profesionales ayudan a los médicos en el diagnóstico, tratamiento y atención de los pacientes en muchas áreas diferentes.

allocating   Apportioning for a specific purpose or to particular persons or things.
distribuir   Asignar a un fin específico o a personas o cosas en particular.

allopathy   A method of treating a disease by introducing a condition that is intended to cause a pathologic reaction that will be antagonistic to the condition being treated.
alopatía   Método de tratar una enfermedad provocando una afección con el fin de causar una reacción patológica, la cual será opuestaa la enfermedad que se está tratando.

allowed charge   The maximum amount of money that many third-party payors will pay for a specific procedure or service.   Often based on the UCR fee.
cargo permitido   Cantidad máxima de dinero que muchos pagadores intermediarios pagan por una práctica o servicio especifico; con frecuencia se basa en el cargo   UCR.

alopecia   Partial or complete lack of hair.
alopecia   Pérdida de cabello, parcial o total.

alphabetic filing   Any system that arranges names or topics according to the sequence of the letters in the alphabet.
archivo alfabético   Cualquier sistema que ordena los nombres o temas siguiendo la secuencia de las letras del alfabeto.

alphanumeric   Systems made up of combinations of letters and numbers.
alfanumérico   Sistema constituido por combinaciones de letras y números.

ambiguous   Capable of being understood in two or more possible senses or ways; unclear.
ambiguo   Que puede entenderse de dos o más maneras; que no es claro.

amblyopia   Reduction or dimness of vision with no apparent organic cause; often referred to as *lazy eye syndrome*.
ambliopía   Reducción o disminución de la visión sin causa orgánica aparente; con frecuencia se conoce como *síndrome del ojo vago*.

ambulatory   Able to walk about and not be bedridden.
ambulatorio   Capaz de caminar y no tiene que estar postrado en la cama.

amenity   Something conducive to comfort, convenience, or enjoyment.
amenidad   Algo que proporciona confort, comodidad o placer.

amino acids   Organic compounds that form the chief constituents of protein and are used by the body to build and repair tissues.
aminoácidos   Compuestos orgánicos que son los constituyentes principales de la proteína y son usados por el cuerpo para formar y reparar tejidos.

amorphous   Lacking a defined shape.
amorfo   Que carece de forma definida.

analyte   The substance or chemical being analyzed or detected in a specimen.
analito   La sustancia o producto químico que se analiza o que se detecta en una muestra.

anaphylaxis   Exaggerated hypersensitivity reaction that in severe cases leads to vascular collapse, bronchospasm, and shock.
anafilaxia   Reacción de hipersensibilidad exagerada, la cual, en casos graves, conduce a colapso vascular, broncospasmo y choque.

anastomosis   The surgical joining together of two normally distinct organs.
anastomosis   Unión quirúrgica de dos órganos normalmente diferentes.

ancillary   Subordinate; auxiliary.
auxiliar   Subordinado, complementario.

ancillary diagnostic services   Services that support patient diagnoses (e.g., laboratory or x-ray).
servicios de diagnóstico auxiliares   Servicios que apoyan el diagnóstico del paciente (como laboratorio o rayos x).

"and" In the context of ICD-9-CM, the word "and" should be interpreted as "and/or."
"y" En el contexto de ICD-9-CM, la palabra "y" debe interpretarse como "y/o."

anemia A condition marked by deficiency of red blood cells.
anemia Enfermedad caracterizada por una deficiencia de glóbulos rojos en la sangre.

angiocardiography Radiography of the heart and great vessels using an iodine contrast medium.
angiocardiografía Radiografía del corazón y los vasos sanguíneos mayores usando un medio de contraste yodado.

angiography Radiography of blood vessels using an iodine contrast medium.
angiografía Radiografía de los vasos sanguíneos usando un medio de contraste yodado.

angioplasty Interventional technique using a catheter to open or widen a blood vessel to improve circulation.
angioplastia Técnica quirúrgica que usa un catéter para abrir o hacer más ancho un vaso sanguíneo a fin de mejorar la circulación.

animate Full of life; to give spirit and support to expressions.
animar Dar vida; dar ánimo y apoyo a las manifestaciones.

annotating To furnish with notes, which are usually critical or explanatory.
anotar Añadir notas, por lo general, críticas o explicatorias.

annotation A note added by way of comment or explanation.
anotación Nota añadida a modo de comentario o explicación.

anomalies Faulty development of the fetus resulting in deformities or deviations from normal.
anomalías Desarrollo defectuoso del feto que tiene como resultado deformidades o desviaciones de lo normal.

anorexia Lack or loss of appetite for food.
anorexia Falta o pérdida del apetito.

anoxia Absence of oxygen in the tissues.
anoxia Ausencia de oxígeno en los tejidos.

anteroposterior (AP) Frontal projection in which the patient is supine or facing the x-ray tube.
anteroposterior (AP) Proyección frontal en la cual el paciente está en posición supina o frente al tubo de rayos x.

antibody Immunoglobulin produced by the immune system in response to bacteria, viruses, or other antigenic substances.
anticuerpo Inmunoglobulina producida por el sistema inmunológico en respuesta a bacterias, virus u otras substancias antigénicas.

anticoagulant A chemical added to the blood after collection to prevent clotting.
anticoagulante Producto químico que se añade a la sangre después de extraerla para que no forme coágulos.

antidiuretic hormone (ADH) A hormone secreted at the posterior pituitary gland that causes water retention in the kidneys and elevates the blood pressure; also known as *vasopressin*.
hormona antidiurética (ADH) Hormona secretada por la glándula pituitaria posterior y que provoca retención de agua en los riñones y aumento de la presión sanguínea. Es conocida también como *vasopresina*.

antigen A foreign substance that causes the production of a specific antibody.
antígeno Substancia extraña que provoca la producción de un anticuerpo específico.

antimicrobial agent A drug that is used to treat infection.
agente antimicrobiano Substancia que se usa para tratar infecciones.

antiseptic Pertaining to substances that inhibit the growth of microorganisms (e.g., alcohol and Betadine).
antiséptico Perteneciente o relativo a las substancias que inhiben el crecimiento de microorganismos como el alcohol y la Betadina.

antiseptic A substance that kills microorganisms.
antiséptico Substancia que mata microorganismos.

antiseptic An agent that inhibits bacterial growth and can be used on human tissue.
antiséptico Agente que inhibe el crecimiento bacteriano y que puede usarse en los tejidos humanos.

aortogram A radiographic image of the aorta made with the use of an iodine contrast medium.
aortograma Radiografía de la aorta usando un medio de contraste yodado.

apnea Absence or cessation of breathing.
apnea Ausencia o cese de la respiración.

appeal A legal proceeding by which a case is brought before a higher court for review of the decision of a lower court.
apelación Procedimiento legal por el cual un caso se lleva ante un tribunal superior para obtener una revisión de la decisión de un tribunal inferior.

appellate Having the power to review the judgment of another tribunal or body of jurisdiction; for example, an appellate court reviews the rulings of a lower court.
de apelación Que tiene el poder de revisar el veredicto de otro tribunal o cuerpo jurídico, como una corte de apelación.

applications Software programs designed to perform specific tasks.
aplicaciones Programas informáticos diseñado para realizar tareas específicas.

appraisal An expert judgment of the value or merit of something; judging as to quality.
evaluación Acción de emitir un juicio experto sobre el valor o mérito de algo; juzgar la calidad de algo; evaluar el rendimiento en el trabajo.

arbitration The hearing and determination of a cause in controversy by a person or persons either chosen by the parties involved or appointed under statutory authority.
arbitraje Vista y resolución de una causa en conflicto por una persona o personas elegida/s por las partes implicadas o designadas por la autoridad establecida por ley.

arbitrator A neutral person chosen to settle differences between two parties in a controversy.
árbitro Persona neutral seleccionada para poner fin a las diferencias entre dos partes involucradas en un conflicto.

archaic Of, relating to, or characteristic of an earlier or more primitive time.
arcaico Perteneciente o relativo a una época anterior o más primitiva; que tiene las características de dicha época.

archive To file or collect records or documents in or as if in an archive.
archivar Guardar o recoger informes o documentos en un archivo o de manera similar.

arrhythmia An abnormality or irregularity in the heart rhythm.
arritmia Anomalía o irregularidad en el ritmo cardiaco.

arteriography Radiography of the arteries in which an iodine contrast medium is used.
arteriografía Radiografía de las arterias usando un medio de contraste yodado.

arthritis Inflammation of a joint.
artritis Inflamación de una articulación.

arthrogram A fluoroscopic image of the soft tissue components of a joint for which a contrast medium is injected directly into the joint capsule.
artrografía Examen fluoroscópico de los componentes de los tejidos blandos de las articulaciones con una inyección directa de un medio de contraste en la cápsula de la articulación.

articular Pertaining to a joint.
articulatorio Perteneciente o relativo a una articulación.

artificial intelligence The aspect of computer science that deals with computers taking on the attributes of humans. An example is an expert system, which is capable of making decisions; this might be software designed to help a physician diagnose an illness when given a set of symptoms. Game-playing programming and programs designed to recognize human language are other examples of artificial intelligence.
inteligencia artificial Parte de la informática que se ocupa de la incorporación de atributos humanos a las computadoras. Un ejemplo de esto es un sistema práctico capaz de tomar decisiones, como los programas informáticos diseñados para ayudar a los médicos a diagnosticar a un paciente dado un conjunto de síntomas. Los programas de juegos y otros programas diseñados para reconocer el lenguaje humano son otros ejemplos.

ASCII (American Standard Code for Information Interchange) A code representing English characters as numbers, with each given a number from 0 to 127.
ASCII (Estándar Americano de Codificación para el-Intercambio de Información) Un código que representa carácteres ingleses como números, en el cual a cada uno se le asigna un número de 0 a-127.

asepsis The process or state of making or keeping something free of infection or infectious materials; the state of being free of pathogens.
asepsia Que está libre del infecciones.

assault An intentional, unlawful attempt to do bodily injury to another by force.
asalto Intento ilícito de causar daño físico a otro usando la fuerza.

assent To agree to something, especially after thoughtful consideration.
asentir Aceptar algo, especialmente cuando se hace tras una detenida reflexión.

asystole Absence of a heartbeat.
asistolia Ausencia de latidos del corazón.

ataxia Failure or irregularity of muscle actions and coordination.

ataxia Fallo o irregularidad del movimiento y coordinación musculare.

atherosclerosis A form of arteriosclerosis distinguished by fatty deposits within the inner layers of larger arterial walls.
aterosclerosis Forma de arteriosclerosis que se distingue por la presencia de depósitos de grasa en las capas internas de las paredes de las arterias mayores.

atria The two upper chambers of the heart.
aurículas Las dos cavidades superiores del corazón.

atrioventricular (AV) node A part of the cardiac conduction system located between the atria and the ventricles.
nódulo aurioventricular (AV) Parte del sistema cardiaco que se encuentra entre las aurículas y los ventrílculos.

atrophy A decrease in the size of a normally developed organ.
atrofia Disminución del tamaño de un órgano desarrollado de forma normal.

atrophy To waste away or decrease in size.
atrofia Desgastado, disminuido en tamaño.

attenuated Weakening or a change in virulence of a pathogenic microorganism.
atenuado Cambio o debilitación en la virulencia de un microorganismo.

audiologist An allied healthcare professional who specializes in the evaluation of hearing function, detection of hearing impairment, and determination of the anatomic site of impairment.
audiólogo Profesional del cuidado de la salud que se especializa en evaluar la función auditiva, detectar las dificultades auditivas y determinar el-lugar físico en el que se produce el problema auditivo.

audit A formal examination of an organization's or individual's accounts or financial situation; a methodic examination and review.
auditoría Análisis formal de las cuentas o estado financiero de una organización o un individuo; examen y revisión sistemáticos.

augment To make greater, more numerous, larger, or more intense.
aumentar Hacer mayor, más numeroso, más grande o más intenso.

aura A peculiar sensation that precedes the appearance of a more definite disturbance.

aura Sensación peculiar que precede a la aparición de un trastorno definido.

authorization A term used by managed care for an approved referral.
autorización Término usado en el cuido administrado para referirse a la aprobación de la referencia de un paciente de un médico a otro profesional del cuidado o de la salud.

autoimmune Referring to the development of an immune response to one's own tissues; action against one's own cells that causes localized and systemic reactions.
autoinmune Desarrollo de una respuesta inmunológica a los propios tejidos; actuar contra sus propias células para originar reacciones sistémicas localizadas.

autoimmune disorder A disturbance in the immune system in which the body reacts against its own tissue. Examples of autoimmune disorders include multiple sclerosis, rheumatoid arthritis, and systemic lupus erythematosus.
trastorno autoinmune Trastorno del sistema inmunológico en el cual el cuerpo reacciona contra sus propios tejidos. Algunos ejemplos de trastornos autoinmunes incluyen la esclerosis múltiple, la artritis reumatoide y el lupus eritematoso sistémico.

axial projection A radiograph taken with a longitudinal angulation of the x-ray beam; sometimes referred to as a *semiaxial projection*.
proyección axial Radiografía que se toma con un ángulo longitudinal del haz de rayos x; a veces se llama *proyección semi-axial*.

azotemia Retention of excessive amounts of nitrogenous wastes in the blood.
azotemia Retención en la sangre de cantidades de desperdicios nitrogenados.

backup Any type of storage of files to prevent their loss in the event of hard disk failure.
copia de seguridad Cualquier tipo de almacenamiento de archivos para evitar que se pierdan en caso de que ocurrra un fallo en el disco duro.

bailiff An officer of some U.S. courts who usually serves as a messenger or usher and keeps order at the request of the judge.
alguacil Funcionario de algunos tribunales estadounidenses que suele servir como mensajero o ujier y que se ocupa de mantener el orden a petición del juez.

bank reconciliation The process of proving that a bank statement and checkbook balance are in agreement.

reconciliación bancaria Proceso por el cual se prueba que un estado bancario y un saldo de una libreta de cheques concuerdan.

banners Also called *banner ads;* advertisements often found on a Web page that can be animated to attract the user's attention in hopes the person will click on the ad, be redirected to the advertiser's home page, and make a purchase from the site or gain information.
viñetas Viñetas o anuncios de viñetas; anuncios, a veces animados, que se hallan, con frecuencia en las páginas web; su fin es atraer la atención del usuario con la esperanza de que éste haga clic en el anuncio, y así sea llevado a la página principal del anunciante para que compre algo en ese sitio o para que obtenga información sobre el mismo.

battery Willful, unlawful use of force or violence on the person of another; offensive touching or use of force on a person without that person's consent.
golpiza Uso de la fuerza o violencia en contra de la persona de otro, de manera intencional e ilegítima. Tocar de manera ofensiva a una persona o usar la fuerza en contra de ella sin su consentimiento.

beneficence The act of doing or producing good, especially performing acts of charity or kindness.
beneficencia Acción de hacer o producir el bien, en especial llevando a cabo obras caritativas o bondadosas.

beneficiary The person who receives the benefits of an insurance policy. The "insured" person on a Medicare claim.
beneficiario Persona que recibe los beneficios de una póliza de seguro. La persona "asegurada" en una reclamación de Medicare.

benefits Services or payments provided under a health plan, employee plan, or some other agreement, including programs such as health insurance, pensions, retirement planning, and many other options, that may be offered to employees of a company or organization.
beneficios Servicio o pago proporcionado bajo un plan de salud, un plan de empleados o algún otro acuerdo, incluyendo programas como seguros de salud, pensiones, planes de retiro y muchas otras opciones que pueden ser ofrecidas a los empleados de una compañía u organización.

benefits The amount payable by the insurance company for a monetary loss to an individual insured by that company, under each coverage.
beneficios Suma que ha de pagar la compañía aseguradora por una pérdida monetaria a un individuo asegurado por dicha compañía, bajo cada cobertura.

benign Not cancerous and not recurring.
benigno No canceroso y no recurrente.

bevel The angled tip of a needle.
bisel Punta de aguja en ángulo.

bifurcate To divide from one into two branches.
bifurcar Dividir una unidad en dos ramas.

bifurcation The point of forking or separation into two branches.
bifurcación Lugar en el que se separan dos ramas.

bilirubin An orange pigment in bile; the accumulation of bilirubin leads to jaundice.
bilirrubina Pigmento de color naranja que se encuentra en la bilis; cuando se acumula produce ictericia.

bilirubinuria The presence of bilirubin in the urine.
bilirrubinuria Presencia de bilirrubina en la orina.

biophysical Pertaining to the science that deals with the application of physical methods and theories to biologic problems.
biofísico Perteneciente o relativo a la ciencia que trata de la aplicación de métodos y teorías físicas a los problemas biológicos.

birthday rule An insurance rule that states that when an individual is covered under two insurance policies, the insurance plan of the policyholder whose birthday comes first in the calendar year (month and day—not year) becomes primary.
regla del cumpleaños Cuando un individuo está cubierto bajo dos pólizas de seguro, el plan de seguro del titular de la póliza cuya fecha de cumpleaños esté antes en el año civil (mes y día, no año) se convierte en el plan primario.

blatant Completely obvious, conspicuous, or obtrusive, especially in a crass or offensive manner; brazen.
flagrante Completamente obvio, notorio o inoportuno, en especial de una manera torpe u-ofensiva; desvergonzado.

bond A durable, formal paper used for documents.
obligación Papel duradero y formal usado para documentos.

bounding pulse A pulse that feels full because of increased power of cardiac contractions or increased blood volume.
pulso saltón Pulso que se siente lleno debido a un aumento de potencia en las contracciones cardiacas o debido a un aumento del volumen de la sangre.

bradycardia A slow heartbeat; a pulse below 60 beats per minute.

bradicardia Latido lento; pulso por debajo de 60 pulsaciones por minuto.

bradypnea Respirations that are regular in rhythm but slower than normal in rate.
bradipnea Respiración que tiene un ritmo regular pero es más lenta de lo normal.

broad-spectrum antimicrobial agent A drug used to treat a broad range of infections.
agente antimicrobiano de amplio espectro Sustancia que se usa para tratar una amplia gama de infecciones.

bronchiectasis Dilation of the bronchi and bronchioles associated with a secondary infection or ciliary dysfunction.
broncoectasia Dilatación de los bronquios y bronquiolos asociada con una infección secundaria o disfunción ciliar.

bronchoconstriction Narrowing of the bronchiole tubes.
broncoconstricción Estrechamiento de los bronquiolos.

bruit An abnormal sound or a murmur heard on auscultation of an organ, vessel, or gland.
ruido Sonido o murmullo anómalo que se oye al auscultar un órgano, vaso sanguíneo o glándula.

bucky A moving grid device that prevents scatter radiation from fogging the radiographic film.
bucky Dispositivo de rejilla móvil que evita que la difusión de la radiación empañe la película.

bundle of His Fibers that conduct electrical impulses from the AV node to the ventricular myocardium.
haz de His Fibras que conducen impulsos eléctricos del nódulo aurioventricular al miocardio ventricular.

burnout Exhaustion of physical or emotional strength or motivation, usually as a result of prolonged stress or frustration.
agotamiento Llegar al fin de la fortaleza o motivación física o emocional, por lo general como resultado un prolongado estado de estrés o frustración.

bursa A fluid-filled, saclike membrane that provides for cushioning and frictionless motion between two tissues.
bursa Membrana con forma de saco llena de fluido que proporciona amortiguación y movimiento sin fricción entre dos tejidos.

byte A unit of data that contains 8 binary digits.
byte Unidad de información que contiene ocho dígitos binarios.

C&S (culture and sensitivity) A procedure performed in the microbiology laboratory in which a specimen is cultured on artifical media to detect bacterial or fungal growth, followed by appropriate screening for antibiotic sensitivity.
C&S (cultivo y sensibilidad) Procedimiento llevado a cabo en el laboratorio de microbiología en el cual se cultiva un espécimen en un medio artificial para detectar el crecimiento de bacterias u hongos y después investigar su sensibilidad los antibióticos.

cache A special high-speed storage area that can be part of the computer's main memory or a separate storage device. One function of the cache is to store in the computer's memory the Web sites visited; this allows faster recall the next time the Web site is requested.
caché Almacenamiento especial de alta velocidad que puede formar parte de la memoria principal de la computadora o puede ser un dispositivo de almacenamiento separado. Una función del caché es almacenar las páginas Web visitadas en la memoria de la computadora para llegar a ellas con mayor rapidez la próxima vez que desee ver la página.

candidiasis An infection, caused by a yeastlike fungus, that typically affects the vaginal mucosa and skin.
candidiasis Infección causada por una levadura (una especie de hongo) que típicamente afecta la mucosa y la piel vaginal.

cannula A rigid tube that surrounds a blunt or a sharp, pointed trocar that is inserted into the body; when the trocar is withdrawn, fluid may escape from the body through the cannula, depending on the insertion site.
cánula Tubo rígido que envuelve un trocar romo o un trocar de punta afilada que se inserta en el cuerpo; cuando se saca, puede salir fluido corporal a través de la cánula, según en donde haya sido insertada.

caption A heading, title, or subtitle under which records are filed.
leyenda Encabezamiento, título o subtítulo bajo el cual se archivan los informes.

carbohydrates Chemical substances that contain only carbon, oxygen, and hydrogen; they include sugars, glycogen, starches, dextrins, and celluloses.
carbohidratos Sustancias químicas, en las que se incluyen azúcares, glucógenos, almidones, dextrinas y celulosas, y están formadas sólo por carbono, oxígeno e hidrógeno.

carcinogenic A substance that is known to cause cancer.
cancerígeno Sustancia que se sabe que produce cáncer.

carcinogens Substances or agents that cause the development or increase the incidence of cancer.
carcinógeno Sustancia o agente que origina el desarrollo de cáncer o aumenta su incidencia.

cardiac arrest Complete cessation of cardiac contractions.
paro cardiaco Detención completa de las contracciones cardiacas.

cardiac arrhythmia An irregular heartbeat caused by a malfunction in the heart's electrical system.
arritmias cardiacas Pulso irregular que es resultado de un mal funcionamiento del sistema eléctrico del corazón.

cardioversion The use of electroshock to convert an abnormal cardiac rhythm to a normal one.
cardioversión Utilización de un electrochoque para normalizar un ritmo cardiaco anómalo.

cartilage The rubbery, smooth, somewhat elastic connective tissue that covers the ends of bones.
cartílago Tejido de unión similar a la goma, suave y un tanto elástico, que cubre los extremos de los huesos.

case management The process of assessing and planning patient care, including referral and follow up, to ensure continuity of care and quality management.
administración de casos Proceso de evaluación y planificación de la atención al paciente, incluyendo envío de pacientes a especialistas y seguimiento del caso para asegurar la continuidad del tratamiento y la calidad de la administración.

cash on delivery (COD) The method of payment used when an article or item is delivered; payment is expected before the item is released.
contra reembolso (COD) Método de pago usado cuando se entrega un artículo u objeto y el destinatario ha de pagar antes de recibirlo.

casts A fibrous or proteinaceous material, molded to the shape of the part in which it accumulated, that is thrown off into the urine in kidney disease.
cálculos Materiales fibrosos o proteínicos que han tomado la forma de la parte del cuerpo en la que han sido acumulados y que se expulsan a través de la orina en los casos de enfermedades renales.

categorically Placed in a specific division of a system of classification.
categorizado Colocado en un lugar específico dentro de una división de un sistema de clasificación.

caustic (1) A sarcastic remark or phrase. (2) A substance that burns or destroys tissue by chemical action.
cáustico (1) Comentario o frase dicha con sarcasmo. (2) Substancia que quema o destruye tejidos por acción química.

CD burner A CD writer that can write data onto a blank CD or copy data from a CD to a blank CD.
grabador de CD Dispositivo que puede escribir datos en un CD en blanco o copiar datos de un CD a otro CD en blanco.

centrifuge An apparatus consisting essentially of a compartment that spins around a central axis to separate contained materials of different specific gravities or to separate colloidal particles suspended in a liquid.
centrifugadora Aparato que consiste básicamente de un compartimiento que gira alrededor de un eje central para separar materiales con diferentes pesos específicos, o para separar partículas coloidales suspendidas en un líquido.

cerebrospinal fluid The fluid within the subarachnoid space, the central canal of the spinal cord, and the four ventricles of the brain.
fluido cerebroespinal Fluido del interior del espacio subaracnoideo, el canal central de la médula espinal y los cuatro ventrículos del cerebro.

certification Attested as being true as represented or as meeting a standard; to have been tested, usually by a third party, and awarded a certificate based on proven knowledge.
certificación Atestiguar que algo es verdadero en cuanto a lo que representa, o al cumplimiento de un estándar; que ha sido examinado, por lo general por una tercera parte, y que se le ha concedido un certificado basándose en el conocimiento del que ha dado prueba.

cerumen A waxy secretion in the ear canal, commonly called *ear wax*.
cerumen Secreción cerosa del canal del oído, comúnmente se conoce como *cera de los oídos*.

cervical Referring to the region of the neck that contains the seven cervical vertebrae.
cervical Región del cuello en la que hay siete vértebras cervicales.

chain of command A series of executive positions in order of authority.
cadena de mando Serie de puestos ejecutivos en orden de autoridad.

channels A means of communication or expression; a way, course, or direction of thought.
canales Medios de comunicación o de expresión; vía, curso o dirección del pensamiento.

characteristic A distinguishing trait, quality, or property.
característica Rasgo, cualidad o propiedad distintiva.

chief complaint The reason for seeking medical care.
problema principal Razón por la cual un paciente solicita atención médica.

chiropractic A medical discipline; the chiropractic physician focuses on the nervous system and manually and painlessly adjusts the vertebral column to affect the nervous system, resulting in healthier patients.
quiropráctica Disciplina médica en la que los médicos quiroprácticos se centran en el sistema nervioso y ajustan la columna vertebral manualmente y sin dolor, para lograr un efecto sobre el sistema nervioso, dando como resultado pacientes más sanos.

cholesterol A substance produced by the liver and also found in plant and animal fats that can cause fatty deposits or atherosclerotic plaques in the blood vessels.
colesterol Ustancia que produce el hígado y que se halla en las grasas animales y vegetales, y que puede producir depósitos grasos o placas ateroscleróticas en los vasos sanguíneos.

chronic Persisting for a prolonged period.
crónico Que persiste por largo tiempo.

chronic bronchitis Recurrent inflammation of the membranes lining the bronchial tubes.
bronquitis crónica Inflamación recurrente de-las membranas que recubren los tubos bronquiales.

chronologic order Of, relating to, or arranged in or according to the order of time.
orden cronológico Perteneciente o relativo al orden en el tiempo; organizado según el orden en el tiempo.

circumvent To manage to avoid something, especially by ingenuity or stratagem.
circunvenir Lograr evitar algo usando ingeniosidad o estratagemas.

cite To quote by way of example, authority, or proof, or to mention formally in commendation or praise.
cita Que se nombra para servir de ejemplo, autoridad o prueba o para hacer una mención formal como recomendación o alabanza.

claims clearinghouse A centralized facility (sometimes called a *third-party administrator*, or TPA) to which insurance claims are transmitted; the clearinghouse checks and redistributes claims electronically to various insurance carriers.
centro de reclamaciones Establecimiento centralizado (algunas veces conocido como *administrador mediador* o TPA) al cual se transmiten las reclamaciones de seguros y que se encarga de verificar y redistribuir las reclamaciones electrónicamente a varias compañías de seguros.

clarity The quality or state of being clear.
claridad Calidad o estado de claro.

clause A group of words containing a subject and a predicate that functions as part of a complex or compound sentence.
cláusulas Conjunto de palabras que incluye un sujeto y un predicado y que funciona como miembro de una oración compuesta.

clean claim An insurance claim form that has been completed correctly (with no errors or omissions) and can be processed and paid promptly.
reclamación limpia Formulario de reclamación de seguro que ha sido llenado correctamente (sin errores ni omisiones) y que puede procesarse y pagarse prontamente.

clearinghouses Networks of banks that exchange checks with one another.
sistema de compensación Redes bancarias que intercambian cheques entres sí.

clinical trials Research studies that test how well new medical treatments or other interventions work in the subjects, usually human beings.
ensayos clínicos Estudio de investigación que prueba cómo actúan los nuevos tratamientos médicos u otras intervenciones en los sujetos, normalmente en los seres humanos.

clitoris The small, elongated, erectile body situated above the urinary meatus at the superior point of the labia minora.
clítoris Órgano eréctil pequeño y alargado situado sobre el meato urinario a la altura de los labios menores.

clubbing Abnormal enlargement of the distal phalanges (fingers and toes) that is associated with cyanotic heart disease or advanced chronic pulmonary disease.
hipocratismo digital (dedos en palillo de tambor) Engrosamiento anómalo de las falanges distales (en los dedos de las manos y de los pies), relacionado con una enfermedad cardiaca cianótica o una enfermedad pulmonar crónica avanzada.

coagulate To form into clots.
coagular Formar coágulos.

"code also" In ICD-9-CM coding, when more than one code is necessary to identify a given condition fully, "code also" or "use additional code" is used.
"código adicional" Cuando se necesita más de un código para identificar por completo una afección (enfermedad) determinado, se usa "código adicional" o "usar código adicional."

Code of Federal Regulations (CFR) The Code of Federal Regulations (CFR) is a coded delineation of the rules and regulations published in the *Federal Register* by the various departments and agencies of the federal government. The CFR is divided into 50 titles, which represent broad subject areas, and further into chapters, which provide specific detail.

Código de Regulaciones Federales (CFR) El Código de Regulaciones Federales (CFR) es un resumen codificado de las normas y regulaciones publicadas en el Registro Federal por los diferentes departamentos y agencias del gobierno federal. El CFR se divide en 50 Títulos que representan amplias áreas temáticas, los cuales, a su vez, se subdividen en capítulos que proporcionan detalles específicos.

cognitive Pertaining to the operation of the mind; the process by which a person becomes aware of perceiving, thinking, and remembering.
cognitivo Perteneciente o relativo a la operación del proceso mental por el cual nos damos cuenta de cómo, percibimos, pensamos y recordamos.

cohesive Sticking together tightly; exhibiting or producing cohesion.
cohesivo El estado de estar estrechamente unidos; mostrar o producir cohesión.

coitus Sexual union between male and female; also known as *intercourse*.
coito Unión sexual entre un macho y una hembra.

collagen The protein that forms the inelastic fibers of tendons, ligaments, and fascia.
colágeno Proteína que forma las fibras no elásticas de los tendones, los ligamentos y la fascia.

collodion A preparation of cellulose nitrate that dries to a strong, thin, protective, transparent film when applied to the skin.
colodión Preparación de nitrato de celulosa que, cuando se aplica a la piel, se seca formando una película fina resistente, protectora y transparente.

colloidal Pertaining to a gluelike substance.
coloidal Perteneciente o relativo a una substancia parecida a la cola.

colostrum The thin, yellow, milky fluid secreted by the mammary glands a few days before and after delivery.
calostro Fluido lácteo poco espeso y amarillo que segregan las glándulas mamarias unos días antes y después del parto.

coma An unconscious state from which the patient cannot be aroused.
coma Estado inconsciente del cual el paciente no puede ser despertado.

comfort zone A mental state in which an individual feels safe and confident.
zona de bienestar Un lugar en la mente en el que un individuo se siente seguro y confiado.

commensurate Corresponding in size, amount, extent, or degree; equal in measure.
equiparable Que es equivalente en tamaño, cantidad o grado; de igual medida.

commercial insurance Plans (sometimes called *private insurance*) that reimburse the insured (or his or her dependents) for monetary losses resulting from illness or injury according to a specific schedule as outlined in the insurance policy and on a fee-for-service basis. Individuals insured under these plans normally are not limited to any one physician and usually can see the healthcare provider of their choice.
seguro comercial Planes (a veces llamados *seguros privados*) que reembolsan al asegurado (o a sus dependendientes) por pérdidas monetarias debidas a enfermedad o lesión siguiendo una escala específica que se explica en la póliza de seguro y cobrando un cargo por cada servicio. Los individuos asegurados bajo estos planes, por lo general, no están limitados a un solo médico y suelen poder acudir al proveedor del cuidado de la salud que elijan.

co-morbidities Pre-existing conditions that, because of their presence with a specific principal diagnosis, increase the length of stay in a healthcare facility by at least 1 day in approximately 75% of cases.
patologías coexistentes Enfermedades preexistentes que, debido a su presencia junto al diagnóstico principal, causan un aumento en la duración de la estadía de al menos un día en aproximadamente 75% de los casos.

competence The quality or state of being competent; having adequate or requisite capabilities.
competencia Capacidad o aptitud de quien es competente en algo; tener las capacidades necesarias o cumplir con los requisitos necesarios para hacer algo.

competent Having adequate abilities or qualities; having the capacity to function or perform in a certain way.
competente Que tiene ciertas capacidades o cualidades; que tiene la capacidad de funcionar o actuar de un modo determinado.

complications Conditions that arise during the hospital stay that prolong the length of stay by at least 1 day in approximately 75% of the cases.
complicaciones Condiciones que surgen durante la permanencia en el hospital que prolongan el tiempo de la estadía en al menos un día en aproximadamente 75% de los casos.

compression The state of being pressed together.
compresión Condición de estar apretado.

computed tomography (CT) A computerized x-ray imaging modality that provides axial and three-dimensional scans.
tomografía asistida por computadora (TAC) Modalidad de formación computarizada de imágenes de rayos x que proporciona imágenes de escáner axiales y tridimensionales.

computer A machine designed to accept, store, process, and give out information.
computadora (u ordenador) Máquina diseñada para aceptar, almacenar, procesar y emitir información.

concise Expressing much in brief form.
conciso Que expresa mucho en forma breve.

concurrently Occurring at the same time.
concurrente Que ocurre al mismo tiempo.

cones Structures in the retina that make the perception of color possible.
conos Estructuras que se encuentran en la retina y que hacen posible la percepción del color.

congruence Consistency between the verbal expression of the message and the sender's nonverbal body language.
congruencia Expresión verbal del mensaje que corresponde al lenguaje corporal no verbal del emisor.

congruent Being in agreement, harmony, or correspondence; conforming to the circumstances or requirements of a situation.
congruente Que está en acuerdo, armonía o correspondencia; conforme a las circunstancias o requisitos de una situación.

connotation An implication; something suggested by a word or thing.
connotación Implicación; lo que sugiere una palabra o una cosa.

contaminate To make impure or unclean; to make unfit for use by the introduction of unwholesome or undesirable elements.
contaminación Volver impuro o sucio; hacer que algo sea inadecuado para el uso por la introducción de elementos insalubres o indeseables.

contaminated Soiled with pathogens or infectious material; nonsterile.
contaminado Manchado con materiales patógenos o infecciosos; no estéril.

contamination Becoming nonsterile through contact with any nonsterile material.
contaminación Pasar al estado de no estéril por contacto con cualquier material no estéril.

continuation pages The second and following pages of a letter.
paginas de continuación En una carta, la segunda página y las siguientes.

continuing education credits (CEUs) Credits for courses, classes, or seminars related to an individual's profession that are designed to promote education and to keep the professional up-to-date on current procedures and trends in the field; CEUs often are required to maintain licensure.
créditos de educación continua (CEU) Créditos por cursos, clases o seminarios relacionados con la profesión de un individuo y que tienen la finalidad de promocionar la educación y mantener al profesional al corriente de los procedimientos y tendencias actuales en su campo; con frecuencia son obligatorios para obtener una licencia.

continuity of care Care that continues smoothly from one provider to another so that care is not interrupted and the patient receives the most benefit.
continuidad de la atención Atención que continúa sin interrupciones de un proveedor a otro, de manera que el paciente recibe los máximos beneficios sin que haya una interrupción de la atención sanitaria.

contralateral Pertaining to the opposite side of the body.
colateral Perteneciente o relativo a la parte opuesta del cuerpo.

contrast media Substances used to enhance visualization of soft tissues in imaging studies.
medios de contraste Substancias usadas para mejorar la visualización de los tejidos blandos en estudios de formación de imágenes.

contributory negligence Statutes in some states that may prevent a party from recovering damages if the person contributed in any way to the injury or condition.
negligencia concurrente Estatutos existentes en algunos estados que impiden que una parte sea recompensada por daños si esta parte ha contribuido en algún modo a provocar la lesión o enfermedad.

cookies Messages sent to the hard drive from the Web server that identify users and allow preparation of custom Web pages for them, possibly displaying their name on return to the site.
cookies Mensaje que se envía al navegador de la red desde el servidor, el cual identifica a los usuarios y puede preparar páginas web especiales para ellos, posiblemente, mostrando su nombre la próxima vez que visiten el sitio.

coordination of benefits The mechanism used in group health insurance to designate the order in which multiple carriers are to pay benefits to prevent duplicate payments.

coordinación de beneficios Mecanismo usado en seguros de enfermedad de grupo para designar el orden en el que varias compañías de seguros tienen que pagar los beneficios para evitar pagos dobles.

co-payment Also called *co-insurance;* a policy provision frequently found in medical insurance whereby the policyholder and the insurance company share the cost of covered losses in a specified ratio (e.g., 80/20: 80% by the insurer and 20% by the insured).
co-pago Un co-pago (o *co-seguro*) es una provisión frecuente de la póliza en los seguros médicos, por la que el titular de la póliza y la compañía aseguradora comparten el costo de las pérdidas cubiertas en una proporción determinada (ej.: 80/20: 80% por parte del asegurador y 20% por parte del asegurado).

COPD (chronic obstructive pulmonary disease) A progressive, irreversible lung condition that results in diminished lung capacity.
COPD (enfermedad pulmonar obstructiva crónica) Enfermedad pulmonar progresiva e irreversible que conlleva una reducción de la capacidad pulmonar.

copulation Sexual intercourse.
copulación Cópula sexual.

coronal plane The plane that divides the body into anterior and posterior parts.
plano coronal Plano que divide el cuerpo en una anterior y una posterior.

corticosteroids Natural or synthetic antiinflammatory hormones.
corticosteroides Hormonas antiinflamatorias, naturales o sintéticas.

costal Pertaining to the ribs.
costal Perteneciente o relativo a las costillas.

coulombs per kilogram (C/kg) The international unit of radiation exposure.
culombios por kilogramo (C/kg) Unidad internacional de exposición a la radiación.

counteroffer A return offer made by one who has rejected an offer or a job.
contraoferta Oferta-respuesta hecha por quien ha rechazado una oferta o trabajo.

creatinine Nitrogenous waste from muscle metabolism that is excreted in the urine.
creatinina Residuo nitrogenado del metabolismo muscular que se excreta en la orina.

credentialing The act of extending professional or medical privileges to an individual; the process of verifying and evaluating that person's credentials.

concesión de credenciales Acción de conceder privilegios profesionales o médicos a un individuo; proceso de verificar y evaluar los credenciales de esa persona.

credibility The quality or power of inspiring belief.
credibilidad Calidad de creíble; facilidad para ser creído.

credit An entry on an account constituting an addition to a revenue, net worth, or liability account; the balance in a person's favor in an account.
crédito Dato que se entra en una cuenta y que constituye una adición a los ingresos, ganancia neta o cuenta de pasivo; saldo a favor de una persona en una cuenta.

crenate Forming notches or leaflike, scalloped edges on an object.
crenar Formar muescas o bordes en forma de concha o de hoja en un objeto.

crepitation A dry, crackling sound or sensation.
crepitación Sonido o sensación seca y crujiente.

critical thinking The constant practice of considering all aspects of a situation when deciding what to believe or what to do.
razonamiento crítico Práctica constante de considerar todos los aspectos de una situación al decidir qué creer o qué hacer.

cross-training Training in more than one area so that a multitude of duties may be performed by one person or so that substitutions of personnel may be made when necessary or in emergencies.
entrenamiento cruzado Entrenamiento en más de un área, de modo que una persona pueda desempeñar varias labores o que se puedan realizar sustituciones de personal cuando sea necesario o en caso de emergencia.

cryosurgery The technique of exposing tissue to extreme cold to produce a well-defined area of cell destruction.
criocirugía Técnica que consiste en exponer los tejidos a un frío extremo para producir una destrucción de células en un área bien definida.

cryptogenic Hidden origin.
criptogénico De origen oculto.

cultivate To foster the growth of; to improve by labor, care, or study.
cultivar Promover el desarrollo; mejorar algo por medio de trabajo, cuidado o estudio.

curettage The act of scraping a body cavity with a surgical instrument, such as a curette.

curetaje Acción de raspar una cavidad corporal con un instrumento quirúrgico, como una cureta o cucharilla cortante.

cursor A symbol that appears on the computer monitor to show where the next character to be typed will appear.
cursor Símbolo que aparece en el monitor y que muestra el lugar donde aparecerá el próximo carácter que se escriba.

curt Marked by rude or peremptory shortness.
cortante Caracterizado por una interrupción ruda o perentoria.

cyanosis A blue discoloration of the mucous membranes and body extremities caused by lack of oxygen.
cianosis Color azul de las membranas mucosas y las extremidades provocado por una falta de oxígeno.

cyberspace The nonphysical space of the online world of computer networks.
ciberespacio Palabra que se usa para describir el espacio no-físico del mundo en linea de las redes informáticas.

cyst A small, capsulelike sac that encloses certain organisms in their dormant or larval stage.
quiste Pequeño saco en forma de cápsula que encierra ciertos organismos en estado letárgico o larval.

damages Loss or harm resulting from injury to person, property, or reputation; monetary compensation imposed by law for losses or injuries.
daños Pérdidas o perjuicios que resultan de injuriar a una persona, atentar contra una propiedad o una reputación; compensación monetaria impuesta por ley en casos de pérdidas o injurias.

database A collection of related files that serves as a foundation for retrieving information.
base de datos Conjunto de archivos relacionados que sirven de base para la recuperación de información.

debit An entry on an account constituting an addition to an expense or asset balance or a deduction from a revenue, net worth, or liability balance.
débito Dato que se entra en una cuenta y que constituye una adición a los gastos o a una cuenta de activo o una deducción de un ingreso, ganancia neta o cuenta de pasivo.

debit card A card similar to a credit card with which money may be withdrawn or the cost of purchases paid directly from the holder's bank account without the payment of interest.
tarjeta de débito Tarjeta similar a la de crédito pero con la cual se puede retirar dinero o pagar compras directamente de la cuenta bancaria del titular sin tener que pagar intereses.

debridement The removal of foreign material and dead, damaged tissue from a wound.
desbridamiento Eliminación de materiales extraños y tejidos muertos y deteriorados de una herida.

decedent A legal term used to represent a deceased person.
difunto Término legal usado para referirse a una persona muerta.

decode To convert, as in a message, into intelligible form; to recognize and interpret.
decodificar Convertir la información, como en un mensaje, de modo que sea inteligible; reconocer e interpretar.

decubitus ulcer A sore or ulcer over a bony prominence caused by ischemia from prolonged pressure; a bed sore.
úlcera por decúbito Llaga o úlcera sobre una prominencia ósea debida a una isquemia por presión prolongada; escara.

deductible A specific amount of money a patient must pay out of pocket, up front, before the insurance carrier begins paying. Often this amount ranges from $100 to $1,000. The deductible amount must be met on a yearly or per incident basis.
deducible Cantidad de dinero específica que un paciente debe pagar de su bolsillo antes de que la compañía de seguros comience a pagar. Con frecuencia esta suma está entre 100 y 1000 dólares. Esta cantidad deducible ha de satisfacerse—anualmente o por caso.

default To fail to pay financial debts, especially a student loan.
incumplimiento Dejar de pagar deudas financieras, especialmente en un préstamo de estudiante.

defense mechanisms Psychological methods of dealing with stressful situations that are encountered in day-to-day living.
mecanismos de defensa Métodos psicológicos de hacer frente a situaciones tensas que surgen en la vida diaria.

deferment A postponement, especially of payment of a student loan.
aplazamiento Postergación de un pago, especialmente en un préstamo de estudiante.

defibrillator A machine used to deliver an electrical shock to the heart through electrodes placed on the chest wall.

desfibrilador Máquina usada para dar un electrochoque al corazón por medio de electrodos colocados en la pared torácica.

deficiencies Conditions caused by a below-normal intake of a particular substance.
deficiencias Estados causados por un consumo menor del normal de una sustancia específica.

demeanor Behavior toward others; outward manner.
conducta Comportamiento hacia los demás; comportamiento que se exterioriza.

demographic The statistical characteristics of human populations (as in age or income), used especially to identify markets.
dato demográfico Característica estadística de la población humana (como edad o ingresos), que se usa sobre todo para identificar mercados.

detrimental Harmful or damaging.
perjudicial Que es obvio que causa daño o perjuicio.

device driver A computer program or set of commands that enables a device connected to the computer to function. For instance, a printer may come equipped with software that must be loaded onto the computer first so that the printer will work.
controlador de dispositivo Programa que controla un dispositivo conectado a una computadora y que hace que dicho dispositivo pueda funcionar. Por ejemplo, una impresora puede estar equipada con un programa que primero ha de cargarse en la computadora para que ésta funcione.

diabetes mellitus type 2 A condition in which the body is unable to use glucose for energy because of a lack of insulin production in the pancreas or because of resistance to insulin on the cellular level.
diabetes mellitus tipo 2 Incapacidad de utilizar la glucosa para producir energía, debido a una falta de producción de insulina en el páncreas o a una resistencia a la insulina en el nivel celular.

diagnose To determine the nature of a disease, injury, or congenital defect.
diagnóstico Determinación del origen de una enfermedad, lesión o defecto congénito.

diagnosis The concise technical description of the cause, nature, or manifestations of a condition or problem. *Initial diagnosis:* The physician's temporary impression, sometimes called a *working diagnosis*. *Differential diagnosis:* A comparison of two or more diseases with similar signs and symptoms. *Final diagnosis:* The conclusion reached by the physician after evaluating all findings, including laboratory and other test results.
diagnóstico Descripción técnica y concisa de la causa, naturaleza o manifestaciones de una enfermedad o problema. *Inicial:* Impresión momentánea del médico, a veces se llama diagnóstico de trabajo. **Diagnóstico diferenciado:** comparación de dos o más enfermedades con signos y síntomas similares. *Final:* Conclusión médica a la que se llega tras evaluar todos los datos, incluyendo los resultados de análisis de laboratorio y otras pruebas.

diaphoresis The profuse excretion of sweat.
diaforesis Excreción profusa de sudor.

diaphysis The middle portion of a long bone, which contains the medullary cavity.
diafisis Parte intermedia de un hueso largo en la que está la cavidad medular.

dictation The act or manner of uttering words to be transcribed.
dictado Acción de pronunciar palabras para que sean transcritas.

diction The choice of words, especially with regard to clearness, correctness, and effectiveness.
dicción Acción de elegir las palabras, especialmente para lograr claridad, corrección y eficacia en el discurso.

digestion The process of converting food into chemical substances that can be used by the body.
digestión Proceso de transformar alimentos en sustancias químicas que pueden ser usadas por el cuerpo.

Digital Subscriber Lines (DSL) High-speed, sophisticated modulation schemes that operate over existing copper telephone wiring systems; often referred to as "last mile technologies" because DSL is used for connections from a telephone switching station to a home or office and not between switching stations.
Línea de Abonado Digital (DSL) Sofisticado sistema de modulación de alta velocidad que opera en sistemas de cableado telefónicos de cobre ya existentes; con frecuencia se habla del DSL como "tecnología de las últimas millas" porque se utiliza para conexiones entre un centro de conmutación telefónica y un hogar u oficina, y no entre centros de conmutación.

Digital Versatile Disk (DVD) An optical disk that holds approximately 28 times more information than a CD and is most commonly used to hold full-length movies. A CD holds approximately 600 megabytes, whereas a DVD can hold approximately 4.7 gigabytes.
Disco Digital Versátil (DVD) El DVD es un disco óptico con capacidad para almacenar unas 28 veces más información que un CD; su uso más común es para guardar películas de larga duración. Mientras que un CD puede almacenar unos 600 megabytes, un DVD tiene una capacidad aproximada de almacenamiento de 4.7 gigabytes.

dilation (1) Opening or widening the circumference of a body orifice with a dilating instrument. (2) The opening of the cervix through the process of labor, measured as 0 to 10 centimeters dilated.
dilatación (1) Proceso de abrir o ensanchar un orificio corporal con un instrumento dilatador. (2) Ensanchamiento del cuello del útero durante el proceso del parto, se mide en centímetros, de 0 a 10.

dilation and curettage (D&C) The procedure in which the cervix is widened and the endometrial wall of the uterus is scraped.
dilatación y curetaje (D&C) Proceso de hacer más ancho el cuello del útero y raspar su pared endometrial.

diluent A liquid used to dilute a specimen or reagent.
diluyente Líquido usado para diluir un espécimen o un reactivo.

dingy claim A claim that is put on hold because it lacks certain adjunction that allows it to be processed, often because of system changes.
reclamación oscura Reclamación en espera de ser procesada debido a que se necesita alguna información o elemento adicional, con frecuencia, debido a cambios en el sistema.

diplopia Double vision.
diplopía Visión doble.

direct filing system A filing system in which materials can be located without consulting an intermediary source of reference.
sistema directo de archivo Sistema de archivo en el cual los materiales pueden ser localizados sin consultar una fuente de referencia intermedia.

dirty claim Claims that contain errors or omissions and that cannot be processed or must be processed by hand because of OCR scanner rejection.
reclamación sucia Reclamación con errores u omisiones que no puede procesarse o que debe procesarse manualmente debido a que el escáner OCR la rechaza.

disbursements Funds paid out.
desembolsos Dinero o fondos que se pagan.

discretion The quality of being discrete; having or showing good judgment or conduct, especially in speech.
discreción Calidad de discreto; tener sensatez o tacto al obrar, especialmente al hablar.

disease A pathologic process having a descriptive set of signs and symptoms.
enfermedad Proceso patológico que tiene una serie descriptiva de signos y síntomas.

disinfection The destruction of pathogens by physical or chemical means.
desinfección Destrucción de agentes patógenos con medios físicos o químicos.

disk A magnetic surface capable of storing computer programs.
disco Superficie magnética capaz de almacenar programas de computadora.

disk drives Devices that load a program or data stored on a disk into the computer.
unidades de discos Dispositivos que cargan en la computadora un programa o datos almacenados en un disco.

disorder Disruption of normal system functions.
trastorno Interrupción de las funciones normales de un sistema.

disparaging Speaking slightingly about something or someone, with a negative or degrading tone.
menospreciar Hablar con desdén de algo o alguien, con un tono negativo o degradante.

disposition The tendency of something or someone to act in a certain manner under given circumstances.
disposición Tendencia de algo o alguien a actuar de un modo específico en determinadas circunstancias.

disruption A breaking down, or throwing into disorder.
disrupción Interrupción o creación de un estado de trastorno.

dissect To cut or separate tissue with a cutting instrument or scissors.
diseccionar Cortar o separar tejidos con tijeras u otro instrumento cortante.

dissection The cutting or separating of a specimen into pieces and exposing the parts for scientific examination.
disección Separar en piezas y dejar las partes a la vista para realizar un estudio científico.

disseminate To disperse throughout.
diseminar Dispersar, esparcir.

disseminate To disburse; to spread around.
diseminado Suelto, esparcido.

diurnal rhythm Patterns of activity or behavior that follow day-night cycles.
ritmo diurno Patrones de actividad o comportamiento que siguen a los ciclos nocturnos.

docket A formal record of judicial proceedings; a list of legal causes to be tried.
orden del día Registro formal de procesos judiciales; lista de causas legales a juzgar.

domestic mail Mail sent within the boundaries of the United States and its territories.
correo nacional Correo que se envía dentro de los límites de Estados Unidos y sus territorios.

dosimeter A badge for monitoring the exposure of personnel to radiation.
dosímetro Placa para controlar la exposición a la radiación del personal.

drawee The bank or facility on which a check is drawn or written.
librado Banco o entidad contra la que se gira o emite un cheque.

due process A fundamental, constitutional guarantee that all legal proceedings will be fair and that one will be given notice of the proceedings and an opportunity to be heard before the government acts to take away life, liberty, or property; a constitutional guarantee that a law will not be unreasonable or arbitrary.
proceso debido Garantía fundamental constitucional de que todos los procesos legales serán justos, que las partes implicadas serán notificadas de los procedimientos y que se les dará la oportunidad de ser escuchados rantes que el gobierno les quite su vida, libertad o propiedad; garantía constitucional de que la ley no irá en contra de la razón ni será arbitraria.

duty Obligatory tasks, conduct, service, or functions that arise from one's position, as in life or in a group.
deber Tareas, conducta, servicio o funciones de carácter obligatorio que conlleva el ocupar un puesto, en la vida o como miembro de un grupo.

dyspnea Difficult or painful breathing.
disnea Respiración difícil o dolorosa.

e-banking Electronic banking via computer modem or over the Internet.
banca electrónica Operaciones bancarias a través del módem de una computadora o en Internet.

ecchymosis A hemorrhagic skin discoloration, commonly called *bruising*.
equimosis Descolorament o hemorrágico de la piel comúnmente conocido como *magulladura*.

e-commerce A term used to describe the sale and purchase of goods and services over the Internet; doing business over the Internet; an abbreviation for *electronic commerce*.

comercio electrónico Expresión que se usa para describir la compra y venta de bienes y servicios a través de Internet; hacer negocios a través de Internet. Se conoce también con la abreviatura de *comercio-e*.

edema An abnormal accumulation of fluid in the interstitial spaces of tissue; swelling between layers of tissue.
edema Acumulación anómala de fluido en los espacios intersticiales de los tejidos; inflamación entre capas de tejidos.

effacement The thinning of the cervix during labor, measured in percentages from 0% to 100% effaced.
borramiento Adelgazamiento del cuello del útero durante el parto. Se mide en porcentaje, borrado de 0 a 100 por ciento.

elastic pulse A pulse with regular alterations of weak and strong beats, without changes in cycle.
pulso elástico Pulso con alteraciones regulares de latidos fuertes y débiles sin cambios en el ciclo.

elastin An essential part of elastic connective tissue that is flexible and elastic when moist.
elastina Parte esencial del tejido conectivo elástico que cuando está húmedo es flexible y elástico.

electrodesiccation Destructive drying of cells and tissue by means of short, high-frequency electrical sparks.
electrodesecación Secado destructivo de células y tejidos por medio de cortas descargas eléctricas de alta frecuencia.

electrolytes Small molecules that conduct an electrical charge. Electrolytes are necessary for proper functioning of muscle and nerve cells.
electrolitos Pequeñas moléculas que conducen una carga eléctrica. Los electrolitos son necesarios para un funcionamiento correcto de los músculos y las células nerviosas.

electronic claims Claims submitted to insurance processing facilities using a computerized medium, such as direct data entry, direct wire, dial-in telephone digital fax, or personal computer download and upload.
reclamación electrónica Reclamaciones enviadas al lugar de procesamiento de la compañía aseguradora usando un sistema computarizado, tales como entrada de datos directa, cable directo, fax digital con marcado telefónico, o a través de una computadora personal.

e-mail Communications transmitted via computer using a modem.

correo electrónico Comunicaciones transmitidas a través de una computadora usando un módem.

emancipated minor A person under legal age who is self-supporting and living apart from parents or a guardian.
menor emancipado Persona que no ha alcanzado la mayoría de edad legal y que se mantiene a sí misma y vive sin la custodia de padres o tutores.

embezzlement Stealing from an employer; appropriation without permission of goods, services, or funds for personal use.
desfalco Robo a un empleador; apropiación sin permiso de bienes, servicios o fondos para uso personal.

embolization An interventional technique in which a catheter is used to block off a blood vessel, thereby preventing hemorrhage.
embolización Técnica de intervención usando un catéter para bloquear un vaso sanguíneo y evitar una hemorragia.

embolus Foreign material that blocks a blood vessel, frequently a blood clot that has broken away from some other part of the body.
émbolo Material extraño que bloquea un vaso sanguíneo, con frecuencia un coágulo de sangre procedente de otra parte del cuerpo.

emetic A substance that causes vomiting.
emético Sustancia que causa vómito.

emisor The person who writes a check.
emisor Persona que emite un cheque.

empathy Sensitivity to the individual needs and reactions of patients.
empatía Sensibilidad ante las necesidades y reacciones individuales de los pacientes.

emphysema The pathologic accumulation of air in the tissues or organs; in the lungs, the bronchioles become plugged with mucus and lose elasticity.
enfisema Acumulación patológica de aire en los tejidos u órganos; en los pulmones, los bronquiolos se obstruyen con mucosidade y pierden elasticidad.

emulsification Dispersion of ingested fats into small globules by bile.
emulsionamiento Dispersión (llevada a cabo por la bilis) en pequeños glóbulos de las grasas ingeridas.

encode To convert from one system of communication to another; to convert a message into code.

codificar Convertir de un sistema de comunicación a otro; convertir un mensaje en un código.

encounter Any contact between a healthcare provider and a patient that results in treatment or evaluation of the patient's condition; not limited to in-person contact.
encuentro Cualquier contacto entre un proveedor de atención sanitaria y un paciente que resulta en un tratamiento o evaluación del estado del paciente; no se limita a un contacto personal.

encroachment To advance beyond the usual or proper limits.
intrusiones Ir más allá de los límites habituales o apropiados.

endemic A disease or microorganism that is specific to a particular geographic area.
endémico Enfermedad o microorganismo que-es específico de una zona geográfica en particular.

endocervical curettage The scraping of cells from the wall of the uterus.
curetaje endocervical Raspado de células de la pared uterina.

endorser The person who signs his or her name on the back of a check for the purpose of transferring title to another person.
endosante Persona que firma en la parte posterior de un cheque a fin de transferir la propiedad del mismo a otra persona.

enteric coated A term referring to a special compound used to coat some oral medications; the coating resists the effects of stomach juices and does not dissolve, releasing the medication, until the tablet is exposed to the fluids of the small intestine.
cubierta entérica Capa exterior que se añade a un medicamento que se toma por vía oral, la cual es resistente a los efectos de los jugos gástricos; recubrimiento diseñado para que la medicina sea absorbida en el intestino delgado; formulación usada en medicinas en la cual las tabletas se recubren con un componente especial que no se disuelve hasta que la tableta es expuesta a los fluidos del intestino delgado.

enunciate To utter articulate sounds; to be very distinct in speech.
articular Pronunciar los sonidos de manera cuidada; hablar de una forma muy clara.

enunciation The utterance of articulate, clear sounds; the act of being very distinct in speech.
articulación Pronunciación cuidada, con sonidos claros.

enzymatic reaction A chemical reaction controlled by an enzyme.
reacción enzimática Reacción química controlada por una enzima.

enzyme Any of several complex proteins that are produced by cells and that act as catalysts in specific biochemical reactions.
enzima Cualquiera de las varias proteínas complejas que producen las células y que actúan como catalíticos en reacciones bioquímicas específicas.

epiphysis The end of a long bone.
epífisis Extremo de un hueso largo.

erythropoietin A substance released from the kidney and the liver that promotes red blood cell formation.
eritropoyetina Sustancia liberada por los riñones y el hígado y que promueve la formación de glóbulos rojos.

essential hypertension Elevated blood pressure of unknown cause that develops for no apparent reason; sometimes called *primary hypertension*.
hipertensión esencial Presión sanguínea alta de causa desconocida que surge sin razón aparente; a veces se llama *hipertensión primaria*.

established patients Patients who are returning to the office and who have previously seen the physician.
pacientes establecidos Pacientes que regresan al consultorio médico que ya han sido atendidos por el médico con anterioridad.

etiology The cause of a disorder, as determined for the purpose of classifying a claim.
etiología Clasificación de una reclamación según la causa del trastorno.

eukaryote A single-cell or multicellular organism in which the cell or cells have a distinct, membrane-bound nucleus.
eucariote Organismo unicelular o multicelular cuyas células tienen un núcleo diferenciado rodeado por una membrana.

euthanasia The act or practice of killing or permitting the death of hopelessly sick or injured individuals in a relatively painless way for reasons of mercy.
eutanasia Acción o práctica de matar o permitir la muerte de enfermos o heridos en estado terminal, de una forma relativamente sin dolor, por razones de piedad.

exacerbation An increase in the seriousness of a disease marked by greater intensity of the signs and symptoms; worsening of disease symptoms.
exacerbación Aumento en la gravedad de una enfermedad, caracterizado por una mayor intensidad de los signos y síntomas. Empeoramiento de los síntomas de una enfermedad.

"excludes" In insurance claims, exclusion terms are always written in italics, and the word "Excludes" is enclosed in a box to draw particular attention to these instructions. Exclusion terms may apply to a chapter, a section, a category, or a subcategory. The applicable code number usually follows the exclusion term.
"excluye" Las expresiones de exclusión siempre se escriben en cursiva y la palabra "Excluye" se encierra en una casilla para llamar la atención acerca de estas instrucciones. Los términos de exclusión pueden ser aplicables a un capítulo, una sección, una categoría o una subcategoría. El número de código correspondiente por lo general sigue al término de exclusión.

expediency Haste or caution; a means of achieving a particular end.
prontitud Situación que requiere actuar con prisa o precaución; un medio de alcanzar un fin específico.

expert witness A person who provides testimony to a court as an expert in a certain field or subject to verify facts presented by one or both sides in a lawsuit. An expert witness often is compensated and is used to refute or disprove the claims of one party.
testigo perito Persona que da testimonio ante un tribunal como perito o experto en cierto campo o tema para verificar los hechos presentados por una o ambas partes en litigio, a menudo, cobrando una retribución económica, y cu yo testimonio suele usarse para refutar o impugnar las demandas de una de las partes.

external noise Noise outside the brain that interferes with the communication process.
ruido externo Ruido producido fuera del cerebro y que interfiere con el proceso de comunicación.

externalization Attribution of an event or occurrence to causes outside oneself.
exteriorización Acción de atribuir a un suceso o acontecimiento causas externas al mismo.

externship/internship A training program that is part of the course of study of an educational institution and that is taken in the actual business setting in that field of study; the two terms often are used interchangeably with regard to medical assisting.
prácticas internas/externas Programa de entrenamiento que es parte de un curso de estudio de una institución educativa y se sigue en un lugar real de trabajo en el campo de estudio; estos términos se intercambian cuando se refieren a los asistentes médicos.

exudates Fluids with a high concentration of protein and cellular debris that has escaped from the blood vessels and has been deposited in tissues or on tissue surfaces.
exudados Fluidos con una alta concentración de proteínas y restos celulares extravasados de los vasos

sanguíneos y depositados en los tejidos o en sus superficies.

familial Occurring in or affecting members of a family more than would be expected to occur by chance.
familiar Que sucede o afecta a miembros de una familia más de lo que podría esperarse por azar.

fascia A sheet or band of fibrous tissue located deep in the skin that covers muscles and body organs.
fascia Lámina o banda de tejido fibroso localizada bajo la piel y que cubre los músculos y los órganos.

fastidious With regard to laboratory cultures, an organism that requires specialized media or growth factors to grow.
exigente Que requiere un medio o factores especiales para crecer.

fat A substance stored as adipose tissue in the body that serves as a concentrated energy reserve.
grasa Sustancia que se almacena como tejido adiposo en el cuerpo y sirve como reserva de energía concentrada.

fax The abbreviation for the term *facsimile;* a document sent using a fax machine.
fax Abreviatura de facsímile; documento que se envía usando una máquina de fax.

febrile Pertaining to an elevated body temperature.
febril Perteneciente o relativo a una temperatura corporal elevada.

fecalith A hard, impacted mass of feces in the colon.
fecaloma Masa de heces endurecidas e impactadas en el colon.

fee profile A compilation or average of physicians' fees over a given period.
perfil de cargos Recopilación o porcentaje de cargos médicos en un periodo de tiempo dado.

fee schedule A compilation of pre-established fee allowances for given services or procedures.
escala de cargos Recopilación de asignaciones de cargos preestablecidos para servicios o procedimientos dados.

feedback The transmission of evaluative or corrective information about an action, event, or process to the original or controlling source.
reacciones y comentarios Envío de información de evaluación o corrección a la fuente original o a la que ejerce el control sobre una acción, suceso o proceso.

felony A major crime, such as murder, rape, or burglary, that is punishable by a more stringent sentence than that given for a misdemeanor, or lesser crime.
crimen Delito mayor, como asesinato, violación o robo; se penaliza con una sentencia más severa que un delito menor o falta.

fermentation An enzymatically controlled transformation of an organic compound.
fermentación Transformación de un compuesto orgánico controlada por enzimas.

fervent Exhibiting or marked by great intensity of feeling.
ferviente Que posee sentimientos de gran intensidad o que da muestra de ellos.

fibrillation Rapid, random, ineffective contractions of the heart.
fibrilación Contracciones cardiacas rápidas, aleatorias e inefectivas.

fidelity Faithfulness to something to which one is bound by pledge or duty.
fidelidad Fe en algo a lo que se está unido por juramento o deber.

filtrate The fluid that remains after a liquid is passed through a membranous filter.
filtrado Fluido que queda después de pasar un líquido a través de un filtro membranoso.

fine A sum imposed as punishment for an offense; a forfeiture or penalty paid to an injured party or the government in a civil or criminal action.
multa Suma impuesta como penalización por un delito menor; suma que se paga a una parte a la que se ha perjudicado o dañado, o al gobierno, en un proceso civil o penal.

fiscal agent An organization or private plan under contract to the government to act as a financial representative in handling insurance claims from providers of health care; also referred to as a *fiscal intermediary*.
agente fiscal Organización o plan privado bajo contrato con el gobierno para actuar como representantes financieros en la administración de reclamaciones de seguros por parte de proveedores de atención sanitaria; también se conoce como *intermediario fiscal*.

fiscal intermediary An organization that contracts with the government and other insuring entities to handle and mediate insurance claims from medical facilities.
intermediario fiscal Organización que establece un contrato con el gobierno y otras entidades aseguradoras para administrar reclamaciones de seguro provenientes de centros médicos y para mediar en ellas.

fissures Narrow slits or clefts in the abdominal wall.

fisuras Grietas o hendiduras estrechas en la pared abdominal.

fistulas Abnormal, tubelike passages within the body tissue, usually between two internal organs or from an internal organ to the body surface.
fístulas Pasajes anómalos en forma de tubos entre los tejidos corporales, por lo general entre dos órganos internos, o de un órgano interno a la superficie del cuerpo.

flagged Marked in some way to serve as a reminder that specific action needs to be taken.
señalado Marcado de alguna forma para recordar que se necesita que se tomen medidas al respeto.

Flash Animation technology often used on the opening page of a Web site to draw the attention of, excite, and impress the user.
Flash Tecnología de imágenes animadas que se usa con frecuencia en la página inicial de un sitio web para llamar la atención del usuario, entusiasmarlo e impresionarlo.

flatus Gas expelled through the anus.
flato Gas expulsado a través del ano.

fluoroscopy Direct observation of an x-ray image in motion.
fluoroscopía Observación directa de una imagen de rayos x en movimiento.

flush Directly abutting or immediately adjacent to, such as set even with the edge of a page or column; having no indention.
alineado Directamente contiguo o inmediatamente adyacente, ordenado de forma regular en relación con un borde de una página o columna; sin sangría o espacios en blanco.

follicle-stimulating hormone (FSH) A hormone secreted by the anterior pituitary that stimulates oogenesis and spermatogenesis.
hormona foliculoestimulante (FSH) Hormona que segrega la pituitaria anterior y que estimula los procesos de formación y desarrollo de óvulos y de espermatozoides.

font A design, as in typesetting, for a set of characters.
fuente tipográfica Diseño similar al de la composición para un conjunto de caracteres.

format To magnetically create tracks on a disk in which information will be stored; formatting usually is done by the manufacturer of the disk.
formatear Crear pistas magnéticas en un disco destinado a almacenar información; por lo general, el fabricante del disco es quien se encarga de hacerlo.

fovea centralis A small pit in the center of the retina that is considered the center of clearest vision.

fóvea central Pequeña concavidad en el centro de la retina que se cree que es el centro de visión más claro.

frontal projection The radiographic view in which the coronal plane of the body or body part is parallel to the film plane; AP or PA.
proyección frontal Vista radiográfica en la cual el plano coronal del cuerpo o de la parte del cuerpo está paralelo al plano de la película; AP o PA.

gait The manner or style of walking.
andares Forma o estilo de caminar.

gamete A mature male or female germ cell, which usually has a haploid chromosome set and can initiate the formation of a new diploid individual.
gameto Célula germinal madura, tanto masculina como femenina, que por lo general tiene un conjunto cromosómico haploide y es capaz de iniciar la formación de un nuevo individuo diploide.

gangrene The death of body tissue, as a result of the loss of nutritive supply, and subsequent bacterial invasion and putrefaction.
gangrena Muerte de tejido corporal debido a la pérdida de suministro de nutrientes por invasión bacteriana y putrefacción.

gantry The doughnut-shaped portion of a scanner than surrounds the patient and functions at least in part to gather imaging data.
gantry Parte de un escáner con forma de rosquilla que rodea al paciente y funciona, al menos en parte, reuniendo datos de formación de imágenes.

generic Not protected by trademark.
genéricas Medicinas que no están protegidas por una marca registrada.

genome The genetic material of an organism.
genoma El material genético de un organismo.

genuineness Expressing sincerity and honest feeling.
autenticidad Expresión de sentimientos sincera y honrada.

germicides Agents that destroy pathogenic organisms.
germicidas Agentes químicos que destruyen o matan organismos patógenos.

gigabyte Approximately 1 billion bytes.
gigabyte Aproximadamente, mil millones de bytes.

girth A measure around a body or item.
contorno Medida alrededor de un cuerpo o artículo.

glean To gather information or material bit by bit; to pick over in search of relevant material.

recopilar   Reunir información o material pedazo a pedazo; examinar en busca de material pertinente.

glucagon   A hormone produced by the alpha cells of the pancreatic islets that stimulates the liver to convert glycogen into glucose.
glucagón   Hormona producida por las células alfa de los islotes pancreáticos; estimula al hígado para que convierta el glucógeno en glucosa.

glucosuria   The abnormal presence of glucose in the urine.
glucosuria   Presencia anómala de glucosa en la orina.

glycogen   The sugar (starch) that is formed from glucose and stored mainly in the liver.
glucógeno   Azúcar (almidón) formado a partir de la glucosa y almacenado principalmente en el hígado.

glycohemoglobin (hemoglobin A_{1c})   A type of hemoglobin that is made slowly during the 120-day life span of the red blood cell (RBC). Glycohemoglobin makes up 3% to 6% of hemoglobin in a normal RBC; in individuals with diabetes mellitus, it makes up to 12%.
glucohemoglobina (hemoglobina A_{1c})   Tipo de hemoglobina que se produce lentamente durante el periodo de los 120 días de vida de los glóbulos rojos (RBC). La glucohemoglobina constituye de un 3% a un 6% de la hemoglobina en un RBC normal; en los casos de diabetes mellitus constituye hasta un 12%.

glycosuria   The presence of glucose in the urine.
glucosuria   Presencia de glucosa en la orina.

goniometer   An instrument used to measure the degrees of motion in a joint.
goniómetro   Instrumento para medir los grados de movimiento de una articulación.

government plan   An insurance or healthcare plan sponsored and/or subsidized by the state or federal government, such as Medicaid and Medicare.
plan del gobierno   Seguro o plan de atención sanitaria patrocinado y subvencionado por el gobierno estatal o federal, como Medicaid y Medicare.

grammar   The study of the classes of words, their inflections, and their functions and relations in a sentence; the study of what is preferred and what should be avoided in inflection and syntax.
gramática   Estudio de las clases de palabras, sus desinencias y sus funciones y relaciones en la oración; estudio del uso que se prefiere y de lo que hay que evitar en cuanto a desinencias y sintaxis.

gray (Gy)   The international unit of radiation dose.
gray (Gy)   Unidad internacional de dosis de radiación.

grief   An unfortunate outcome; deep distress caused by bereavement.

pesar   Resultado desafortunado; profunda aflicción causada por la pérdida de un ser querido.

group policy   Insurance written under a policy that covers a number of people under a single master contract, which is issued to their employer or to an association with which they are affiliated.
póliza de grupo   Seguro contratado bajo una póliza que cubre a varias personas bajo un único contrato maestro establecido con su empleador o con una asociación a la que estén afiliados.

growth hormone (GH)   The hormone that stimulates tissue growth and restricts tissue glucose dependence when nutrients are not available; also called *somatotropic hormone*.
hormona del crecimiento (GH)   También llamada *hormona somatotrópica,* estimula el crecimiento de los tejidos y restringe la dependencia de la glucosa de los tejidos cuando no hay nutrientes disponibles.

guarantor   A person who makes or gives a guarantee of payment for a bill.
garante   Persona que paga una factura o que garantiza su pago.

guardian ad litem   The legal representative of a minor.
tutor ad litem   Representante legal de un menor.

hard copy   The readable paper copy or printout of information.
copia impresa   Copia impresa en papel o impresión de la información.

harmonious   Marked by accord in sentiment or action; having the parts agreeably related.
armonioso   Caracterizado por una armonía en los sentimientos o acciones; partes de un todo relacionadas de forma agradable.

health insurance   Protection, in return for periodic premiums, that provides reimbursement of monetary losses resulting from illness or injury. Included under this heading are various types of insurance, such as accident insurance, disability income insurance, medical expense insurance, and accidental death and dismemberment insurance. Also known as *accident and health insurance* or *disability income insurance*.
seguro de enfermedad   Cobertura a cambio del pago de primas periódicas, la cual proporciona el reembolso de las pérdidas monetarias debidas a enfermedad o lesión. Bajo este nombre se incluyen varios tipos de seguros como seguro de accidente, seguro de incapacidad, seguro de gastos médicos y seguro en caso de muerte y pérdida de extremidades. También se conoce como *seguro de accidente y enfermedad* o *seguro de incapacidad*.

hematemesis   Vomiting of bright red blood, which indicates rapid upper gastrointestinal bleeding and is associated with esophageal varices or a peptic ulcer.

hematemesis Vómito de sangre roja brillante que indica hemorragia rápida del sistema gastrointestinal superior, relacionado con varices esofágicas o úlcera péptica.

hematocrit The percentage by volume of packed red blood cells in a given sample of blood after centrifugation; the volume percentage of erythrocytes in whole blood.
hematocrito Porcentaje por volumen de glóbulos rojos en una muestra de sangre dada después de ser centrifugada. Porcentaje del volumen de eritrocitos en la sangre completa.

hematoma A sac filled with blood that may be the result of trauma.
hematoma Saco lleno de sangre que puede ser el resultado de una lesión.

hematuria Blood in the urine.
hematuria Sangre en la orina.

hemoconcentration A condition in which the concentration of blood cells is increased in proportion to the plasma.
hemoconcentración Situación en la cual la concentración de glóbulos rojos ha aumentado en proporción al plasma.

hemoglobin A protein in erythrocytes that transports molecular oxygen in the blood.
hemoglobina Proteína que se encuentra en los eritrocitos que transportan el oxígeno en la sangre.

hemolysis The destruction or dissolution of red blood cells, with subsequent release of hemoglobin.
hemolisis Destrucción o disolución de los glóbulos rojos, con la subsiguiente liberación de hemoglobina.

hemolyzed A term used to describe a blood sample in which the red blood cells have ruptured.
hemolizado Término usado para describir una muestra de sangre en la cual los glóbulos rojos se han roto.

hepatomegaly Abnormal enlargement of the liver.
hepatomegalia Agrandamiento anómalo del hígado.

hereditary Pertaining to a characteristic, condition, or disease transmitted from parent to offspring on the DNA chain.
hereditario Perteneciente o relativo a una característica, estado o enfermedad transmitida de padres a hijos en la cadena de ADN.

hermetically sealed Sealed such that no air may enter or escape.
herméticamente sellado Sellado de forma que el aire no pueda entrar o escapar.

HMO An organization that provides a wide range of comprehensive healthcare services for a specified group at a fixed periodic payment. HMOs may be sponsored by the government, medical schools, hospitals, employers, labor unions, consumer groups, insurance companies, and hospital medical plans.
HMO Organización que proporciona una amplia gama de servicios completos de atención sanitaria para un grupo específico por un pago periódico fijado. Las HMO puedes estar patrocinadas por el gobierno, facultades de medicina, hospitales, patronos, sindicatos laborales, grupos de consumidores, compañías aseguradoras y planes médico-hospitalarios.

holder The person who presents a check for payment.
portador Persona que presenta un cheque para cobrarlo.

holistic Related to or concerned with all of the body's systems as a whole, rather than as separate parts.
holístico Relacionado con todos los sistemas corporales y no dividido en partes.

homeostasis The maintenance of constant internal ambient conditions compatible with life.
homeostasis Mantenimiento de unas condiciones ambientales internas constantes compatibles con la vida.

homeostatic Maintaining a constant internal environment.
homeostático Que mantiene un ambiente interno constante.

hormone A substance, usually a peptide or steroid, produced by one tissue and conveyed by the bloodstream to another to effect physiologic activity, such as growth or metabolism; a chemical transmitter produced by the body and transported to a target tissue or organs by the bloodstream.
hormona Sustancia química transmisora, por lo general un péptido o un esteroide, que es producida por un tejido y transportada por la corriente sanguínea hasta el tejido u órgano—objetivo para provocar un efecto en la actividad fisiológica, como el crecimiento o el metabolismo.

HTML Abbreviation for *hypertext markup language,* the language used to create documents for the Internet.
HTML Abreviatura de *lenguaje de marcas de hipertexto,* que es el lenguaje que se emplea para crear documentos destinados a usarse en Internet.

HTTP Abbreviation for *hypertext transfer protocol,* which designates how messages are defined and transmitted over the Internet; when a URL is entered into the computer, an HTTP command tells the Web server to retrieve the requested Web page.
HTTP Abreviatura de *protocolo de transporte de hipertexto,* que define cómo se interpretan y transmiten los mensajes en Internet; cuando un URL entra en la computadora, una orden de HTTP manda la señal al servidor web para que busque la página web que se solicita.

hub A common connection point for devices in a network containing multiple ports; it often is used to connect segments of an LAN.
nodo Punto de conexión común para dispositivos en una red de conexiones de varios puertos; suele usar se para conectar segmentos de una LAN (red de área local).

hydrocephaly Enlargement of the cranium caused by the abnormal accumulation of cerebrospinal fluid in the cerebral system.
hidrocefalia Agrandamiento del cráneo causado por una acumulación anómala de fluido cerebroespinal en el interior del sistema cerebral.

hydrogenated Combined with, treated with, or exposed to hydrogen.
hidrogenado Combinado con hidrógeno, tratado con él o expuesto a él.

hyperlipidemia An excess of fats or lipids in the blood plasma.
hiperlipemia Exceso de grasas o lípidos en el plasma sanguíneo.

hyperplasia An increase in the number of cells.
hiperplasia Aumento del número de células.

hyperpnea An increase in the depth of breathing.
hiperpnea Aumento en la profundidad de la respiración.

hypertension High blood pressure (i.e., a systolic pressure consistently above 140 mm Hg and a diastolic pressure above 90 mm Hg).
hipertensión Presión sanguínea alta (presión sistólica continuamente por encima de 140 mm Hg y presión diastólica por encima de 90 mm Hg).

hyperventilation Abnormally prolonged and deep breathing, usually associated with acute anxiety or emotional tension.
hiperventilación Respiración profunda anómalamente prolongada, que suele estar asociada con una ansiedad aguda o con tensión emocional.

hypotension Blood pressure that is below normal (i.e., a systolic pressure below 90 mm Hg and a diastolic pressure below 50 mm Hg).
hipotensión Presión sanguínea que está por debajo de lo normal (presión sistólica por debajo de 90 mm Hg y presión diastólica por debajo de 50 mm Hg).

icon A picture, often on the desktop of a computer, that represents a program or an object. By clicking on the icon, the user is directed to the program.
icono Dibujo, con frecuencia colocado en el escritorio de la computadora, que representa un programa o un objeto. Al hacer clic sobre el icono, el usuario es llevado a dicho programa.

idealism The practice of forming ideas or living under the influence of ideas.
idealismo Práctica de formarse ideas o vivir bajo la influencia de ideas.

idiopathic Of unknown cause.
idiopático Causa desconocida.

ileocecal valve The valve at the opening between the ileum and the cecum; also called the *ileocolic valve*.
válvula ileocecal Válvula que controla la abertura entre el íleo y el intestino ciego; también se llama *válvula ileocólica*.

ileostomy The surgical formation of an opening of the ileum onto the surface of the abdomen, through which fecal material is emptied.
ileostomía Formación quirúrgica de una abertura del íleo en la superficie del abdomen, a través de la cual se vacían los materiales fecales.

immigrant A person who comes to a country to take up permanent residence.
inmigrante Persona que va a un país para vivir allí de forma permanente.

immunotherapy The administration of repeated injections of diluted extracts of a substance that causes an allergic reaction; also called *desensitization*.
inmunoterapia Administración de repetidas inyecciones de extractos diluidos de la substancia que provoca una alergia; también se conoce como *desensibilización*.

impenetrable Incapable of being penetrated or pierced; not capable of being damaged or harmed.
impenetrable Que no puede ser penetrado o traspasado; que no puede ser dañado o perjudicado.

implied consent Presumed consent, such as when a patient offers an arm for a phlebotomy procedure.
consentimiento tácito Consentimiento que se supone que ha sido dado, como cuando un paciente presenta el brazo para que se le extraiga sangre.

in vitro Refers to conditions outside of a living body.
in-vitro Expresión que se refiere a condiciones exteriores de un ser vivo.

incentive Something that incites or spurs to action; a reward or reason for performing a task.
incentivo Algo que incita o impulsa a actuar; recompensa o razón para llevar a cabo una tarea.

"includes" In insurance claims, when this term appears under a subdivision such as a category (three digit) code or a two-digit procedure code, this indicates that the code and title include these terms. Other terms also classified to that particular code and title are listed in the Alphabetic Index.

"incluye" La presencia de esta expresión, cuando aparece bajo una subdivisión, como una categoría (código de tres dígitos) o como un código de procedimiento de dos dígitos, indica que el código y el título incluyen estos términos. En los Índices alfabéticos se enumeran otros términos también clasificados para este código específico.

incontinence The inability to control excretory functions.
incontinencia Incapacidad de controlar las funciones excretoras.

indemnity plan The traditional health insurance plan that pays for all or a share of the cost of covered services, regardless of which doctor, hospital, or other licensed healthcare provider is used. Policyholders of indemnity plans and their dependents choose when and where to get healthcare services.
plan de indemnización Plan de seguro de enfermedad tradicional que paga todo o parte del costo de los servicios que cubre, sin importar a qué médico, hospital u otro proveedor de atención sanitaria licenciado se acuda. Los titulares de pólizas de planes de indemnización y las personas que dependen de estos titulares escogen cuándo y dónde recibir atención médica.

indicators An important point or group of statistical values that, when evaluated, indicates the quality of care provided in a healthcare institution.
indicadores Importante punto o grupo de valores estadísticos que al ser evaluados indican la calidad del servicio que se proporciona en una institución de atención sanitaria.

indict To charge with a crime by the finding or presentment of a jury according to due process of law.
acusado Que se le imputa con un cargo criminal por conclusión o acusación de un jurado con el proceso legal debido.

indigent Totally lacking in something necessary.
indigente Que carece totalmente de algo necesario.

indirect filing system A filing system in which an intermediary reference, such as a card file, must be consulted to locate specific files.
sistema indirecto de archivo Sistema de archivo en el cual debe consultarse una fuente de referencia intermedia, como un fichero, para localizar documentos específicos.

individual policy An insurance policy designed specifically for the use of one person (and his or her dependents); a policy that is not associated with the amenities of a group policy, such as lower premiums. Often referred to as "personal insurance."

póliza individual Póliza de seguros destinada específicamente a ser usada por una persona (y quienes dependan de ella) y que no conlleva los beneficios de una póliza de grupo y tiene primas más altas. Con frecuencia se le llama "seguro—personal."

induration An abnormally hard, inflamed area.
induración Área anómalamente dura, inflamada.

infarction Area of tissue that has died because of lack of blood supply.
infarto Área de tejido que ha muerto debido a una falta de suministro de sangre.

infection Invasion of body tissues by microorganisms, which then proliferate and damage tissues.
infección Invasión de los tejidos corporales por microorganismos, los cuales entonces proliferan y dañan los tejidos.

infertile Not fertile or productive; not capable of reproducing.
estéril Que no es fértil o productivo; que no tiene la capacidad de reproducirse.

inflammation A tissue reaction to trauma or disease that includes redness, heat, swelling, and pain.
inflamación Reacción de los tejidos ante una lesión o enfermedad que incluye enrojecimiento, calentamiento, hinchazón y dolor.

inflection A change in the pitch or loudness of the voice.
inflexión Cambio en el tono o volumen de la voz.

informed consent Consent given because the patient understands the proposed treatment and the risks involved, the reasons it should be done, and alternative treatments available (including no treatment) and their attendant risks.
consentimiento informado Consentimiento que implica la comprensión del tratamiento al que se va a ser sometido y de los riesgos que conlleva, del porqué de dicho tratamiento, así como la comprensión de los tratamientos alternativos disponibles (incluyendo la ausencia de tratamiento) y los riesgos que conllevan.

infraction A minor offense against rules or regulations.
infracción Incumplimiento de la ley; delito menor contra las normas establecidas.

initiate To introduce; to cause or start something.
iniciativa El causar o facilitar el comienzo de algo; el hacer que algo comience a ocurrir.

innate Existing in, belonging to, or determined by factors present in an individual since birth.
innato Que existe en un individuo, que le pertenece o que está determinado por factores existentes en ese individuo desde el momento de su nacimiento.

input Information entered into a computer and used to produce output.
entrada Información introducida en una computadora y que la computadora utiliza.

instigate To goad or urge forward; to provoke.
instigar Incitar, exhortar, provocar.

insubordination Disobedience to authority.
insubordinación Desobediencia a la autoridad.

insulin A hormone secreted by the beta cells of the pancreatic islets in response to increased levels of glucose in the blood.
insulina Hormona que segregan las células beta de los islotes pancreáticos en respuesta a la presencia de altos niveles de glucosa en la sangre.

insured A person or organization covered by an insurance policy, along with any other parties for whom protection is provided under the policy terms.
asegurado Persona u organización que está cubierta por una póliza de seguro junto con cualquier otro a quien se proporcione cobertura bajo los términos de la póliza.

intangible Incapable of being perceived, especially by touch; incapable of being precisely identified or realized by the mind.
intangible Que no se puede percibir, especialmente que no se puede tocar; que no puede ser identificado con precisión ni ser comprendido por la mente.

integral Essential; an indispensable part of a whole.
integral Esencial; parte indispensable de un todo.

interaction A two-way communication; mutual or reciprocal action or influence.
interacción Comunicación bidireccional; acción o influencia recíproca o mutua.

intercom A two-way communication system with a microphone and loudspeaker at each station for localized use.
intercomunicador Sistema de comunicación bidireccional con un micrófono y un altavoz en cada estación para uso local.

intermittent Coming and going at intervals; not continuous.
intermitente Que va y viene a intervalos; de forma no continua.

intermittent claudication Recurring cramping in the calves caused by poor circulation of blood to the muscles of the lower leg.
cojera intermitente Calambres recurrentes en las pantorrillas causados por una mala circulación de la sangre de los músculos de la parte inferior de la pierna.

intermittent pulse A pulse in which beats occasionally are skipped.
pulso intermitente Pulso en el cual de vez en cuando se salta algún latido.

internal noise Noise inside the brain that interferes with the communication process.
ruido interno Ruido en el interior del cerebro que interfiere con el proceso de comunicación.

International Classification of Diseases, Ninth Revision, Clinical Modification (ICD-9-CM) A system for classifying diseases to facilitate the collection of uniform, comparable health information for statistical purposes and for indexing medical records for data storage and retrieval.
Clasificación Internacional de Enfermedades, Novena Revisión, Modificación clínica (ICD-9-CM) Sistema de clasificación de enfermedades para facilitar la recopilación de información médica uniforme, tanto para fines estadísticos como para indexar informes médicos a fin de almacenar y recuperar datos.

International Classification of Diseases, Tenth Revision (ICD-10) A system marked by the greatest number of changes in the ICD's history. To allow more specific reporting of diseases and newly recognized conditions, the ICD-10 has approximately 5,500 more codes than the ICD-9.
Clasificación Internacional de Enfermedades, Décima Revisión (ICD-10) Sistema que contiene el mayor número de cambios en la historia de la ICD. Para permitir elaborar informes más precisos de las enfermedades y de los estados patológicos que se conocen sólo recientemente, la ICD-10 incluye aproximadamente 5,500 códigos más que la ICD-9.

international mail Mail sent outside the boundaries of the United States and its territories.
correo internacional Correo que se envía fuera de los límites de Estados Unidos y sus territorios.

interval The length of time between events.
intervalo Espacio de tiempo entre dos sucesos.

intolerable Not tolerable or bearable.
intolerable Que no se puede tolerar o soportar.

intravenous urogram (IVU) A radiographic examination of the urinary tract that uses intravenous injection of an iodine contrast medium.
urograma intravenoso (IVU) Examen radiográfico del tracto urinario usando una inyección intravenosa de un medio de contraste yodado.

intrinsic Belonging to the essential nature or constitution of a thing; indwelling, inward.
intrínseco Que pertenece a la naturaleza o constitución básica de una cosa; inherente, interno.

introspection An inward, reflective examination of one's own thoughts and feelings.
introspección Examen de nuestros propios pensamientos y sentimientos.

invariably Consistently; without changing or being capable of change.
invariablemente De forma constante; que no cambia ni puede cambiar.

invasive A term that refers to entry into the living body, as by incision or insertion of an instrument.
invasivo Que entra en un organismo vivo, como por incisión o inserción de un instrumento.

ipsilateral Pertaining to the same side of the body.
isolateral Perteneciente a la misma parte del cuerpo.

irregular pulse A pulse that varies in force and frequency.
pulso irregular Pulso que varía en fuerza y frecuencia.

ischemia Decreased blood flow to a body part or organ, caused by constriction or plugging of the supplying artery; a temporary interruption in blood supply to a tissue or organ.
isquemia Disminución del flujo sanguíneo a una parte del cuerpo u órgano provocada por la constricción o atasco de la arteria suministradora; interrupción temporal del suministro de sangre a un tejido u órgano.

islets (of Langerhans) Cells of the pancreas that produce insulin (beta cells) and glucagon (alpha cells); also called *pancreatic islets*.
islotes (de Langerhans) Células del páncreas que producen insulina (células beta) y glucagón (células alfa); también llamados *islotes pancreáticos*.

jargon The technical terminology or characteristic idiom of a particular group or special activity.
jerga Terminología técnica o lenguaje característico de un grupo específico o una actividad especial.

jaundice Yellowness of the skin and mucous membranes caused by deposition of bile pigment. Jaundice is not itself a disease, but rather a sign of a number of diseases, especially liver disorders.
ictericia Coloración amarilla en la piel y las membranas mucosas causada por deposición del pigmento biliar. No es una enfermedad pero es un síntoma de muchas enfermedades, sobre todo de trastornos hepáticos.

Java An object-oriented, high-level programming language commonly used and well suited for the Internet.
Java Lenguaje de programación de alto nivel y orientado a objetos que es usado ampliamente y es muy adecuado para Internet.

judicial Of or relating to a judgment, the function of judging, the administration of justice, or the judiciary.
judicial Perteneciente o relativo al juicio, los procesos jurídicos, la administración de justicia o a la judicatura.

jurisdiction A power constitutionally conferred on a judge or magistrate to decide cases according to law and to carry sentence into execution. Jurisdiction is *original* when it is conferred on the court in the first instance (original jurisdiction); it is *appellate* when an appeal is given from the judgment of another court (appellate jurisdiction).
jurisdicción Poder constitucional otorgado a un juez o magistrado para resolver casos de acuerdo con la ley y hacer que se cumplan las sentencias. Es jurisdicción *original* cuando se otorga en un tribunal de primera instancia; es jurisdicción en *apelación* cuando existe una apelación al juicio de otro tribunal.

jurisprudence The science or philosophy of law; a system or body of law or the course of court decisions.
jurisprudencia Ciencia o filosofía que trata sobre la ley; sistema o cuerpo legal; línea de decisiones de los tribunales.

keratin A very hard, tough protein found in the hair, nails, and epidermal tissue.
queratina Proteína muy dura que se encuentra en el pelo, uñas y tejidos epidérmicos.

keratinocytes Any one of the skin cells that synthesize keratin.
queratinocitos Cualquiera de las células de la piel que sintetizan queratina.

ketosis The abnormal production of ketone bodies in the blood and tissues as a result of fat catabolism in cells. Ketones accumulate in large quantities when fat, instead of sugar, is used as fuel for energy in cells.
quetosis Producción anormal de cuerpos de quetosis en la sangre y tejidos como resultado de un catabolismo graso en las células. Los quetones se acumulan en grandes cantidades cuando se usa grasa, en lugar de azúcar, como combustible para las células.

kyphosis An abnormal convex curvature of the thoracic spine region.
cifosis Curvatura convexa anómala de la región espinal torácica.

lacrimation The secretion or discharge of tears.
lagrimeo Secreción o descarga de lágrimas.

language barrier Any type of interference that inhibits the communication process and is related to the difference in languages spoken by the people attempting to communicate.
barrera del idioma Cualquier tipo de interferencia que inhibe el proceso de comunicación y que está relacionado con la diferencia en los idiomas que hablan las personas que intentan comunicarse.

laryngoscopy Visual examination of the voice box area through an endoscope equipped with a light and mirrors for illumination.
laringoscopia Examen visual de la laringe por medio de un endoscopio equipado con una luz y espejos.

latent image Invisible changes in exposed film that become a visible image when the film is processed.
imagen latente Cambios invisibles en la película que se convertirán en una imagen visible cuando se procese la película.

law A binding custom or practice of a community; a rule of conduct or action prescribed or formally recognized as binding or enforceable by a controlling authority.
ley Costumbre o práctica obligatoria de una comunidad; norma de comportamiento o proceder prescrita o reconocida formalmente como norma obligatoria o que se puede hacer cumplir por una autoridad encargada.

learning style The way a person perceives and processes information to learn new material.
estilo de aprendizaje Forma en la que un individuo percibe y procesa la información para aprender cosas nuevas.

leukoderma White patches on the skin.
leucodermia Manchas blancas en la piel.

liable Obligated according to law or equity; responsible for an act or circumstance.
responsable Que tiene alguna obligación según la ley o el derecho lato; responsable de un acto o circunstancia.

libel A written defamatory statement or representation that conveys an unjustly unfavorable impression.
libelo Escrito difamatorio que produce una impresión desfavorable injusta.

ligament A tough connective tissue band that holds joints together by attaching to the bones on either side of the joint.
ligamento Banda de tejido conectivo resistente que sostiene las articulaciones uniendo los huesos de cada lado de la articulación.

ligation The process of tying off something to close it (e.g., a blood vessel during surgery) with a tie called a *ligature*.
ligado Proceso de atar algo, por ejemplo, un vaso sanguíneo durante una cirugía, con una atadura llamada *ligadura*.

limited radiography A limited-scope radiography practice, usually in an outpatient setting, that does not require the same credentials as those for professional radiologic technology; also called *practical radiography*.
radiografía limitada Práctica radiográfica de alcance limitado que se suele usar con pacientes externos y que no requiere las mismas credenciales que se necesitan para la tecnología radiográfica profesional. También se llama radiografía práctica.

lithotripsy A procedure for eliminating a stone (as in the bladder) by crushing or dissolving it in situ with high-intensity sound waves.
litotripsia Procedimiento para eliminar una piedra rompiéndola o disolviéndola in-situ por medio del uso de ondas sonoras de alta intensidad.

litigious Prone to engage in lawsuits.
litigioso Propenso a iniciar pleitos y litigios.

loading dose A double dose of medication administered as the first dose. Loading doses usually are given in antibiotic therapy to reach therapeutic drug levels in the blood quickly.
dosis de ataque Dosis doble de una medicación ladministrada como primera dosis. Suele hacerse con terapia antibiótica para alcanzar rápidamente los niveles terapéuticos en sangre.

lordosis An abnormal concave curvature of the cervical and lumbar spines.
lordosis Curvatura cóncava anómala de la espina cervical y lumbar.

lower GI series A fluoroscopic examination of the colon that usually involves rectal administration of barium sulfate (also called a *barium enema*) as a contrast medium.
serie GI inferior Examen fluoroscópico del colon, por lo general usando una administración rectal de

sulfato de bario (también llamado *enema de bario*) como medio de contraste.

lumbar   The area of the lower back containing the five lumbar vertebrae.
lumbar   Región posterior inferior en la que hay cinco vértebras lumbares.

lumen   The open space within a hollow tube such as a blood vessel, the intestine, a needle, or an examining instrument.
lumen   Espacio abierto, como en el interior de un vaso sanguíneo, el intestino, una aguja, un tubo o un instrumento para examinar.

luteinizing hormone (LH)   A hormone produced by the pituitary gland that promotes ovulation.
hormona luteinizante (LH)   Hormona que produce la glándula pituitaria y que promueve la ovulación.

luxation   Dislocation of a bone from its normal anatomic location.
luxación   Dislocación de un hueso de su ubicación anatómica normal.

lymphadenopathy   Any disorder of the lymph nodes or lymph vessels.
linfadenopatía   Cualquier trastorno de los nódulos o de los vasos linfáticos.

macromolecules   The molecules needed for metabolism: carbohydrates, lipids, proteins, and nucleic acids.
macromoléculas   Moléculas que se necesitan para el metabolismo: carbohidratos, lípidos, proteínas y ácidos nucleicos.

magnetic resonance imaging (MRI)   An imaging modality that uses a magnetic field and radiofrequency pulses to create computer images of both bones and soft tissues in multiple planes.
formación de imágenes por resonancia magnética (MRI)   Modalidad de formación de imágenes en la que se usa un campo magnético y pulsos de radiofrecuencia para crear imágenes computarizadas, tanto de huesos como de tejidos blandos, en planos múltiples.

major diagnostic categories (MDCs)   Broad clinical categories differentiated from all others on the basis of body system involvement and cause of disease.
categorías de diagnosis principales (MDCs)   Amplias categorías clínicas que se diferencian de todas las demás en base a la inclusión del sistema corporal y la etiología de la enfermedad.

maker (of a check)   Any individual, corporation, or legal party who signs a check or any type of negotiable instrument.

signatario (de un cheque)   Cualquier individuo, corporación o parte legal que firma un cheque o cualquier tipo de instrumento negociable.

malignant   Cancerous.
maligno   Canceroso.

managed care   An umbrella term for all healthcare plans that provide health care in return for preset monthly payments and that offer coordinated care through a defined network of primary care physicians and hospitals.
atención administrada   Término que engloba todos los planes de atención sanitaria que proporcionan atención médica a cambio de pagos mensuales preestablecidos y atención coordinada a través de una red definida de médicos de cabecera y hospitales.

mandated   Required by an authority or law.
obligatorio   Que lo exige una autoridad o la ley.

mandatory   Containing or constituting a command.
obligatorio   Que contiene una orden o que es una orden en sí mismo.

manifestation   Something easily understood or recognized by the mind.
manifestación   Algo que puede ser comprendido o reconocido por la mente con facilidad.

manipulation   Moving or exercising a body part by an externally applied force.
manipulación   Mover o ejercitar una parte del cuerpo por medio de la aplicación de una fuerza externa.

mastectomy   Surgical removal of the breast, usually including the excision of lymph nodes in the axillary region.
mastectomía   Eliminación quirúrgica del seno que por lo general incluye la escisión de los nódulos linfáticos de la región axilar.

matrix   Something in which a thing originates, develops, takes shape, or is contained; a base on which to build.
matriz   Algo donde las cosas se originan, desarrollan, toman forma o están contenidas; base sobre la cual construir.

m-banking   Banking through the use of wireless devices, such as cellular phones and wireless Internet services.
banca-m   Operaciones bancarias a través de dispositivos inalámbricos, como teléfonos celulares y servicios de comunicaciones inalámbricas.

media   The term applied to agencies of mass communication, such as newspapers, magazines, and telecommunications.

medios de comunicación Término que se aplica a las agencias de noticias o de comunicación de masas, como periódicos, revistas y telecomunicaciones.

mediastinum The space in the center of the chest, under the sternum.
mediastino Espacio en el centro del pecho, bajo el esternón.

medical savings account A tax-deferred bank or savings account combined with a low-premium, high-deductible insurance policy, designed for individuals or families who choose to fund their own healthcare expenses and medical insurance.
cuenta de ahorros para gastos médicos Cuenta bancaria o de ahorros de impuestos diferidos combinada con una póliza de seguro con primas bajas y deducibles altos destinada a individuos o familias que eligen financiar ellos mismos sus gastos de atención sanitaria y su seguro médico.

medically indigent An individual who can afford to pay for his or her normal daily living expenses but cannot afford adequate healthcare.
médicamente indigente Individuo que puede pagar sus gastos normales de la vida cotidiana pero que no puede abordar el pago de un servicio de atención sanitaria adecuado.

medically necessary Criteria used by third-party payers to decide whether a patient's symptoms and diagnosis justify specific medical services or procedures; also known as *medical necessity*.
médicamente necesario Criterio usado por pagadores intermediarios para decidir si los síntomas y el diagnóstico de un paciente justifican el uso de procedimientos o servicios médicos específicos; también se conoce como *necesidad médica*.

Medigap A term sometimes applied to private insurance products that supplement Medicare insurance benefits.
Medigap Término que se aplica algunas veces a seguros privados que complementan los beneficios del seguro Medicare.

medullary cavity The inner portion of the diaphysis that contains the bone marrow.
cavidad medular Porción interna de la diáfisis que contiene la médula ósea.

megabyte Approximately 1 million bytes.
megabyte Aproximadamente, un millón de bytes.

megahertz (MHz) A measuring unit for microprocessors. A megahertz is 1 million cycles of electromagnetic current alternation per second; it is used as a unit of measure for the clock speed of computer microprocessors. The hertz is a unit of measure named after Heinrich Hertz, a German physicist.
megahercio (MHz) Unidad de medida para microprocesadores, abreviada MHz. Un megahercio es un millón de ciclos de alternancia de corriente electromagnética por segundo y se usa como unidad de medida para la velocidad de los—microprocesadores de computadoras. El hercio recibe su nombre de Heinrich Hertz, un físico alemán.

melena A black, tarry stool containing digested blood; it usually is the result of bleeding in the upper GI tract.
melena Deposición negra y alquitranada que contiene sangre digerida y por lo general es le resultado de una hemorragia en el tracto gastrointestinal superior.

mentor A trusted counselor or guide.
mentor Consejero o guía de confianza.

metabolite A substance produced by metabolism.
metabolito Sustancia producida por el metabolismo.

meticulous Marked by extreme or excessive care in the consideration or treatment of details.
meticuloso Caracterizado por una atención exagerada o excesiva a los detalles.

microcephaly Abnormally small head size in relation to the rest of the body.
microcefalia Tamaño pequeño de la cabeza en relación con el resto del cuerpo.

microfilm A film bearing a photographic record of printed or other graphic matter on a reduced scale.
microfilm Película que contiene una fotografía de un documento impreso u otro elemento gráfico a escala reducida.

microorganism An organism of microscopic or submicroscopic size.
microorganismo Organismo de tamaño microscópico o sub-microscópico.

MIDI The abbreviation for *musical instrument digital interface*. A MIDI interface allows computers to record and manipulate sound.
MIDI Abreviatura para *interfaz digital para instrumentos musicales*. Una interfaz MIDI permite a las computadoras grabar y manipular sonido.

miotic Any substance or medication that causes contraction of the pupil.
miótico Cualquier sustancia o medicamento que produce una contracción de la pupila.

misdemeanor A minor crime punishable by fine or imprisonment in a city or county jail rather than in a penitentiary.

falta Delito menor, por oposición a delito mayor, se penaliza con multa o prisión en una cárcel de una ciudad o condado más bien que con prisión en una penitenciaría.

mock To imitate or practice.
simular Imitar o practicar.

modem The acronym for *modulator demodulator;* a device that allows information to be transmitted over phone lines at speeds measured in bits per second (bps).
módem Abreviatura para modulador desmodulador, un dispositivo que permite transmitir información a través de las líneas telefónicas a velocidades que se miden en bits por segundos (bps).

molecule A group of like or different atoms held together by chemical forces.
molécula Grupo de átomos iguales o diferentes que se mantiene unido por fuerzas químicas.

monochromatic Having or consisting of one color or hue.
monocromático Que tiene un solo color o tonalidad.

mononuclear white blood cell A leukocyte with an unsegmented nucleus, particularly monocytes and lymphocytes.
glóbulo blanco mononuclear Leucocito que tiene un núcleo sin segmentar; en particular los monocitos y linfocitos.

mons pubis The fat pad that covers the symphysis pubis.
monte del pubis Almohadilla de grasa que cubre la sínfisis púbica.

morale The mental and emotional condition (e.g., enthusiasm, confidence, or loyalty) of an individual or group with regard to the function or tasks at hand.
moral Estado mental y emocional (como entusiasmo, lealtad o confianza) de un individuo o grupo en cuanto al puesto que desempeña o el trabajo que realiza.

motivation The process of inciting a person to some action or behavior.
motivación Proceso de incitar a una persona a hacer algo o a comportarse de una forma determinada.

multimedia The presentation of graphics, animation, video, sound, and text on a computer in an integrated way or all at once. CD-ROMs are the most effective multimedia devices.
multimedia Presentación de gráficos, imágenes animadas, video, sonido y texto en una computadora de forma integrada o simultánea. Los CD ROM son los dispositivos de multimedia más eficaces.

multiparous Pertaining to women who have had two or more pregnancies.

multípara Perteneciente o relativo a la mujer que ha tenido dos o más embarazos.

multitasking Performing multiple tasks at one time.
multitarea Realización de varias tareas diferentes al mismo tiempo.

municipal court A court that sits in some cities and larger towns and that usually has civil and criminal jurisdiction over cases arising within the municipality.
Municipal corte Se aplica al juzgado con sede en algunas ciudades y pueblos grandes y que suele tener jurisdicción civil y penal sobre casos que surgen dentro de la municipalidad.

murmur An abnormal sound heard on auscultation of the heart; it may or may not be pathologic.
murmullo Sonido anómalo que se escucha al auscultar el corazón y que puede ser patológico o no.

myelography A fluoroscopic examination of the spinal canal involving spinal injection of an iodine contrast medium.
mielografía Examen fluoroscópico del canal espinal con una inyección espinal de un medio de contraste yodado.

myelomeningocele A herniation of part of the spinal cord and its meninges that protrudes through a congenital opening in the vertebral column.
mielomeningocele Hernia de una parte de la médula espinal y sus meninges que sale hacia fuera a través de una abertura congénita en la columna vertebral.

myocardial Pertaining to the heart muscle.
miocárdico Perteneciente o relativo al músculo cardiaco.

myocardium The heart muscle.
miocardio Músculo cardiaco.

myoglobinuria The abnormal presence of a hemoglobin-like chemical of muscle tissue in the urine; it occurs as a result of muscle deterioration.
mioglobinuria Presencia anómala en la orina de una susbtancia química del tejido muscular parecida a la hemoglobina; es el resultado de una deterioración muscular.

mysticism The experience of seeming to have direct communication with God or the ultimate reality.
misticismo Experiencia de parecer tener comunicación directa con Dios o una realidad superior.

nanometer One billionth ($1/10^{-9}$) of a meter.
nanómetro Una mil millonésima parte (10^{-9}) de metro.

naturopathy An alternative to conventional medicine in which holistic methods are used, as well as herbs and natural supplements, in the belief that the body will heal itself. Currently, naturopathic physicians can be licensed in 12 states.
naturopatía Alternativa a la medicina convencional en la que se usan métodos holísticos, así como hierbas y suplementos naturales, con la creencia de que el cuerpo sanará por sí mismo. En la actualidad, los médicos naturópatas pueden obtener la licencia en doce estados.

necrosis Pertaining to the death of cells or tissue.
necrosis Perteneciente o relativo a la muerte de células o tejidos.

negative feedback mechanism A homeostatic mechanism that responds as a regulator to counteract a change.
mecanismo de respuesta negativa Mecanismo homeostático que responde como regulador para contrarrestar un cambio.

negligence Failure to exercise the care that a prudent person usually exercises; implied inattention to one's duty or business; implied want of due or necessary diligence or care.
negligencia Falta de cuidado en algo que se hace; falta implícita de atención en el deber o trabajo; deseo implícito de una diligencia o cuidado necesario o merecido.

negotiable Legally transferable to another party.
negociable Que se puede transferir legalmente a otra parte.

networking The exchange of information or services among individuals, groups, or institutions; meeting and getting to know individuals in the same or similar career fields and sharing information about available opportunities.
interconexión Intercambio de información o servicios entre individuos, grupos o instituciones; conocer a individuos del mismo campo profesional o de campos similares y compartir información acerca de oportunidades de empleo.

neural tube defect Any of a group of congenital anomalies involving the brain and spinal column that are caused by failure of the neural tube to close during embryonic development.
defecto del tubo neural Cualquiera de las anomalías congénitas que afectan al cerebro y a la médula espinal y que tienen su origen en que el tubo neural no logró cerrarse durante el desarrollo embrionario.

nodule A small lump, lesion, or swelling that is felt when the skin is palpated.
nódulo Pequeña protuberancia, herida o hinchazón que se siente al tocar la piel.

nomogram A graph on which variables are plotted so that a particular value can be read on the appropriate line.
nomograma Gráfica en la que las variables están presentadas de tal manera que se puede leer un valor específico en la línea adecuada.

nonmaleficence Refraining from the act of causing harm or doing evil.
ausencia de maleficencia No hacer el mal.

no-show A person who fails to keep an appointment without giving advance notice.
no-acudió Persona que no acude a una cita médica sin dar previo aviso.

nosocomial infection An infection acquired during hospitalization or in a healthcare setting. These infections often are caused by *Escherichia coli,* hepatitis viruses, *Pseudomonas* organisms, and staphylococci.
infección nosocomial Infección adquirida en un establecimiento de atención sanitaria o durante una hospitalización. Con frecuencia se debe a *E. coli,* virus de hepatitis, pseudomonas y estafilococos.

nosocomial Pertaining to or originating in the hospital; a term for an infection that either was not present or was incubating before the patient was admitted to the hospital.
nosocomial Perteneciente o relativo al hospital, incubado en el hospital, dícese de la infección que no estaba presente ni en estado de incubación antes de ser ingresado al hospital.

"note" In coding manuals, notes are found in both the Alphabetic Index and the Tabular Index as instructions or guides for classification assignments; they define the category content or the use of subdivision codes.
"nota" Las notas se encuentran tanto en los Índices alfabéticos como en las instrucciones o guías en las Asignaciones de clasificación, para definir el contenido de la categoría o el uso de los códigos de subdivisión.

NSAIDs Nonsteroidal antiinflammatory drugs.
NSAIDs Medicamentos antiinflamatorios no esterioides.

nuclear medicine An imaging modality that uses radioactive materials injected or ingested into the body to provide information about the function of organs and tissues.
medicina nuclear Modalidad de la formación de imágenes que usa materiales radioactivos inyectados en el cuerpo o ingeridos para obtener información acerca del funcionamiento de órganos y tejidos.

obesity An excessive accumulation of body fat (usually defined as a weight more than 20% above the recommended body weight).

obesidad Acumulación excesiva de grasa en el cuerpo (se suele definir como más del 20% del peso recomendado).

objective information Information gathered by watching or observing a patient.
información objetiva Información que se recoge vigilando u observando a un paciente.

oblique projection The radiographic view in which the body or part is rotated so that the projection is neither frontal nor lateral.
proyección oblicua Vista radiográfica en la cual que cuerpo o parte del cuerpo se gira de forma que la proyección no es frontal ni lateral.

obliteration Making something indecipherable or imperceptible by obscuring or wearing away.
obliterar Hacer algo indescifrable o imperceptible oscureciéndolo o desgastándolo.

obturator A disk or plate that closes an opening.
obturador Disco o placa que cierra una abertura.

obturator A metal rod with a smooth, rounded tip that is placed inside hollow instruments to reduce damage to body tissues during insertion of the instrument.
obturador Varilla de metal con un extremo redondeado que se coloca en el interior de instrumentos huecos para disminuir la destrucción de los tejidos corporales durante su inserción.

occlusion The complete blocking off of an opening.
oclusión Cierre completo de una abertura.

"omit code" In insurance claims, a term used primarily in volume 3 of the ICD-9-CM when a procedure is the method of approach for an operation.
"omitir código" Esta expresión se usa sobre todo en el tomo 3 cuando el procedimiento es el método de acercamiento a una operación.

opaque Not translucent or transparent.
opaco Que no es translúcido ni transparente.

OPIM (other potentially infectious material) Substances or material other than blood (e.g., body fluids, such as urine and semen) that have the potential to carry infectious pathogens.
OPIM (otras materias potencialmente peligrosas) Sustancias o materias además de la sangre (como, por ejemplo, los fluidos corporales, la orina, el semen).

opinion A formal expression of judgment or advice by an expert; the formal expression of the legal reasons and principles on which a legal decision is based.

opinión Expresión formal de un juicio o consejo dado por un experto; expresión formal de las razones y principios legales sobre los que se basa una decisión legal.

opportunistic infection An infection caused by a normally nonpathogenic organism in a host whose resistance has been decreased.
infección oportunista Infección en una persona con una resistencia a las enfermedades más baja de lo normal, provocada por un organismo que en condiciones normales no resulta patógeno.

optic disc The region at the back of the eye where the optic nerve meets the retina. It is considered the blind spot of the eye, because it contains only nerve fibers and no rods or cones and therefore is insensitive to light.
papila óptica Región en la parte posterior del ojo donde el nervio óptico se une con la retina. Se considera el punto ciego del ojo, ya que allí sólo hay fibras nerviosas y no bastoncillos ni conos, y por tanto es insensible a la luz.

optic nerve The second cranial nerve, which carries impulses for the sense of sight.
nervio óptico Segundo nervio del cráneo que transporta impulsos para el sentido de la vista.

optical character recognition (OCR) Electronic scanning of printed items as images, followed by the use of special software to recognize these images (or characters) as ASCII text.
reconocimiento óptico de caracteres (OCR) Proceso de escanear electrónicamente documentos impresos como si fueran imágenes y después, usando un programa de computadora especial, reconocer esas imágenes (o caracteres) como texto ASCII.

ordinance An authoritative decree or direction; a law set forth by a governmental authority, specifically a municipal regulation.
ordenanza Decreto u orden de la autoridad; ley definida por una autoridad gubernamental, específicamente, una regulación municipal.

organelle A differentiated structure within a cell (e.g., a mitochondrion, vacuole, or chloroplast) that performs a specific function.
organelo Estructura diferenciada dentro de una célula, como un mitocondrio, vacuola o cloroplasto que realiza una función específica.

orthopnea Difficulty breathing in the supine position. The individual must sit or stand to breathe comfortably.
ortopnea Dificultad para respirar estando en posición supina. El individuo debe estar sentado o de pie para respirar con comodidad.

orthostatic (postural) hypotension   A temporary fall in blood pressure when a person rapidly changes from a recumbent position to a standing position.
hipotensión ortostática (relacionada con la postura)   Baja temporal de la presión sanguínea cuando una persona cambia con rapidez de una posición recostada a una posición en pie.

osteopathy   A medical discipline based primarily on the manual diagnosis and holistic treatment of impaired function resulting from loss of movement in all kinds of tissues.
osteopatía   Disciplina médica que se basa primordialmente en el diagnóstico manual y el tratamiento holístico de funciones deterioradas como resultado de la pérdida de movilidad en todo tipo de tejidos.

osteoporosis   A condition of loss of bone density; lack of calcium intake is a major factor in its development.
osteoporosis   Disminución de la densidad de los huesos. La falta de consumo de calcio es uno de los factores principales de su desarrollo.

otitis externa   Inflammation or infection of the external auditory canal.
otitis externa   Inflamación o infección del canal auditivo externo.

otosclerosis   The formation of spongy bone in the labyrinth of the ear, often causing the auditory ossicles to become fixed and unable to vibrate when sound enters the ears.
otosclerosis   Formación de huesos parecidos a esponjas en el laberinto del oído, a menudo causando que los huesecillos auditivos queden fijos y que no puedan vibrar cuando el sonido entra en los oídos.

ototoxic   Pertaining to a substance or medication that damages the eighth cranial nerve or the organs of hearing and balance.
ototóxico   Perteneciente o relativo a una sustancia o medicamento que daña el octavo nervio craneal o los órganos auditivos y del equilibrio.

OUTfolder   A folder used to provide space for the temporary filing of materials.
Carpeta OUT   Carpeta que se usa para proporcionar espacio para archivar materiales de forma temporal.

OUTguide   A heavy guide used to replace a folder that has been temporarily moved from the filing space.
Guía OUT   Guía grande que se usa para reemplazar una carpeta que ha sido retirada temporalmente del archivo.

output   Information processed by the computer and transmitted to a monitor, printer, or other device.
salida   Información procesada por la computadora y enviada a un monitor, impresora u otro dispositivo.

over-the-counter drugs   Medications legally sold without a prescription.
medicinas de venta libre   Medicinas que se venden sin receta legalmente.

oxytocin   A hormone secreted by the posterior pituitary gland that stimulates smooth muscle contractions of the uterus or mammary glands.
oxitocina   Hormona que segrega la glándula pituitaria posterior y que estimula las contracciones del útero o de las glándulas mamarias.

palliative   An agent that relieves or alleviates symptoms without curing the disease; something that alleviates or eases a painful situation without curing it.
paliativo   Agente que calma o alivia los síntomas sin curar la enfermedad; algo que alivia o hace más soportable una situación dolorosa sin curarla.

pandemic   Affecting most of the people in a country or a number of countries.
pandémico   Que afecta a la mayoría de la población de un país o de varios países.

paper claims   Hard copies of insurance claims that have been completed and sent by surface mail.
reclamaciones de papel   Copias impresas de reclamaciones de seguros que han sido completadas y enviadas por correo ordinario.

papilledema   Bulging of the optic disc and dilated retinal veins, which are seen through ophthalmoscopic examination of the retina. Papilledema is a sign of increased intracranial pressure.
edema papilar   Abultamiento de la papila óptica y de las venas retinianas dilatadas que se ven en un examen oftalmoscópico de la retina. La emeda papilar es una señal de un aumento en la presión intracraneal.

paraphrased   Pertaining to a text, passage, or work that has been restated to give the meaning in another form.
parafraseado   Perteneciente o relativo a un texto, selección u obra que ha sido expresado nuevamente para dar su significado de otra forma.

paraphrasing   Expressing an idea in different wording in an effort to enhance communication and clarify meaning.
parafrasear   Expresar una idea con palabras diferentes para mejorar la comunicación y hacer más claro su significado.

parenteral   Referring to injection or introduction of substances into the body through any route other than the digestive tract (e.g., subcutaneous, intravenous, or intramuscular administration).

parenteral Inyección o introducción de sustancias en el cuerpo a través de cualquier otra vía que no sea el tracto digestivo, como administración subcutánea, intravenosa o intramuscular.

paresthesia An abnormal sensation of burning, prickling, or stinging.
parestesia Sensación anómala de ardor, escozor o aguijoneo.

paroxysmal Pertaining to a sudden, recurrent spasm of symptoms.
paroxístico Perteneciente o relativo a espasmos repentinos recurrentes o a sus síntomas.

participating provider A physician or other healthcare provider who enters into a contract with a specific insurance company or program and by doing so agrees to abide by certain rules and regulations set forth by that particular third-party payer.
proveedor participante Médico u otro proveedor de atención sanitaria que establece un contrato con una compañía o programa de seguro específico, y al hacerlo acepta respetar ciertas normas y regulaciones establecidas por ese pagador intermediario.

parturition The act or process of giving birth to a child.
parto Acción o proceso de dar a luz un niño.

patency The condition of a body cavity or canal that is open or unobstructed.
abertura Estado abierto de un cuerpo, cavidad o canal.

pathogen An agent that causes disease, especially a living microorganism such as a bacterium or fungus; a disease-causing microorganism.
patógeno Agente que causa enfermedades, especialmente microorganismos vivos como bacterias u hongos; microorganismos causantes de enfermedades.

pathogenic Pertaining to disease-causing microorganisms.
patogénico Perteneciente o relativo a los microorganismos causantes de enfermedades.

pathophysiology The study of biologic and physical manifestations of disease as they are related to system abnormalities and physiologic disturbances.
patofisiología Estudio de las manifestaciones biológicas y físicas de las enfermedades y cómo se relacionan con las anomalías del sistema y las alteraciones fisiológicas.

payables The balance due to a creditor on an account.
pendiente de pago Saldo que se le debe al acreedor en una cuenta.

payee The person named on a draft or check as the recipient of the amount shown.
beneficiario Persona que se nombra en una letra de cambio o en un cheque como receptor de la cantidad indicada.

payer The person who writes a check to be cashed by the payee.
pagador Persona que emite el cheque a ser cambiado por el beneficiario.

peer review organization A group of medical reviewers who contract with the Health Care Financing Administration (HCFA) to ensure quality control and the medical necessity of services provided by a facility.
organizacione de revisión colegial Grupo de revisores médicos contrata dos por HCFA para garantizar el control de calidad y la necesidad médica de los servicios ofrecidos por un establecimiento.

pegboard system A method of tracking patient accounts that allows the figures to be proven accurate by using mathematic formulas; also called the "write it once" system.
sistema de tablero perforado Método de controlar las cuentas de los pacientes que permite la demostración de la exactitud de las cifras por medio de fórmulas matemáticas; también conocido como sistema "escríbelo una vez."

perceiving The process by which an individual looks at information and sees it as real.
percibir Proceso en el cual un individuo mira la información y la ve como real.

perception A quick, acute, and intuitive cognition; the capacity for comprehension; an awareness of the elements of the environment.
percepción Conocimiento rápido, agudo e intuitivo; capacidad de comprensión; conocimiento de los elementos del medio ambiente.

pericardium The membranous sac that encloses the heart.
pericardio Saco membranoso que envuelve el corazón.

periosteum The thin, highly innervated, membranous covering of a bone.
periostio Membrana fina y sin nervios que recubre un hueso.

peristalsis The wavelike movement by which the gastrointestinal tract moves food downward.
peristalsis Movimiento ondulatorio por el cual el tracto gastrointestinal mueve la comida hacia abajo.

perjured testimony Testimony involving the voluntary violation of an oath or vow, either by swearing to what is untrue or by failing to do what has been promised under oath; false testimony.

perjuro Testimonio que comprende la violación voluntaria de un juramento o promesa, ya sea jurando algo que es falso o no cumpliendo lo que se ha prometido bajo juramento; falso testimonio.

"perks" Perquisites; extra advantages or benefits from working in a specific job that may or may not be commonplace in that particular profession.
beneficios adicionales Ventajas o beneficios adicionales del trabajar en un puesto de trabajo específico que pueden ser o no comunes a esa profesión en particular.

permeable Allowing a substance to pass or soak through.
permeable Permite el paso o penetración de una sustancia.

persona An individual's social facade or front that reflects the role the individual is playing in life; the personality a person projects in public.
persona Lo que vemos de un individuo, la imagen social que refleja el papel que dicho individuo tiene en la sociedad; la personalidad que una persona proyecta en público.

pertinent Having a clear, decisive relevance to the matter at hand.
pertinente Que tiene una importancia clara y decisiva en el asunto que se está tratando.

petechiae Small, purplish hemorrhagic spots on the skin.
petequia Pequeñas manchas en la piel, hemorrágicas y de color violeta.

phenylalanine An essential amino acid found in milk, eggs, and other foods.
fenilalanina Aminoácido esencial que se encuentra en la leche, los huevos y otros alimentos.

philanthropist An individual who makes an active effort to promote human welfare.
filántropo Individuo que se ocupa activamente de promover el bienestar humano.

philosopher A person who seeks wisdom or enlightenment; an expounder of a theory in a certain area of experience.
filósofo Persona que busca la sabiduría o el esclarecimiento; persona que expone una teoría en cierta área de experiencia.

phlebotomy The invasive procedure used to obtain a blood specimen for testing, experimentation, or diagnosis of disease.
flebotomía Procedimiento invasivo que se usa para obtener un espécimen de sangre para analizar, experimentar o diagnosticar una enfermedad.

phonetic Referring to an alteration of ordinary spelling that better represents the spoken language, that uses only characters of the regular alphabet, and that is used in a context of conventional spelling.
escritura fonética Alteración de la escritura normal que representa mejor el lenguaje hablado, emplea sólo caracteres del alfabeto normal y se usa en un contexto de escritura convencional.

phosphors Fluorescent crystals that give off light when exposed to x-rays.
fósforos Cristales fluorescentes que alumbran cuando se exponen a los rayos x.

photometer An instrument for measuring the intensity of light, specifically to compare the relative intensities of different lights or their relative illuminating power.
fotómetro Instrumento para medir la intensidad de la luz, específicamente para comparar las intensidades relativas de luces diferentes o su poder de iluminación relativo.

photophobia Abnormal visual sensitivity to light.
fotofobia Sensibilidad visual anómala a la luz.

physiologic noise Physiologic interference with the communication process.
ruido fisiológico Interferencia fisiológica con el proceso de comunicación.

pipet A cylindric glass or plastic tube used to deliver fluids.
pipeta Tubo cilíndrico de vidrio o plástico que se usa para distribuir fluidos.

pitch The property of a sound, especially a musical tone, that is determined by the frequency of the waves producing it; the highness or lowness of sound; the relative level, intensity, or extent of some quality or state.
tono Propiedad de un sonido, especialmente de un tono musical, que está determinada por la frecuencia de las ondas que lo producen; cualidad alta o baja de un sonido; nivel, intensidad o extensión relativos de alguna cualidad o estado.

plaque An abnormal accumulation of a fatty substance.
placa Acumulación anómala de una sustancia grasa.

plasma The liquid portion of whole blood that contains active clotting agents.
plasma Parte líquida de la sangre completa que contiene agentes coagulantes activos.

policyholder The person who pays a premium to an insurance company (and in whose name the policy is written) in exchange for the protection provided by a policy of insurance.

titular de la póliza   Persona que paga una prima a una compañía aseguradora (y a cuyo nombre se contrata la póliza) a cambio de la cobertura que proporciona una póliza de seguro.

polycythemia vera   A condition marked by an abnormally large number of red blood cells in the circulatory system.
policitemia vera   Afección que se caracteriza por una cantidad anómalamente elevada de glóbulos rojos en el sistema circulatorio.

polydipsia   Excessive thirst.
polidipsia   Sed excesiva.

polymorphonuclear white blood cells   Leukocytes with a segmented nucleus; also known as *polymorphonuclear neutrophils* (PMNs) or *segmented neutrophils*.
glóbulos blancos polimorfonucleares   Leucocitos que tienen un núcleo segmentado; también se conocen como *neutrófilos polimorfonucleares* (PMN) o *neutrófilos segmentados*.

polyphagia   Excessive appetite.
polifagia   Aumento del apetito.

polyps   Tumors on stems; they are frequently found in or on mucous membranes and in the mucosal lining of the colon.
pólipos   Tumores en racimos que se encuentran con frecuencia en las membranas mucosas y en el recubrimiento mucoso del colon.

polyuria   Excessive urine production; excretion of an unusually large amount of urine.
poliuria   Producción y excreción de orina excesivas.

portal hypertension   Increased venous pressure in the portal circulation caused by cirrhosis or compression of the hepatic vascular system.
hipertensión portal   Aumento de la presión venosa en la circulación portal causado por cirrosis o compresión del sistema vascular hepático.

portfolio   A set of pictures, drawings, documents, or photographs either bound in book form or loose in a folder.
portafolio   Conjunto de ilustraciones, dibujos, documentos o fotografías, organizadas ya sea archivadas en forma de libro, o sueltas en una carpeta.

posteroanterior (PA)   A frontal projection in which the patient is prone or facing the x-ray film or image receptor.
posterioanterior (PA)   Proyección frontal en la que el paciente está boca abajo o de frente a la película de rayos x o al receptor de imagen.

post   To transfer or carry from a book of original entry to a ledger; to enter figures in an accounting system.
asentar   Transferir o traer desde un libro de entradas originales a un libro mayor; entrar cifras en un sistema de contabilidad.

postmortem   Done, collected, or occurring after death.
postmortem   Hecho, recogido o sucedido después de la muerte.

power of attorney   A legal instrument authorizing a person to act as the attorney or agent of the grantor. The authority may be limited to the handling of specific procedures. The person authorized to act as the agent is known as the *attorney in fact*.
potestad legal   Instrumento legal que autoriza a una persona a actuar como abogado o agente de la persona que le concede el poder. La autorización puede estar limitada al manejo de procedimientos específicos. La persona autorizada a actuar como agente se conoce como *abogado de hecho*.

precedence   Superiority in rank, dignity, or importance; the condition of being, going, or coming ahead or in front of another.
precedencia   Superioridad en rango, dignidad o importancia; condición de estar, ir o venir primero o antes.

precedent   A person or thing that serves as a model; something done or said that may serve as an example or rule to authorize or justify a subsequent act of the same kind.
precedente   Persona o cosa que sirve como modelo; algo hecho o dicho anteriormente y que puede servir como ejemplo o norma para autorizar o justificar un acto subsiguiente del mismo tipo.

pre-existing condition   A physical condition of an insured person that existed before the issuance of the insurance policy.
afección preexistente   Afección física de una persona asegurada que ya existía antes de la emisión de la póliza de seguro.

premium   The consideration paid for a contract of insurance; the periodic (monthly, quarterly, or annual) payment of a specific sum of money to an insurance company that in return agrees to provide certain benefits.
prima   Pago por un contrato de seguro; pago periódico (mensual, trimestral o anual) de una suma específica de dinero a una compañía aseguradora, la cual, a cambio, acepta proporcionar ciertos beneficios.

preponderance   A superiority or excess in number or quantity; majority.
preponderancia   Superioridad o mayor número o cantidad; mayoría.

preponderance of the evidence   Evidence that is of greater weight or more convincing than the evidence

offered in opposition to it; evidence that, as a whole, shows that the fact sought to be proven is more probable than not.
preponderancia de evidencia Evidencia que tiene mayor peso o que es más convincente que la evidencia con la que se confronta; evidencia que, en conjunto, muestra que el hecho que se pretende probar es más posible que imposible.

prerequisite Something that is necessary to achieve a result or to carry out a function.
requisito previo Algo que es necesario para obtener un resultado o para desempeñar una función.

present illness The chief complaint, written in chronologic sequence with dates of onset.
enfermedad actual Problema principal, descrito en secuencia cronológica con las fechas de cada acceso.

preservatives Substances added to a specimen to prevent deterioration of cells or chemicals.
preservativos Sustancias añadidas a un espécimen para prevenir el deterioro de células o sustancias químicas.

pressboard A strong, highly glazed composition board resembling vulcanized fiber; heavy card stock.
cartón prensado Cartón de composición resistente y muy satinado que se parece a la fibra vulcanizada; cartulina de gran resistencia.

primary diagnosis The condition or chief complaint for which a patient is treated in outpatient medical care (e.g., the physician's office or a clinic).
diagnóstico primario Afección o problema principal por el cual se trata a un paciente con atención médica externa (en un consultorio médico o una clínica).

principal A capital sum of money due as a debt or used as a fund, for which interest is either charged or paid.
principal Capital o suma de dinero que se debe como deuda o que se usa como fondo, por el cual se cargan o se cobran intereses.

principal diagnosis A condition, established after study, that is chiefly responsible for the admission of a patient to the hospital. It is used in coding inpatient hospital insurance claims.
diagnóstico principal Enfermedad o lesión que, tras su estudio, se determina que es la causa principal por la que un paciente ingresa en el hospital. Es usado en la codificación de reclamaciones de seguros de pacientes hospitalizados.

privately owned laboratories (POLs) Laboratories owned by a private individual or corporation, such as a freestanding laboratory or the laboratory inside a physician's office.
laboratorios privados (POLs) Laboratorios cuyo propietario es un individuo o una corporación privada, como el laboratorio dentro de un consultorio médico o un laboratorio independiente.

processing The way an individual internalizes new information and makes it his or her own.
procesar Forma en la que un individuo interioriza y asimila la información nueva.

procrastination Intentionally putting off doing something that should be done.
procrastinación Dejar a un lado o retrasar, de manera intencional, algo que debe hacerse.

professional behaviors Actions that identify the medical assistant as a member of a healthcare profession, including dependability, respectful patient care, initiative, positive attitude, and teamwork.
comportamientos profesionales Características que identifican al asistente médico como profesional de la atención sanitaria, incluyendo confiabilidad, trato respetuoso a los pacientes, iniciativa, actitud positiva y disposición para trabajar en equipo.

professional courtesy The reduction or omission of a fee for professional associates.
cortesía profesional Reducción o supresión de un cargo para los asociados profesionales.

professionalism Characterizing or conforming to the technical or ethical standards of a profession; exhibiting a courteous, conscientious, and generally businesslike manner in the workplace.
profesionalismo Actitud que se caracteriza por cumplir o actuar de acuerdo con los estándares técnicos y éticos de una profesión; dar muestras de cortesía, meticulosidad y, en general, mostrar un comportamiento adecuado en el lugar de trabajo.

proficiency Competency as a result of training or practice.
pericia Estado de competencia en algo, que se alcanza por medio de entrenamiento o práctica.

profit sharing An offer of part of the company's profits to employees or other designated individuals or groups.
participación en los beneficios Oferta de parte de los beneficios de la compañía a los empleados u otros individuos o grupos designados.

progress notes Notes entered in a patient's chart to track the individual's progress and condition.
notas del progreso Notas escritas en historial médico del paciente para seguir el progreso y estado del mismo.

prokaryote A unicellular organism that lacks a membrane-bound nucleus.
procaryota Organismo unicelular cuyo núcleo no está unido por una membrana.

prolactin (PRL) A hormone secreted by the anterior pituitary gland that stimulates the development of the mammary gland.
prolactina (PRL) Hormona que segrega la glándula pituitaria anterior y que estimula el desarrollo de la glándula mamaria.

proofread To read text and mark corrections.
corregir pruebas Leer un texto y marcar correcciones.

prosthesis An artificial replacement for a body part.
prótesis Pieza artificial para reemplazar una parte del cuerpo.

proteins Organic compounds in plants and animals that contain the major elements carbon, hydrogen, oxygen, and nitrogen and the amino acids essential to maintain life.
proteínas Compuestos orgánicos que existen en plantas y animales y que contienen los elementos principales: carbón, hidrógeno, oxígeno y nitrógeno y los aminoácidos esenciales para el mantenimiento de la vida.

provider An individual or company that provides medical care and services to patients or the public.
proveedor Individuo o compañía que proporciona atenciones y servicios médicos pacientes o al público.

provisional diagnosis A temporary diagnosis made before all test results have been received.
diagnóstico provisional Diagnóstico temporal llevado a cabo antes de recibir todos los resultados de las pruebas.

proxemics The study of the nature, degree, and effect of the spatial separation individuals naturally maintain.
proxemia Estudio de la naturaleza, grado y efecto de la separación espacial que los individuos mantienen de forma natural.

prudent Marked by wisdom or judiciousness; shrewd in the management of practical affairs.
prudente Caracterizado por poseer sabiduría o sensatez; hábil en el manejo de los asuntos prácticos.

psoriasis A usually chronic, recurrent skin disease marked by bright red patches covered with silvery scales.
psoriasis Enfermedad recurrente de la piel, por lo general crónica, caracterizada por manchas de color rojo brillante cubiertas por escamas plateadas.

psychosocial Pertaining to a combination of psychological and social factors.
psicosocial Perteneciente o relativo a una combinación de factores psicológicos y sociales.

public domain The realm embracing property rights that belong to the community at large, are unprotected by copyright or patent, and are subject to appropriation by anyone.
dominio público Campo que abarca los derechos de propiedad que pertenecen a la comunidad en general, que no están protegidos por leyes de derechos de autor ni por patentes y están sujetos a apropiación por parte de cualquiera.

pulmonary consolidation In pneumonia, the process by which the lungs become solidified as they fill with exudates.
solidificación pulmonar Proceso por el cual los pulmones se vuelven rígidos a medida que se llenan con exudados en los casos de pulmonía.

pulse deficit A condition in which the radial pulse is less than the apical pulse. It may indicate a peripheral vascular abnormality.
déficit del pulso Cuando el pulso radial es menor que el apical. Puede indicar una anomalía vascular periférica.

pulse pressure The difference between the systolic and the diastolic blood pressures (less than 30 points or more than 50 points is considered normal).
presión del pulso Diferencia entre las presiones sanguíneas sistólica y diastólica (menos de 30 puntos o más de 50 puede considerarse normal).

pure culture A bacterial or fungal culture that contains a single organism.
cultivo puro Cultivo de bacterias u hongos que contiene un solo organismo.

putrefaction The decomposition of organic matter, which produces a foul smell.
putrefacción Descomposición de materia orgánica que da como resultado un olor fétido.

pyemia The presence of pus-forming organisms in the blood.
piemia Presencia en la sangre de organismos formadores de pus.

quackery The pretense of curing disease.
curanderismo Práctica del que finge curar enfermedades.

quality control An aggregate of activities designed to ensure adequate quality, especially in manufactured products or in the service industries.
control de calidad Conjunto de actividades destinadas a garantizar la calidad adecuada, en especial en productos manufacturados o en las industrias de servicios.

queries Requests for information from a database.
consultas Peticions de información de una base de datos.

rad The conventional unit of absorbed radiation dose.
rad Unidad convencional de dosis de radiación absorbido.

radiograph An x-ray image.
radiografía Imagen obtenida con el uso de rayos-x.

radiographer A person qualified to perform radiographic examinations.
técnico de radiología Persona cualificada para realizar exámenes radiológicos.

radiography Making diagnostic images using x-rays.
radiografía Proceso de diagnosticar imágenes usando rayos x.

radiologist A physician who specializes in medical imaging and/or therapeutic applications of radiation.
médico radiólogo Médico especialista en formación de imágenes o en aplicaciones terapéuticas de la radiación.

radiolucent Referring to a substance that is easily penetrated by x-rays; these substances appear dark on radiographs.
transparente a la radiación Término que se aplica a una substancia que puede ser penetrada con facilidad por los rayos x; estas substancias aparecen oscuras en las radiografías.

radiopaque Referring to a substance that can be easily seen on an x-ray image (i.e., is is not easily penetrated by x-rays); these substances appear light on radiographs.
opaco a la radiación Sustancia que puede visualizarse con facilidad en la imagen de rayos x. Término que se aplica a una substancia que no puede ser penetrada con facilidad por los rayos x; estas substancias aparecen claras en las radiografías.

rales Abnormal or crackling breath sounds during inspiration.
estertores Sonidos respiratorios o crujidos anómalos durante la inspiración.

ramifications Consequences produced by a cause or following from a set of conditions.
ramificaciones Consecuencias producidas por una causa o que siguen a una serie de estados.

rapport A relationship of harmony and accord between the patient and the healthcare professional.
concordia Relación de armonía y acuerdo entre el paciente y el profesional de la atención sanitaria.

Raynaud's phenomenon Intermittent attacks of ischemia in the extremities that result in cyanosis, numbness, tingling, and pain.
fenómeno de Raynaud Ataques intermitentes de isquemia en las extremidades, resultando en cianosis, entumecimiento, picazón y dolor.

RBRVS (resource-based relative value system) A fee schedule designed to provide national uniform payment of Medicare benefits after adjustment to reflect the differences in practice costs across geographic areas.
RBRVS (sistema de valor relativo basado en recursos) Escala de cargos diseñada para proporcionar un pago de beneficios de Medicare uniforme a nivel nacional después de haber sido ajustado para reflejar las diferencias en los costos prácticos a través de áreas geográficas.

ream A quantity of paper consisting of 20 quires or variously 480, 500, or 516 sheets.
resma Una cantidad de papel que consiste de 20 manos o que varía entre 480, 500 o 516 hojas.

reasonable doubt Doubt based on reason and arising from evidence or lack of evidence; not doubt that is imagined or conjured up, but doubt that would cause reasonable persons to hesitate before acting in a manner important to themselves.
duda razonable Duda basada en la razón o que surge de evidencia o falta de evidencia; no es una duda imaginaria ni inventada, sino una duda que puede hacer que una persona razonable vacile antes de dar un paso importante.

receipts Amounts paid on patients' accounts.
recibos Sumas pagadas en las cuentas de los pacientes.

recipient The receiver of something.
receptor El que recibe un artículo u objeto.

rectify To correct by removing errors.
rectificar Corregir eliminando errores.

reduction The return of a structure to its correct anatomic position, as in the reduction of a fracture.
reducción Regreso a la posición anatómica correcta, como en el caso de reducción de una fractura.

referral (reference) laboratory A private or hospital-based laboratory that performs a wide variety of tests, many of them specialized. Physicians often send specimens collected in the office to referral laboratories for testing.
laboratorio de referencia Laboratorio privado o de un hospital que realiza una amplia gama de análisis, muchos de ellos especializados. Con frecuencia los médicos envían especímenes recogidos en la consulta a estos laboratorios para ser analizados.

reflection The process of considering new information and internalizing it to create new ways of examining information.

reflexión Proceso de estudiar información nueva e interiorizarla para crear formas nuevas de examinar información.

refractile Capable of causing light rays to bend, thus altering or distorting an image.
refractante Capaz de provocar la refracción de la luz, desviación alterando o distorcionando una imagen.

registered dietitian (RD) A professionally certified person with a bachelor's degree in food and nutrition who is concerned with the maintenance and promotion of health and the treatment of diseases through proper diet.
dietista registrado (RD) Profesional certificado persona con titulación universitaria en alimentos y nutrición y que se preocupa del mantenimiento y la promoción de la salud y el tratamiento de las enfermedades a través de la dieta adecuado.

relapse The recurrence of disease symptoms after apparent recovery.
recaída Recurrencia de los síntomas de una enfermedad tras una aparente recuperación.

relevant Having a significant and demonstrable bearing on the matter at hand.
pertinente Que tiene una relación importante y demostrable con el asunto que se está tratando.

rem The dose of ionizing radiation equivalent to 1 roentgen of x-ray exposure.
rem La dosis de radiación ionizante equivalente a un roentgen de exposición a rayos x.

remission A decrease in the severity of a disease or symptoms; the partial or complete disappearance of the clinical and subjective characteristics of a chronic or malignant disease.
remisión Disminución de la gravedad de una enfermedad o sus síntomas; desaparición parcial o total de las características clínicas y subjetivas de una enfermedad crónica o maligna.

remittent fever A fever in which a patient's temperature fluctuates greatly but never falls to the normal level.
fiebre remitente Fiebre en la cual la temperatura fluctúa mucho pero nunca baja al nivel normal.

renal threshold The level above which a substance cannot be reabsorbed by the renal tubules and therefore is excreted in the urine.
umbral renal Nivel por encima del cual una sustancia no puede ser reabsorbida por los túbulos renales y por lo tanto es excretada en la orina.

reparations The act of making amends, offering atonement, or giving satisfaction for a wrong or injury.
reparaciones Acción de enmendar u ofrecer compensaciones por un error o un daño.

reprimands Criticisms for a fault; a severe or formal reproof.
reprimendas Críticas por una falta; reprobación severa o formal.

reproach An expression of rebuke or disapproval; a cause or occasion for blame, discredit, or disgrace.
reproche Expresión de crítica o desaprobación; causa o motivo de culpa, descrédito u oprobio.

requisites Things considered essential or necessary.
requisitos Cosas que se consideran esenciales o necesarias.

resolution The ability of the eye to distinguish two objects that are very close together; the sharpness of an image.
resolución Capacidad del ojo para distinguir dos objetos que están muy cerca uno del otro; nitidez de una imagen.

retention Keeping something in possession or use; to keep someone's pay or service.
retención El hecho de mantener en posesión o en uso; mantener a alguien a su servicio o como empleado.

retention schedule A method or plan for retaining or keeping track of medical records and their movement from active to inactive to closed filing.
plan de retención Método o plan para retener o guardar expedientes médicos, y el paso de los mismos del estado de expediente activo a pasivo y a cerrado.

retribution The giving or receiving of reward or punishment; something given or exacted in recompense.
retribución Acto de dar o recibir una recompensa o castigo; algo que se da o se cobra como recompensa.

rhinitis Inflammation of the mucous membranes of the nose.
rinitis Inflamación de las membranas mucosas de la nariz.

rhonchi Abnormal rumbling sounds during expiration that indicate airway obstruction caused by thick secretions or spasms; a continuous, dry rattling in the throat or bronchial tube resulting from partial obstruction.
ronquido Ruido sordo y anómalo durante la expiración que indica obstrucción de las vías respiratorias debido a secreciones espesas o a espasmos; ruido seco y continuo en la garganta o en el tubo bronquial debido a una obstrucción parcial.

rider A special provision or group of provisions added to an insurance policy to expand or limit the benefits otherwise payable. A rider may increase or decrease benefits, waive a condition or coverage, or in any other way amend the original contract.

cláusula adicional Provisión o conjunto de provisiones especiales añadidas a una póliza de seguro para ampliar o limitar los beneficios que de otro modo se pueden pagar. Puede aumentar o disminuir beneficios, anular una condición o cobertura o puede enmendar el contrato original de otra manera.

robotics Technology dealing with the design, construction, and operation of robots in automation.
robótica Tecnología de la automatización que se ocupa del diseño, construcción y operación de robots.

rods Structures in the retina of the eye that form the light-sensitive elements.
bastoncillos Estructuras que están en la retina del ojo y constituyen los elementos sensibles a la luz.

Roentgen (R) The conventional unit of radiation exposure.
Roentgen (R) Unidad convencional de exposición a radiación.

router A device used to connect any number of LANs that communicate with other routers and determine the best route between any two hosts.
direccionador Dispositivo usado para conectar cualquier cantidad de LAN que se comunican con otros direccionadores para determinar la mejor ruta entre dos computadoras conectadas a una red.

sagittal plane The plane that divides the body into right and left halves.
plano sagital Plano que divide el cuerpo en la mitad derecha y la mitad izquierda.

salutation Words or gestures that express greeting, good will, or courtesy.
saludo Expresión de saludo, buenos deseos o cortesía por medio de palabras o gestos.

sanitization Reduction of the number of potentially harmful microorganisms to a relatively safe level.
saneamiento Reducción del número de microorganismos a un nivel relativamente seguro.

sarcasm A sharp or satiric response or ironic utterance designed to cause pain.
sarcasmo Respuesta aguda y frecuentemente satírica o declaración irónica destinada a burlarse o a lastimar.

scanner A device that reads text or illustrations on a printed page and translates the information into a form the computer can understand.
escáner Dispositivo que lee texto o ilustraciones de una página impresa y traduce esa información a un formato comprensible para la computadora.

sclera The white part of the eye that encloses the eyeball.
esclerótica Parte blanca del ojo que encierra el globo ocular.

scleroderma An autoimmune disorder that affects the blood vessels and connective tissue, causing fibrous degeneration of the major organs.
esclerodermia Trastorno autoinmune que afecta a los vasos sanguíneos y los tejidos conectivos provocando degeneración en las fibras de los órganos principales.

sclerotherapy The injection of sclerosing (hardening) solutions to treat hemorrhoids, varicose veins, or esophageal varices.
escleroterapia Inyección de soluciones de esclerosis (endorecedores) para tratar hemorroides, venas varicosas o varices esofágicas.

scoliosis An abnormal lateral curvature of the spine.
escoliosis Curvatura lateral anómala de la columna.

scored tablet A drug tablet manufactured with an indentation that allows the tablet to be broken or cut into equal parts.
tableta con hendidura Tableta que se fabrica con una hendidura que permite dividirla o romperla en partes iguales.

screen Something that shields, protects, or hides; to select or eliminate products or applicants by comparing them with a set of desired criteria.
pantalla Algo que actúa como escudo, que protege u oculta para permitir un proceso de selección.

search engines Computer programs that search documents for keywords and return a list of documents containing those words.
buscadores Programas de computadoras que buscan documentos a partir de palabras clave y proporcionan una lista de los documentos que contienen esas palabras.

seborrhea An excessive discharge of sebum from the sebaceous glands, forming greasy scales on the skin or cheesy plugs in skin pores.
seborrea Descarga excesiva de sebo de las glándulas sebáceas, formando escamas de grasa en la piel o tapones con aspecto de queso en los poros de la piel.

secondary hypertension Elevated blood pressure caused by another medical condition.
hipertensión secundaria Presión sanguínea elevada causada por otra enfermedad o afección médica.

"see" In coding manuals, an instruction to the coder to look in another place; found in volumes 2 and 3 of the Alphabetic Index, this instruction must always be followed.
"ver" Instrucción que se le da a la persona encargada de la codificación para que consulte en

otro lugar. Siempre debe seguirse esta instrucción; la expresión se encuentra en el Índice alfabético, tomos 2 y 3.

"see also" In coding manuals, an instruction to the coder to look elsewhere if the main term or subterm(s) for an entry are not sufficient for coding the information. If a code number follows, "see also" is enclosed in parentheses; if there is no code number, "see also" is preceded by a dash.
"ver también" Instrucción que se le da a la persona encargada de la codificación para que consulte en algún otro lugar si el término o subtérminos principales para una entrada no son suficientes para codificar la información. Si "ver también" va seguido por un número de código, dicho código va entre paréntesis; si no hay número de código, "ver también" va precedido por un guión.

"see category" In coding manuals, an instruction to the coder to refer to a specific category (three-digit code); it must always be followed.
"ver categoría" Instrucción que se le da a la persona encargada de la codificación para que consulte una categoría específica (código de tres dígitos); Siempre debe seguirse.

self-insured plans Insurance plans funded by organizations with a large enough employee base that they can afford to fund their own insurance program.
planes de autoaseguración Planes de seguros implementados por organizaciones con un número de empleados lo suficientemente grande como para permitirles financiar su propio programa de seguros.

sequentially Happening in relation to or by arrangement in a sequence.
secuencial Aquello que ocurre relativo a una secuencia o que es ordenado en secuencia.

serous Pertaining to a thin, watery, serumlike drainage.
seroso Perteneciente o relativo a una materia poco espesa, acuosa, parecida al suero.

serum The portion of whole blood that remains liquid after the blood has clotted.
suero La porción de la sangre que queda líquida después de la coagulación.

service benefit plan A plan that provides benefits in the form of certain surgical and medical services rendered rather than in cash. A service benefit plan is not restricted to a fee schedule.
plan de beneficios de servicio Plan que proporciona beneficios en forma de ciertos servicios médico-quirúrgicos en vez de con dinero en metálico. Un plan de servicio de beneficio no está restringido por una escala de cargos.

sheath The covering surrounding the axon of the nerve cell that acts as an electrical insulator to speed conduction of nerve impulses.
película Recubrimiento que rodea los axones de la célula nerviosa y que se comporta como aislante eléctrico para aumentar la velocidad de conducción del impulso nervioso.

shingling A method of filing whereby each new report is laid on top of the previous report, resembling the shingles of a roof.
laminado Método de archivo en el cual cada informe nuevo se coloca encima del informe anterior, del mismo modo que se colocan las tejas en un techo.

Sievert (Sv) The international unit of radiation dose equivalent.
Sievert (Sv) Unidad internacional de dosis equivalentes de radiación.

sinoatrial (SA) node The pacemaker of the heart, located in the right atrium.
nódulo sinoauricular (SA) Marcapasos del corazón que se halla en la aurícula derecha.

sinus arrhythmia An irregular heartbeat that originates in the sinoatrial (pacemaker) node.
arritmia de seno Ritmo cardiaco irregular que tiene su origen en el nódulo sinoauricular (marcapasos).

socioeconomic Relating to a combination of social and economic factors.
socioeconómico Perteneciente o relativo a una combinación de factores sociales y económicos.

sociologic Oriented or directed toward social needs and problems.
sociologico Que se orienta o dirige hacia las necesidades y problemas sociales.

sonography An imaging modality that uses sound waves to produce images of soft tissues; also called *diagnostic ultrasound*.
sonografía Modalidad de formación de imágenes que usa ondas sonoras para producir imágenes de los tejidos blandos; también se conoce como *ultrasonido de diagnóstico*.

sound card A device that allows a computer to output sound through speakers connected to the main circuitry board (motherboard).
tarjeta de sonido Dispositivo que le permite a una computadora emitir sonido a través de altavoces conectados a la tarjeta principal del circuito.

specimen A sample of body fluid, waste product, or tissue that is collected for analysis and diagnosis.
espécimen Muestra de un fluido corporal, residuo o tejido que se usa para análisis y diagnósticos.

spirometer An instrument that measures the volume of inhaled and exhaled air.
espirómetro Instrumento que sirve para medir el volumen del aire inhalado y exhalado.

spores Thick-walled reproductive cells formed within bacteria and capable of withstanding unfavorable environmental conditions; they are very resistant to disinfection measures.
esporas Células reproductoras de paredes gruesas que se forman dentro de las bacterias y son capaces de resistir condiciones ambientales adversas; tipos de bacterias letárgicas de paredes gruesas que son muy resistentes a las medidas de desinfección.

staff privileges Authorization for a healthcare professional to practice within a specific facility.
privilegios del personal Autorización para un profesional de atención sanitaria, para ejercer la práctica dentro de unas instalaciones específicas.

standards Items or indicators used to measure quality or compliance with a statutory or accrediting body's policies and regulations.
estándares Artículos o indicadores usados para medir la calidad o cumplimiento de las pólizas y-regulaciones de un cuerpo normativo o acreditativo.

stat A medical term meaning "immediately" or "at this moment"; an order found on a laboratory requisition that indicates that the test must be done immediately (from the Latin word *statin,* meaning "at once").
stat Abreviatura usada en medicina que significa inmediatamente o ahora mismo. Orden encontrada en un pedido de laboratorio que indica que el análisis debe llevarse a cabo inmediatamente (de la palabra latina statin, que significa "ahora"); inmediatamente.

stationers Sellers of writing paper.
dependientes de papelería Vendedores de artículos de papelería.

statute A law enacted by the legislative branch of a government.
estatuto Ley sancionada por la rama legislativa de un gobierno.

stereotactic An x-ray procedure to guide the insertion of a needle into a specific area of the breast.
estereotáctico Procedimiento de rayos x para guiar la inserción de una aguja en zonas específicas del pecho.

stereotype Something conforming to a fixed or general pattern; a standardized mental picture that is held in common by many and represents an oversimplified opinion, prejudiced attitude, or uncritical judgment.
estereotipo Algo que se ajusta a un patrón fijado o general; imagen mental estandarizada que tienen en común muchas personas y que representa opiniones simplificadas, actitudes con prejuicios o razonamientos carentes de sentido crítico.

sterilization Complete destruction of all forms of microbial life.
esterilización Destrucción total de toda forma de vida microbiana.

stertorous Referring to a strenuous respiratory effort marked by a snoring sound.
estertóreo Esfuerzo respiratorio penoso que tiene el sonido de un ronquido.

stipulate To specify as a condition or requirement of an agreement or offer; to make an agreement or covenant to do or forbear from doing something.
estipular Especificar como condición o requisito de un acuerdo u oferta; establecer un acuerdo o prometer hacer, o dejar de hacer, algo.

stock option An offer of stocks for purchase to a certain individual or to certain groups, such as employees of a for-profit hospital.
opción sobre acciones Oferta de venta de acciones que se le hace a un ciertos individuos o grupos, como a los empleados de un hospital.

stressors Stimuli that cause stress.
estresantes Dícese de los estímulos que causan estrés.

stridor A shrill, harsh respiratory sound heard during inhalation during laryngeal obstruction.
estridor Sonido respiratorio estridente que se oye durante la inhalación en los casos de obstrucción laríngea.

stroke Sudden paralysis and/or loss of consciousness caused by extreme trauma or injury to an artery in the brain.
apoplejía Súbita pérdida de conocimiento y parálisis causada por una lesión o daño grave de una arteria del cerebro.

stylus A metal probe inserted into or passed through a catheter, needle, or tube to clear the device or to facilitate its passage into a body orifice.
punzón Sonda metálica que se inserta o pasa por medio de un catéter, aguja o tubo y que se usa para limpiar o para facilitar el paso a un orificio del cuerpo.

subjective information Information gained by questioning the patient or taking it from a form.
información subjetiva Información obtenida haciendo preguntas al paciente o tomándola de un formulario.

subluxation Incomplete dislocation of a bone from its normal anatomic location.
subluxación Dislocación incompleta de un hueso desde su posición anatómica normal.

subluxations Slight misalignments of the vertebrae or partial dislocations.
subluxaciones Alineamientos ligeramente defectuosos o dislocaciones parciales de las vértebras.

subordinate Submissive to or controlled by authority; placed in or occupying a lower class, rank, or position.
subordinado Que está sometido a una autoridad o controlado por ella; que ostenta un cargo u ocupa una clase, rango o puesto inferior.

subpoena A writ or document commanding a person to appear in court under penalty for failure to appear.
subpoena Documento escrito ordenando a una persona comparecer en el juzgado bajo penalidad en caso de no comparecencia.

substance number A number based on the weight of a ream of paper containing 500 sheets.
número de sustancia Número basado en el peso de una resma de papel de 500 hojas.

subtle Difficult to understand or perceive; having or marked by keen insight and the ability to penetrate deeply and thoroughly.
sutil Difícil de comprender o percibir; que tiene perspicacia y la capacidad de penetrar a fondo y en toda su extensión en un asunto.

succinct Marked by compact, precise expression without wasted words.
sucinto Caracterizado por una expresión precisa y concisa sin palabras inútiles.

superfluous Exceeding what is sufficient or necessary.
superfluos Que exceden aquello que es suficiente o necesario.

suppurative Forming and/or discharging pus.
supuración Formación o emisión de pus.

surrogate A substitute; something put in place of another.
subrogado Sustituto; puesto en lugar de otro.

switch In networks, a device that filters information between LAN segments, reduces overall network traffic, and increases the speed and efficiency of bandwidth use.
conmutador En las redes de comunicación, dispositivo que filtra información entre segmentos de LAN y disminuye el tráfico global de la red, aumentando la velocidad y la eficacia en el uso del ancho de banda.

syncope Fainting; a brief lapse in consciousness.
síncope Desmayo; lapso breve en estado de consciencia.

syndrome A group of signs and symptoms related to a common cause or presenting a clinical picture of a disease or an inherited abnormality.
síndrome Conjunto de signos y síntomas relacionados con una causa común o que presentan el cuadro clínico de una enfermedad o una anomalía heredada.

synopsis A condensed statement or outline.
sinopsis Declaración resumida; resumen.

synovial fluid Clear fluid found in joint cavities that facilitates smooth movement and nourishes joint structures.
fluido sinovial Fluido claro que se halla en las cavidades de las articulaciones y que facilita los movimientos suaves y nutre las estructuras articulatorias.

tachycardia A rapid but regular heart rate; one that exceeds 100 beats per minute.
taquicardia Ritmo cardiaco rápido pero regular que sobrepasa los 100 latidos por minuto.

tachypnea Respiration that is rapid and shallow; hyperventilation.
taquipnea Respiración rápida y profunda; hiperventilación.

tactful Having a keen sense of what to do or say to maintain good relations with others or avoid offense.
tacto Tener un sentido de lo que se debe hacer o decir para mantener buenas relaciones con los demás y evitar ofenderlos.

target organ The organ affected by a particular hormone.
órgano objetivo Órgano afectado por una hormona específica.

target tissue A group of cells affected by a particular hormone.
tejido objetivo Grupo de células afectadas por una hormona específica.

targeted to Directed toward a specific desire, position, or effect.
dirigido a Dirigido a un fin o meta específico, usado hacia un fin; dirigido hacia un deseo o un puesto específico.

TCP/IP Abbreviation for *transmission control protocol/Internet protocol;* a suite of communications protocols used to connect users or hosts to the Internet.

TCP/IP Abreviatura de *protocolo de control de transmisión/protocolo Internet*; conjunto de protocolos de comunicación que se usa para conectar usuarios o computadoras a Internet.

tedious Tiresome because of length or dullness.
tedioso Que cansa porque es demasiado largo o aburrido.

telecommunications The science and technology of communication by transmission of information from one location to another via telephone, television, telegraph, or satellite.
telecomunicaciones Ciencia y tecnología de la comunicación basada en la transmisión de información de un lugar a otro por teléfono, televisión, telégrafo o satélite.

telemedicine The use of telecommunications in the practice of medicine, allowing great distances between healthcare professionals, colleagues, patients, and students.
telemedicina Uso de las telecomunicaciones en la práctica médica, permitiendo la comunicación entre profesionales de atención sanitaria, colegas, pacientes y estudiantes que se hallan a grandes distancias.

teleradiology The use of telecommunications devices to enhance and improve the results of radiologic procedures.
telerradiología Uso de dispositivos de telecomunicación para mejorar y perfeccionar los resultados de procedimientos radiológicos.

tendon A tough band of connective tissue that connects muscle to bone.
tendón Banda resistente de tejido conectivo que conecta los músculos con los huesos.

teratogen Any substance that interferes with normal prenatal development.
teratógeno Cualquier sustancia que interfiere con el desarrollo prenatal normal.

teratogenic A substance known to cause birth defects.
teratogénico Sustancia que se sabe que provoca defectos de nacimiento.

testimony A solemn declaration usually made orally by a witness under oath in response to interrogation by a lawyer or an authorized public official.
testimonio Declaración solemne, por lo general oral, hecha por un testigo bajo juramento como respuesta a una pregunta (o preguntas) de un abogado o un funcionario público autorizado.

thanatology The description or study of the phenomena of death and of psychological methods of coping with death.
tanatología Descripción o estudio del fenómeno de la muerte y de los métodos psicológicos para hacerle frente.

third-party payer An entity (usually an insurance company) that makes a payment on an obligation or debt but is not a party to the contract that created the debt.
pagador mediador Entidad (por lo general una compañía aseguradora) que hace un pago de una obligación o deuda pero que no es parte del contrato que ha creado dicha deuda.

third-party payer Someone other than the patient, spouse, or parent who is responsible for paying all or part of the patient's medical costs.
pagador mediador Alguien ajeno al paciente, cónyuge, padre o madre que es responsable del pago de todo o parte de los gastos médicos del paciente o de parte de ellos.

thixotropic gel A material that appears to be a solid until subjected to a disturbance, such as centrifugation, when it becomes a liquid.
gel tisotrópico Material que parece ser sólido hasta el momento en que se somete a una alteración como la centrifugación, cuando se convierte en líquido.

thoracic Pertaining to the region between the neck and low back that contains the 12 thoracic vertebrae.
torácica Perteneciente o relativo a región de la espalda entre el cuello y la región lumbar inferior en la que hay 12 vértebras torácicas.

thready pulse A pulse that is scarcely perceptible.
pulso débil Pulso que es apenas perceptible.

thrombus A blood clot.
trombo Coágulo de sangre.

thyroid-stimulating hormone (TSH) A hormone secreted by the anterior lobe of the pituitary gland that stimulates the secretion of hormones produced by the thyroid gland.
hormona estimulante de la tiroides (TSH) Hormona que segrega el lóbulo anterior de la glándula pituitaria y que estimula la secreción de hormonas producidas por la glándula tiroides.

tickler file A chronologic file used as a reminder that something must be taken care of on a certain date.
archivo cronológico Archivo que se usa para recordar que algo que debe llevarse a cabo en una fecha determinada.

tinea A fungal skin disease that results in scaling, itching, and inflammation.
tinea Enfermedad de la piel causada por hongos y que produce descamación, picazón e inflamación.

tissue culture The technique or process of keeping tissue alive and growing in a culture medium.
cultivo de tejidos Técnica o proceso de mantener un tejido vivo y en fase de crecimiento en un medio de cultivo.

toxemia An abnormal condition of pregnancy characterized by hypertension, edema, and protein in the urine.
toxemia Característica anómala del embarazo, con presencia de hipertensión, edema y proteínas en la orina.

tracer A radioactive substance administered to a patient undergoing a nuclear medicine imaging procedure.
trazador Sustancia radioactiva que se administra al paciente para someterlo a procedimientos de formación de imágenes en medicina nuclear.

tracheostomy A surgical opening through the neck into the trachea that is made to facilitate breathing.
traqueotomía Abertura realizada quirúrgicamente en el cuello a la altura de la tráquea para facilitar la respiración.

transaction An exchange or transfer of goods, services, or funds.
transacción Intercambio o transferencia de bienes, servicios o fondos.

transcription A written copy made either in longhand or by machine.
transcripción Copia escrita de algo, hecha a mano, o con la ayuda de una máquina.

transducer The part of the sonography machine in contact with the patient that sends high-frequency sound waves and receives the sound echoes that return from the patient's body.
transductor Parte de una máquina de sonografía que está en contacto con el paciente envía ondas sonoras de alta frecuencia y recibe los ecos de los sonidos que regresan del cuerpo del paciente.

transection A cross-section; division by cutting across.
sección transversal División cortando a través.

transient ischemic attack A condition of temporary neurologic symptoms caused by gradual or partial occlusion of a cerebral blood vessel.
ataque isquémico transitorio Síntomas neurológicos temporales causados por una oclusión gradual o parcial de un vaso sanguíneo del cerebro.

transillumination Inspection of a cavity or an organ by passing light through its walls.
diafanoscopia Inspección de una cavidad u órgano haciendo pasar luz a través de sus paredes. **transport medium** A medium used to keep an organism alive during transport to the laboratory. **medio para transporte** Medio usado para mantener un organismo vivo durante el transporte al laboratorio.

transverse plane The plane that divides the body into superior and inferior parts.
plano transversal Plano que divide el cuerpo en parte superior e inferior.

trauma A physical injury or wound caused by an external force or by violence.
trauma Lesión física o herida causada por una fuerza externa o violencia.

treatises Systematic expositions or arguments in writing, including methodic discussion of the facts and principles involved and the conclusions reached.
tratados Exposiciones sistemáticas o argumentos escritos que incluyen una descripción metódica de los hechos y principios involucrados y las conclusiones a las que se ha llegado.

triage A process of responding to requests for immediate care and treatment after evaluating the urgency of the need and prioritizing the treatment; the sorting and allocation of treatment to patients according to a system of priorities designed to maximize the number of survivors and treat the sickest patients first.
criterio de selección Responder a peticiones de atención y tratamiento inmediato tras evaluar la urgencia de la necesidad y establecer prioridades de tratamiento. Clasificación y asignación de tratamiento a pacientes según un sistema de prioridades destinado a maximizar el número de sobrevivientes y tratar primero a los pacientes más enfermos.

triglycerides Fatty acids and glycerols that are bound to proteins and form high- and low-density lipoproteins.
triglicéridos Ácidos grasos y gliceroles que se unen a las proteínas y forman lipoproteínas de alta y baja densidad.

truss An elastic, canvas, or metallic device for retaining a reduced hernia within the abdominal cavity.
braguero Malla elástica o dispositivo metálico para retener una hernia reducida dentro de la cavidad abdominal.

turgor The resistance of the skin to being grasped between the fingers and released; normal skin tension, which is reduced with dehydration and increased with edema.
turgor Resistencia de la piel a ser pellizcada; tensión normal de la piel que disminuye con la deshidratación y aumenta con el edema.

type and cross-match Tests performed to assess the compatibility of blood intended for transfusion with the person's own blood.

prueba de tipo y RH Análisis que se realizan para evaluar la compatibilidad de la sangre que va a ser usada en una transfusión.

unequal pulses Pulses in which the beats vary in intensity.
pulso desigual Pulso en el cual los latidos varían en intensidad.

Uniform Commercial Code A unified set of rules covering many business transactions; often referred to simply as the UCC, it has been adopted in all 50 states, the District of Columbia, and most U.S. territories.
Código de Comercio Uniforme Conjunto de normas unificadas que cubren muchas transacciones comerciales; se conoce simplemente como UCC y ha sido adoptado en los 50 estados, el Distrito de Columbia y la mayoría de los territorios estadounidenses.

unique identifiers Codes used as part of a method of anonymous HIV testing in which the code is used, instead of a name, to protect the patient's confidentiality.
identificadores únicos Método de prueba de VIH (HIV) anónimo en el cual se usa un código en lugar de nombres, para proteger la confidencialidad del paciente.

unit-dose A method used by a pharmacy to prepare individual doses of medications.
dosis unitaria Método usado por la farmacia para preparar dosis individuales de medicamentos.

universal claim form The form developed by the HCFA (now known as the Centers for Medicare and Medicaid Services [CMS]) and approved by the American Medical Association (AMA) for use in submitting all government-sponsored claims.
formulario de reclamación universal Formulario desarrollado por la Administración financiera de la atención sanitaria (HCFA, ahora conocida como Centros de servicios de Medicare y Medicaid, o CMS) y aprobado por AMA para usarse al someter todas las reclamaciones subvencionadas por el gobierno.

upper GI series Fluoroscopic examination of the esophagus, stomach, and duodenum in which orally administered barium sulfate is used a contrast medium.
serie GI superior Examen fluoroscópico del esófago, estómago y duodeno usando una administración oral de sulfato de bario como medio de contraste.

urea The major nitrogenous end product of protein metabolism and the chief nitrogenous component of the urine.
urea Principal producto final nitrogenado del metabolismo de las proteínas y el principal componente nitrogenado de la orina.

urease An enzyme that catalyzes the hydrolysis of urea to form ammonium carbonate.
ureasa Enzima que cataliza la hidrólisis de la urea para formar carbonato de amonio.

uremia A toxic renal condition characterized by an excess of urea, creatinine, and other nitrogenous end products in the blood.
uremia Enfermedad renal tóxica que se caracteriza por un exceso de urea, creatinina y otros productos finales en la sangre.

urgency A sudden, compelling desire to urinate and the inability to control the release of urine.
urgencia Deseo repentino y apremiante de orinar y la incapacidad de controlarlo.

URL Abbreviation for *uniform resource locator;* the global address of documents or information on the Internet. The URL provides the IP address and the domain name for the Web page, such as "microsoft.com."
URL Abreviatura de *localizador universal de recursos;* la dirección a nivel mundial, de documentos o de información en Internet. El URL proporciona la dirección IP y el nombre del dominio de una página web, como por ejemplo: "microsoft.com."

urticaria A skin eruption marked by inflamed wheals; hives.
urticaria Erupción cutánea que produce ampollas imflamadas.

"use additional code" In coding manuals, this term appears only in volume 1 of the ICD-9-CM in those subdivisions where the user should add further information by means of an additional code to give a more complete picture of the diagnosis. In some cases, "if desired" follows the term. However, "if desired" is not used for coding in military medical treatment facilities; in these cases, when the term "use additional code... if desired" appears, "if desired" is disregarded and the appropriate additional code is assigned.
"usar código adicional" Esta expresión aparece sólo en el tomo 1, en aquellas subdivisiones en las que el usuario debe añadir más información por medio de un código adicional para proporcionar un cuadro más completo del diagnóstico. En algunos casos, se verá "si se desea" tras el término. En la codificación en establecimientos militares de tratamiento médico, no se usará la expresión "si se desea." Por lo tanto, cuando aparezca el término "usar código adicional... si se desea," no se tendrá en cuenta "si se desea" y se asignará el código adicional correspondiente.

utilization review The review of individual cases by a committee to make sure that services are medically necessary and to study how providers use medical care resources.

revisión de utilización Revisión de casos individuales por un comité, para asegurarse de que los servicios son médicamente necesarios y estudiar cómo los proveedores usan los recursos de cuidados de salud.

Valsalva's maneuver A maneuver that occurs when a person strains to defecate and urinate, uses the arms and upper trunk muscles to move up in bed, or strains during laughing, coughing, or vomiting. It causes blood to become trapped in the great veins, preventing it from entering the chest and right atrium, which may cause a heart attack and death.
maniobra de Valsalva Ocurre cuando uno hace fuerza para defecar y orinar, usa los brazos y los músculos de la parte superior del tronco para levantarse de la cama, o hace fuerza al reír, toser o vomitar. Causa una retención de sangre en las venas mayores, impidiendole que entre en el pecho y la aurícula derecha y puede provocar un ataque al corazón y la muerte.

vasodilation An increase in the diameter of a blood vessel.
vasodilatación Aumento en el diámetro de un vaso sanguíneo.

vector An organism, such as an insect or a tick, that transmits the causative organisms of disease.
vector Organismos, tales como un insecto o garrapata, que transmite los organismos que provocan enfermedades.

ventricles The two lower chambers of the heart.
ventrículos Las dos cavidades inferiores del corazón.

veracity Devotion to or conformity with the truth.
veracidad Compromiso o conformidad con la verdad.

verdict The finding or decision of a jury on a matter submitted to it in trial.
veredicto Conclusión o decisión de un jurado en un asunto sometido a juicio.

versatile Embracing a variety of subjects, fields or skills; having a wide range of abilities.
versátil Que abarca diferentes sujetos, campos o destrezas; que tiene una amplia gama de destrezas.

vertigo Dizziness; a sensation of faintness or an inability to maintain normal balance.
vertigo Mareo; sensación de desmayo o de incapacidad de mantener el equilibrio normal.

vested Granted or endowed with a particular authority, right, or property; having a special interest in something.

conferirido Concedido o dotado con una autoridad, derecho o propiedad particular; que tiene un interés especial en algo.

viable Capable of living, developing, or germinating under favorable conditions.
viable Capaz de vivir, desarrollarse o germinar bajo condiciones favorables.

virtual reality An artificial environment experienced by a computer user, often by using special gloves, earphones, and goggles to enhance the experience, that feels as if it were a real environment.
realidad virtual Entorno artificial que experimenta el usuario de una computadora, muchas veces usando guantes especiales, audífonos y lentes para mejorar la experiencia, y que parece ser un ambiente real.

virulent Exceedingly pathogenic, noxious, or deadly.
virulento Excesivamente patógeno, nocivo o mortal.

viscosity The quality of being thick and lacking the capability of easy movement.
viscosidad Cualidad de espeso e incapaz de moverse con facilidad.

vocation The work in which a person is regularly employed.
profesión Trabajo en el que una persona está empleada regularmente.

volatile Referring to a flammable substance's capacity to vaporize at a low temperature; easily aroused; tending to erupt in violence.
volátil Referente a la capacidad de una sustancia flamable para evaporarse a baja temperatura. Que reacciona con facilidad y tiene tendencia a entrar en erupción de forma violenta.

vulva The external female genitalia, which begins at the mons pubis and terminates at the anus.
vulva Zona genital exterior femenina que comienza en el monte púbico y termina en el ano.

watermark A mark in paper resulting from differences in thickness usually produced by pressure from a projecting design in the mold or on a processing roll; it is visible when the paper is held up to the light.
filigrana Marca en un papel que resulta de diferencias de espesor, por lo general se produce presionando un diseño en relieve en el molde o en un rodillo de procesamiento, y es visible por transparencia.

wet mount A slide preparation in which a drop of liquid specimen is protected by a coverslip and observed with a microscope.
montaje húmedo Preparación de una lámina en la que una gota de espécimen líquido por ejemplo, se

protege con una cubierta de vidrio y se observa con un microscopio.

wheal A localized area of edema or a raised lesion.
roncha Área localizada de un edema o una lesión protuberante.

"with" In ICD-9-CM coding, the term "with," "with mention of," or "associated with" in a title dictates that both parts of the title must be present in the statement of the diagnosis to assign the particular code.
"con" En el contexto de la ICD-9-CM, las expresiones "con", "con mención de" y "asociado con" en un título exigen que ambas partes del título estén presentes en la descripción del orden de diagnóstico para asignar el código específico.

workers' compensation Insurance against liability imposed on certain employers to pay benefits and furnish care to injured employees and to pay benefits to dependents of an employee killed in the course of or in a situation arising out of the worker's employment.
compensación laboral Seguro contra la responsabilidad impuesta a ciertos patrones para pagar beneficios y proporcionar atenciones a los trabajadores lesionados, y pagar beneficios a las personas que dependan de trabajadores que mueran en el trabajo o a causa de él.

Zip drive A small, portable disk drive that is used primarily for backing up information and archiving computer files; a 100-megabyte Zip disk holds the equivalent of about 70 floppy disks.
unidad Zip Unidad de un disco pequeño y portátil que se usa principalmente para hacer copias de seguridad de información y para guardar archivos electrónicos. Un disco Zip de 100 megabytes tiene una capacidad equivalente a la de unos 70 disquetes.

NOTES

NOTES

NOTES

NOTES

NOTES